Evidence-based Clinical Chinese Medicine

Volume 22
Urinary Tract Infection

Evidence-based Clinical Chinese Medicine

Print ISSN: 2529-7562
Online ISSN: 2529-7554

Series Co Editors-in-Chief

Charlie Changli Xue *(RMIT University, Australia)*
Chuanjian Lu *(Guangdong Provincial Hospital of Chinese Medicine, China)*

Published

More information on this series can also be found at https://www.worldscientific.com/series/ebccm

Evidence-based Clinical Chinese Medicine

Co Editors-in-Chief

Charlie Changli Xue
RMIT University, Australia

Chuanjian Lu
Guangdong Provincial Hospital of Chinese Medicine, China

Volume 22
Urinary Tract Infection

Lead Authors

Meaghan Coyle
RMIT University, Australia

Xindong Qin
Guangdong Provincial Hospital of Chinese Medicine, China

World Scientific

NEW JERSEY · LONDON · SINGAPORE · BEIJING · SHANGHAI · HONG KONG · TAIPEI · CHENNAI · TOKYO

Published by

World Scientific Publishing Co. Pte. Ltd.

5 Toh Tuck Link, Singapore 596224

USA office: 27 Warren Street, Suite 401-402, Hackensack, NJ 07601

UK office: 57 Shelton Street, Covent Garden, London WC2H 9HE

Library of Congress Cataloging-in-Publication Data

Names: Xue, Charlie Changli, author. | Lu, Chuan-jian, 1964–   author.
Title: Evidence-based clinical Chinese medicine / Charlie Changli Xue, Chuanjian Lu.
Description: New Jersey : World Scientific, 2016. | Includes bibliographical references and index.
Identifiers: LCCN 2015030389| ISBN 9789814723084 (v. 1 : hardcover : alk. paper) |
    ISBN 9789814723091 (v. 1 : paperback : alk. paper) |
    ISBN 9789814723121 (v. 2 : hardcover : alk. paper) |
    ISBN 9789814723138 (v. 2 : paperback : alk. paper) |
    ISBN 9789814759045 (v. 3 : hardcover : alk. paper) |
    ISBN 9789814759052 (v. 3 : paperback : alk. paper)
Subjects: | MESH: Medicine, Chinese Traditional--methods. | Clinical Medicine--methods. |
    Evidence-Based Medicine--methods. | Psoriasis. | Pulmonary Disease, Chronic Obstructive.
Classification: LCC RC81 | NLM WB 55.C4 | DDC 616--dc23
LC record available at http://lccn.loc.gov/2015030389

Volume 22: Urinary Tract Infection
ISBN 978-981-122-316-7 (hardcover)
ISBN 978-981-122-317-4 (ebook for institutions)
ISBN 978-981-122-318-1 (ebook for individuals)

British Library Cataloguing-in-Publication Data
A catalogue record for this book is available from the British Library.

For any available supplementary material, please visit
https://www.worldscientific.com/worldscibooks/10.1142/11907#t=suppl

Disclaimer

The information in this book is based on systematic analyses of the best available evidence for Chinese medicine interventions both historical and contemporary. Every effort has been made to ensure accuracy and completeness of the data herein. This book is intended for clinicians, researchers and educators. The practice of evidence-based medicine consists of consideration of the best available evidence, practitioners' clinical experience and judgment, and patients' preference. Not all interventions are acceptable in all countries. It is important to note that some of the substances mentioned in this book may no longer be in use, may be toxic, or may be prohibited or restricted under the provisions of the Convention on International Trade in Endangered Species of Wild Fauna and Flora (CITES). Practitioners, researchers and educators are advised to comply with the relevant regulations in their country and with the restrictions on the trade in species included in CITES appendices I, II and III. This book is not intended as a guide for self-medication. Patients should seek professional advice from qualified Chinese medicine practitioners.

Foreword

Since the late 20th century, Chinese medicine, including acupuncture and herbal medicine, has been increasingly used throughout the world. The parallel development and spread of evidence-based medicine has provided challenges and opportunities for Chinese medicine. The opportunities have been evidence-based medicine's emphasis on the effective use of the best available clinical evidence, incorporating the clinicians' clinical experience, subject to patients' preference. Such practices have a patient focus which reflects the historical nature of Chinese medicine practice. However, the challenges are also significant due to the fact that, despite the long-term development and very rich literature accumulated over 2,000 years, there is an overall lack of high-level clinical evidence for many of the interventions used in Chinese medicine.

To address this knowledge gap, we need to generate clinical evidence through high-quality clinical studies and to evaluate evidence to enable effective use of such available evidence to promote evidence-based Chinese medicine practice.

Modern Chinese medicine is rooted in its classical literature and the legacies of ancient doctors, grounded in the practice of expert clinicians and increasingly informed by clinical and experimental research efforts. In recognition of the unique features of Chinese medicine, for each of the conditions in this series a 'whole-evidence' approach is used to provide a synthesis of different types and levels of evidence to enable practitioners to make clinical decisions informed by the current best evidence.

There are four main components of this 'whole-evidence' approach. In the first component, we present the current approaches to the diagnosis, differentiation and treatment of each condition based on expert consensus in published textbooks and clinical guidelines. This provides an overview of how the condition is currently managed. The second component provides an analysis of the condition in historical context based on systematic searches of the *Zhong Hua Yi Dian* 中华医典, which includes the full texts of more than 1,000 classical medical books. These analyses provide objective views on how the condition has been treated over two millennia, reveal continuities and discontinuities between traditional and modern practice, and suggest avenues for future research.

The third component is the assessment of evidence derived from modern clinical studies of Chinese medicine interventions. The methods established by the *Cochrane Collaboration* are used as the basis for conducting systematic reviews and undertaking meta-analyses of outcome data for randomised controlled trials (RCTs). In addition, the clinical relevance of meta-analysis data is enhanced by examining the herbal formulas, individual herbs and acupuncture treatments that were assessed in the RCTs and the evidence base is broadened by the inclusion of data from controlled clinical trials and non-controlled studies. The fourth component is to determine how the herbal medicine interventions may achieve the effects indicated by the clinical trials. Thus, for each of the most frequently used herbs, we provide reviews of their effects in pre-clinical models and their likely mechanisms of action.

For each condition, this 'whole-evidence' approach links clinical expertise, historical precedent, clinical research data and experimental research to provide the reader with assessments of the current state of the evidence for the efficacy, effectiveness and safety of Chinese medicine interventions using herbal medicines, acupuncture and moxibustion, and other health care practices such as *taichi* 太极.

Since these books are available in Chinese and English, they can benefit patients, practitioners and educators internationally and enable practitioners to make clinical decisions informed by the current best evidence.

These publications represent a major milestone in the development of Chinese medicine and make a significant contribution to the development of evidence-based Chinese medicine globally.

Co-Editors-in-Chief
Distinguished Professor Charlie Changli Xue,
RMIT University, Australia

Professor Chuanjian Lu, Guangdong Provincial Hospital of Chinese Medicine, China

Purpose of This Book

This book is intended for clinicians, researchers and educators. It can be used to inform tertiary education and clinical practice by providing systematic, multidimensional assessments of the best available evidence for using Chinese medicine to manage each common clinical condition.

How to Use This Book

Some Definitions

A glossary is included, containing terms and definitions which frequently appear in the book. It also describes the definitions of statistical tests, methodological terms, evaluation tools and interventions. For example, in this book, integrative medicine refers to the combined use of a Chinese medicine treatment with conventional medical management, and combination therapies refer to two or more Chinese medicines from different therapy groups (Chinese herbal medicine, acupuncture or other Chinese medicine therapies) administered together. Terminology used throughout the book is based on the World Health Organization's *Standard Terminologies on Traditional Medicine in the Western Pacific Region* (2007) where possible or is from the cited reference.

Data Analysis and Interpretation of Results

In order to synthesise the clinical evidence, a range of statistical analysis approaches are used. In general, the effect size for dichotomous data is reported as a risk ratio (RR) with 95% confidence intervals (CI), and for continuous data, they are reported as mean difference (MD) with 95% CI. Statistically significant effects are indicated with an asterisk*. Readers should note that statistical significance does not necessarily correspond with a clinically important effect. Interpretation of results should take into consideration the clinical significance, quality of studies (expressed as 'high', 'low' or 'unclear' risk of bias in this book) and heterogeneity amongst the studies. Tests for heterogeneity are conducted using the I^2 statistic. An I^2 score greater than 50% may indicate substantial heterogeneity.

Use of Evidence in Practice

The Grading of Recommendations Assessment, Development and Evaluation (GRADE) approach was used to summarise the results and certainty of the evidence for critical and important comparisons and outcomes. Due to the diverse nature of Chinese medicine practice, treatment recommendations are not included with the summary of findings tables. Therefore, readers will need to interpret the evidence with reference to the local practice environment.

Limitations

Readers should note some of the methodological limitations of the classical literature and the clinical evidence.

- Search terms used to search the *Zhong Hua Yi Dian* 中华医典 database may not include all terms that have been used for the condition, which may alter the findings.
- Chinese language has changed over time. Citations have been interpreted for analysis, and such interpretations may be subject to disagreement.
- Chinese medicine theory has evolved over time. As such, concepts described in classical Chinese medical literature may no longer be found in contemporary works.
- Symptoms described in citations may be common to many conditions, and a judgment was required to determine the likelihood of

the citation being related to the condition. This may have introduced some bias due to the subjective nature of the judgment.

- The vast majority of the clinical evidence for Chinese medicine treatments has come from China. The applicability of the findings to other populations and other countries requires further assessment.
- Many studies included participants with varying disease severity. Where possible, subgroup analyses were undertaken to examine the effects in different subpopulations. As this was not always possible, the findings may be limited to the population included, and not to subpopulations.
- The potential risk of bias found in many included studies suggested methodological limitations. The findings for GRADE assessments based on studies of very low- to moderate-certainty evidence should be interpreted accordingly.
- Nine major English- and Chinese-language databases were searched to identify clinical studies, in addition to clinical trial registers. Other studies may exist which were not identified through searches, and which may alter the findings.
- The calculation of frequency of herbal formula use was based on formula names. It is possible that studies evaluated herbal treatments with the same or similar herb ingredients, but which were given different formula names. Due to the complexity of herbal formulas, it was considered not appropriate to make a judgment as to the similarity of formulas for analysis. As such, the frequency of formulas reported in Chapter 5 may be underestimated.
- The most frequently utilised herbs which may have contributed to the treatment effect have been described in Chapter 5. These herbs may provide leads for further exploration. Calculation of the herbs with potential effect is based on frequency of formulas reported in the studies, and does not take into consideration the clinical implications and functions of every herb in a formula.

Authors and Contributors

CO-EDITORS-IN-CHIEF
Distinguished Prof. Charlie Changli Xue (*RMIT University, Australia*)
Prof. Chuanjian Lu (*Guangdong Provincial Hospital of Chinese Medicine, China*)

CO-DEPUTY EDITORS-IN-CHIEF
Assoc. Prof. Anthony Lin Zhang (*RMIT University, Australia*)
Dr. Brian H May (*RMIT University, Australia*)
Prof. Xinfeng Guo (*Guangdong Provincial Hospital of Chinese Medicine, China*)
Prof. Zehuai Wen (*Guangdong Provincial Hospital of Chinese Medicine, China*)

LEAD AUTHORS
Dr. Meaghan Coyle (*RMIT University, Australia*)
Dr. Xindong Qin (*Guangdong Provincial Hospital of Chinese Medicine, China*)

CO-AUTHORS
RMIT University (Australia):
Dr. Mary Xinmei Zhang
Dr. Kevin Kaiyi Wang
Assoc. Prof. Anthony Lin Zhang
Distinguished Prof. Charlie Changli Xue

Guangdong Provincial Hospital of Chinese Medicine (China):
Prof. Chuanjian Lu
Dr. Lihong Yang
Dr. Jueyao Liang
Prof. Wei Mao
Prof. Xinfeng Guo
Prof. Xusheng Liu

Members of Advisory Committee and Panel

CO-CHAIRS OF PROJECT PLANNING COMMITTEE
Prof. Peter J Coloe (*RMIT University, Australia*)
Prof. Yubo Lyu (*Guangdong Provincial Hospital of Chinese Medicine, China*)
Prof. Dacan Chen (*Guangdong Provincial Hospital of Chinese Medicine, China*)

CENTRE ADVISORY COMMITTEE (IN ALPHABETICAL ORDER)
Prof. Keji Chen (*The Chinese Academy of Sciences, China*)
Prof. Aiping Lu (*Hong Kong Baptist University, China*)
Prof. Caroline Smith (*University of Western Sydney, Australia*)
Prof. David F Story (*RMIT University, Australia*)

METHODOLOGY EXPERT ADVISORY PANEL (IN ALPHABETICAL ORDER)
Prof. Zhaoxiang Bian (*Hong Kong Baptist University, China*)
Prof. Lixing Lao (*The University of Hong Kong, China*)
The Late Prof. George Lewith (*University of Southampton, United Kingdom*)
Prof. Jianping Liu (*Beijing University of Chinese Medicine, China*)
Prof. Frank Thien (*Monash University, Australia*)
Prof. Jialiang Wang (*Sichuan University, China*)

CONTENT EXPERT ADVISORY PANEL (IN ALPHABETICAL ORDER)
Prof. David Johnson (*Australasian Kidney Trials Network,
University of Queensland, Princess Alexandra Hospital,
Translational Research Institute, Australia*)
Dr. George Wu (*Credit Valley Hospital, Canada*)
Prof. Daji Xu (*Hong Kong Baptist University, China*)
Prof. Peiqing Zhang (*Heilongjiang Provincial Academy of Traditional
Chinese Medicine, China*)

Distinguished Professor Charlie Changli Xue

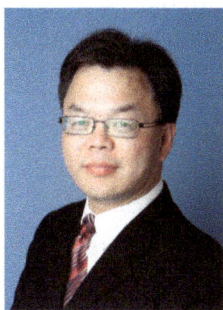

Distinguished Professor Charlie Changli Xue holds a Bachelor of Medicine (majoring in Chinese Medicine) from Guangzhou University of Chinese Medicine, China (1987) and a PhD from RMIT University, Australia (2000). He has been an academic, researcher, regulator and practitioner for almost three decades. Professor Xue has made significant contributions to evidence-based educational development, clinical research, regulatory framework and policy development, and provision of high-quality clinical care to the community. Professor Xue is recognised internationally as an expert in evidence-based traditional medicine and integrative health care.

Professor Xue is the Inaugural National Chair of the Chinese Medicine Board of Australia appointed by the Australian Health Workforce Ministerial Council (in 2011), and he was reappointed for a second term in 2014. Since 2007, he has been a Member of the World Health Organization (WHO) Expert Advisory Panel for Traditional and Complementary Medicine, Geneva. Professor Xue is also an Honorary Senior Principal Research Fellow at the Guangdong Provincial Academy of Chinese Medical Sciences, China.

At RMIT, Professor Xue is Executive Dean, School of Health and Biomedical Sciences. He is also Director, WHO Collaborating Centre for Traditional Medicine.

Between 1995 and 2010, Professor Xue was Discipline Head of Chinese Medicine at RMIT University. He leads the development of five successful undergraduate and postgraduate degree programmes in Chinese Medicine at RMIT University which is now a global leader in Chinese medicine education and research.

Professor Xue's research has been supported by research grants of over AUD 15 million including six project grants from the Australian Government's National Health and Medical Research Council (NHMRC) and two Australian Research Council (ARC) grants. He has contributed over 200 publications and has been frequently invited as keynote speaker for numerous national and international conferences. Professor Xue has contributed to over 300 media interviews on issues related to complementary medicine education, research, regulation and practice.

Professor Chuanjian Lu

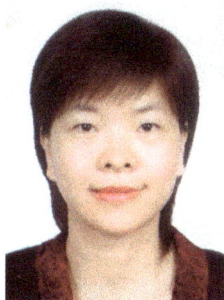

Professor Chuanjian Lu is the Vice-president of Guangdong Provincial Hospital of Chinese Medicine (Guangdong Provincial Academy of Chinese Medical Sciences, Second Clinical Medical College of Guangzhou University of Chinese Medicine). She is also the Chair of the Guangdong Traditional Chinese Medicine (TCM) Standardisation Technical Committee, and the Vice-chair of the Immunity Specialty Committee of the World Federation of Chinese Medicine Societies (WFCMS).

Professor Lu has engaged in scientific research into TCM, clinical practice and teaching for some 25 years. Her research has been devoted to integrating traditional and conventional medicine. She has edited and published 12 monographs and 120 academic research articles as first author and corresponding author with over 30 articles being included in SCI journals.

She has received widespread recognition for her achievements, with awards for Excellent Teacher of South China, National Outstanding Women TCM Doctor and National Outstanding Young Doctor of TCM. She also received the Science and Technology Star of the Association of Chinese Medicine, the National Excellent Science and Technology Workers of China Award and the Five-continent Women's Scientific Awards of China Medical Women's Association.

Professor Lu has won the Award of Science and Technology Progress over ten times from Guangdong Provincial Government, China Association of Chinese Medicine and Chinese Hospital Association.

Acknowledgements

The authors and contributors would like to acknowledge the valuable contributions of the following people who assisted with database searches, data extraction, data screening, data assessment, translation of documents, editing and/or administrative tasks: Dr. Jhodie Duncan, Ms. Huanyu Liu, Mr. Jiahao Zeng, Ms. Lu Zeng, Ms. Meifang Liu, Ms. Qing Zhang, Mr. Xianlong Zhang, Ms. Yanmei Zhang, Ms. Yenan Mo and Ms. Ziqi Xu.

Contents

Contents

Contents

List of Figures

List of Tables

1

Introduction to Urinary Tract Infection

OVERVIEW

Urinary tract infections are common in late adolescence and early adulthood, and the incidence increases again in advancing age. Typical symptoms of lower urinary tract infection include dysuria, increased urinary frequency and urgency, haematuria and suprapubic pain, while upper urinary tract infection may also include fever, flank pain and costovertebral tenderness. Antibiotics are the key to successful treatment, although many patients experience recurrence that can be difficult to predict and control.

Definition of Urinary Tract Infection

Uncomplicated urinary tract infection (UTI) is a bacterial infection in the absence of structural or functional abnormalities, or other chronic diseases.[1] Infection can occur in the urethra (urethritis), bladder (cystitis), ureters or kidney (pyelonephritis). Various classification systems exist, and clinical guidelines frequently categorise UTIs as uncomplicated or complicated.[2] The European Association of Urology defines uncomplicated UTIs as 'acute, sporadic or recurrent lower (uncomplicated cystitis) and/or upper (uncomplicated pyelonephritis) UTI, limited to non-pregnant, pre-menopausal women with no known relevant anatomical and functional abnormalities within the urinary tract or comorbidities'.[2,Pt.3.1] Uncomplicated UTIs occur more frequently in females, children and the elderly.[3] Urinary tract infections in males are usually attributed to anatomical or functional changes in the urinary tract, procedures such as catheterisation, and obstruction such as benign prostatic hypertrophy.[4] Complicated UTIs are usually associated with indwelling catheters, structural or functional abnormalities, immune suppression or antibiotic exposure,[3] and are beyond the scope of this book.

Persistent UTIs are those that are not resolved after seven to 14 days of antibiotic treatment.[5] Recurrence of UTIs refers to new symptomatic infection following adequate treatment and confirmed resolution of a previous infection.[5] Several definitions for recurrence exist, such as a frequency of at least two UTIs in six months, or at least three in one year.[2,4,6] The latter is the more commonly accepted definition.[7]

Recurrence can be further categorised into relapse and reinfection. Relapse refers to a UTI with the same organism following adequate treatment.[5] Reinfection refers to a UTI from a different organism, or an infection with the same pathogen despite previous negative urine culture.[8] Reinfections are thought to be more common than relapses.[9]

Clinical Presentation

Signs and symptoms can differ according to the location of infection. Urethritis often presents with dysuria, but dysuria needs to be differentiated from other conditions such as vaginitis.[10] Urethritis presents with a gradual onset of mild symptoms, and haematuria is rarely present.[11] Cystitis typically presents with sudden onset of dysuria with, or without, increased urinary frequency or urgency, suprapubic pain or haematuria.[10,11] Clinical presentation of pyelonephritis can range from mild symptoms to sepsis.[11] In addition to positive urinalysis or culture, pyelonephritis may present with fever and chills, nausea, vomiting, flank pain and costovertebral angle tenderness; the symptoms of cystitis may also be present.[12]

Most cases of UTI present with multiple signs or symptoms. In a survey of 2,715 European women with recurrent UTI, the mean number of symptoms was five.[1] The most common symptom was frequent urination (reported by 90.5% of women), followed by burning pain (82.6%), urinary urgency (78.4%) and bladder pain (77.4%).

However, urinary symptoms and bacteriuria (presence of bacteria in the urine) may not present simultaneously. Bacteriuria may be present in the absence of urinary signs and symptoms, and some cases that present with symptoms are negative for bacteriuria.[13,14] After resolution of the initial infection, recurrence typically occurs within three months and may occur in clusters.[15] The chance of reinfection within six months is higher when uropathogenic *E. coli* (UPEC) was the cause of the initial infection.[16]

Epidemiology

Uncomplicated bacterial UTI is one of the most common infections seen in the community,[17] and is the most common outpatient infection in the United States.[18] Uncomplicated symptomatic UTI is most common in women aged 18 to 29 years.[19] Uncomplicated cystitis is more common than pyelonephritis,[10] with one case of pyelonephritis for every 28 cases of cystitis in Finnish women.[20] Urinary tract infections are more common in women,[3] likely due to the female anatomy with a shorter distance between the anus and urethra and shorter length of urethra.[4] Estimates in 1993 suggest 150 million people experience a UTI per year worldwide.[21]

Prevalence in the United States has been estimated at 0.7%.[18] Based on registry data for 2,339 cases of women with a UTI in the United States, Taur and Smith (2007) extrapolated that there were 7 million visits to health practitioners per year between 1998 and 2001.[22] The number of visits for UTI symptoms was higher in 2007, with 10.5 million visits to health practitioners and 2.2 million visits to hospital emergency departments.[18]

Approximately 11% of American women reported at least one UTI in the previous year, and the incidence was highest in women aged between 18 and 24 years.[19] Despite reports that the incidence increases to approximately 20% in women aged 65 years or more,[8,23] self-reported incidence in this age group was less than 10% in research by Foxman *et al.* (2000).[19] Recurrent UTI is common among women, affecting between 27% and 44% of women who have experienced a UTI previously.[20,24]

Uncomplicated cystitis is the second most common infection in the community setting in Europe.[4] In Australia, UTIs accounted for 1.2% of the problems managed in general practice between 2015 and 2016.[25] In China, 50% of hospital-acquired infections are UTIs,[26] while few studies have examined community-acquired infections such as UTIs.[27]

Burden

Urinary tract infections incur a personal, social and economic burden. In a study of the natural course of acute UTI in women, symptoms lasted on average 3.83 days, and longer when the uropathogen was resistant to antibiotic treatment or when treatment was not provided.[28] Estimates from the United States suggest health care costs, including costs of consultation and treatment, and work absenteeism due to UTI, are USD 3.5 billion per year.[3]

In additional to physical symptoms, the personal burden of recurrent UTI includes anxiety and depression, and feelings of guilt about being unable to perform daily activities.[23] Repeated urine testing or imaging studies for recurrent UTI can impact on health-related quality of life and poses a financial burden for patients.[23] A recent multinational study of 1,941 European women with recurrent UTI found 47.4% had experienced at least six UTIs in the previous year, and 14.4% suffered at least 13 infections, resulting in a mean of 2.78 doctor visits.[1] The mean number of antibiotic prescriptions was 2.89, with an estimated cost of at least €54.57 per person per year. Women in this study took an average of 3.1 sick days each year.

A systematic review by Bermingham *et al.* (2012)[29] found few studies had examined the impact of UTI on health-related quality of life. Some studies found poorer quality of life on general wellbeing scales in people with UTI, compared with those without UTI, while others showed no difference. None of the included studies used disease-specific quality of life scales. The multinational study by Wagenlehner *et al.* (2018)[1] also examined the impact of recurrent UTI on quality of life using the Rand 12-item Short Form Health Survey (SF-12). Women with an active infection during the survey had lower physical and mental health scores than women who were in remission. Women in remission had lower scores on the mental health domain, indicating poorer quality of life, compared with US population norms.

Risk Factors

Women are more likely to experience a UTI than men.[30] Risk factors that predispose people to UTI and host defence factors that affect bacterial virulence have been identified. Behavioural risk factors include a new sexual partner within one year, sexual intercourse and use of spermicide/condom/diaphragm.[30,31] Previous antibiotic use increases the risk of UTI. This has been postulated to alter the normal microbiota of the vagina and gut, and may contribute to the development of drug-resistant bacteria.[3]

Biological factors include structural or function abnormalities, urinary obstruction, residual urine, atrophic vaginitis, urinary incontinence, prior history of UTI, use of catheters, and health conditions such as diabetes mellitus, pregnancy, kidney transplant, vaginal infection and obesity.[30,31] Trauma or manipulation may also contribute to UTI.[30]

Non-modifiable host factors include female gender, genetics and innate immune responses.[32] Genetic factors also play a role in the susceptibility to UTI. People who are non-secretors of ABH blood group antigen are more likely to develop a UTI, as are those with compromised immunity.[33] Increased numbers of adhesin receptors in the bladder epithelium increases the likelihood of bacterial colonisation.[31] Vaginal *Lactobacilli* contribute to maintaining vaginal pH. A decline in oestrogen during menopause reduces vaginal *Lactobacilli*, which creates an opportunity for uropathogens.[33] Risk factors for recurrent UTI are similar to those for sporadic UTI.[34] In addition, childhood and maternal history of UTI increase the risk of recurrent infections.[10,34]

Pathological Processes

The most common bacterial species in both complicated and uncomplicated UTI is *Escherichia coli* (*E. coli*),[3,23] accounting for between

75% and 95% of uncomplicated UTI cases.[10] Uropathogenic *E. coli* is a subset of extraintestinal *E. coli* that is specifically associated with uncomplicated UTI.[10,32] Other species that cause UTI include *Klebsiella pneumoniae, Enterococcus* species, group B *Streptococcus, Proteus mirabilis* and other *Proteus* species, *Staphylococcus saprophyticus, Pseudomonas aeruginosa, Staphylococcus aureus* and *Candida* species.[3,35]

Many uncomplicated UTIs develop when bacteria from the perineum, vagina or gastrointestinal tract invade the urethra.[3,36] Several protective factors act to prevent bacteria establishment (colonising) in the urinary tract. Uropathogens are flushed from the urethra or vagina during urination, and the normal bacterial flora resident in the perineal area act to resist uropathogens.[36] Furthermore, the acidic environment of the vagina inhibits bacterial growth.[37] When these protective mechanisms fail, bacteria have the opportunity to colonise the urinary tract.

The mechanisms by which bacteria cause infections in the urinary tract are generally well understood, with some differences in mechanisms according to the uropathogen. Most UTIs are caused by periurethral contamination by bacteria that live in the gut.[3] Uropathogenic *E. coli*, the cause of most UTIs, leave the gastrointestinal tract, and are exposed to the external environment. Exposure to oxygen initiates expression of adhesive fibres on the cell surface called pili.[38] Flagella on the cell surface allow movement of bacteria up the urethra to the bladder.[39] Pili facilitate the adhesion of many bacteria to the epithelial cells of the bladder (uroepithelial cells), and type 1 pili are key for UPEC adhesion.[3] FimH adhesin found at the end of type 1 pili allows UPEC to bind to uroplakins, the protein component of the apical membrane of uroepithelial cells.[3,31] The $\alpha_3\beta_1$ integrins expressed at the surface of the uroepithelial cell also act as receptors for UPEC.[3] Once attached, the bacterium invades the uroepithelial cell.

Bacterial invasion triggers the innate immune response. Lipopolysaccharide (LPS) secreted by UPEC is detected by Toll-like receptor 4 (TLR4) expressed by uroepithelial cells.[40] Once activated, TLR4 stimulates the enzyme adenylyl cyclase 3 to produce cyclic adenosine monophosphate (cAMP).[41] The increased level of intracellular cAMP induces exocytosis of intracellular UPEC through the cell membrane.[41] Toll-like receptor 4 also induces expression of the pro-inflammatory cytokine interleukin (IL)-6 and C-X-C motif chemokine ligand (CXCL)-8.[42] The inflammatory response also results in neutrophil infiltration to remove extracellular bacteria.[32] The ability of bacteria to colonise the urinary tract depends on the outcome of this inflammatory process.[3]

Some bacteria can avoid exocytosis and escape into the host cell cytoplasm.[3,42] Bacteria release toxins and proteases that damage host cells and allow for the release of nutrients that help bacteria to grow, and produce siderophores to obtain iron.[3] Once inside, bacteria can multiply and develop intracellular bacterial communities (IBCs),[42] with a biofilm-like barrier to antibiotics.[3] Uropathogenic *E. coli* and other uropathogens change shape to allow them to become resistant to neutrophils in order to survive.[3]

When mature, IBCs assume a filamentous cellular shape to exit the cell and invade other host cells, thus continuing the cycle.[3,42] Shedding of the superficial epithelial cells exposes transitional cells below. Bacteria can then invade these immature cells.[43] The small size of transitional cells and abundance of actin filaments appear to restrict bacterial multiplication.[43] Unable to replicate, bacteria establish quiescent intracellular reservoirs that can remain viable for several months.[3] It is hypothesised that bacteria are reactivated when actin filaments rearrange during transitional cell differentiation into uroepithelial cells, leading to recurrent infections.[42,43] Bacteria can also migrate to, and colonise, the kidney to cause pyelonephritis.[42] The mechanisms of other bacteria in establishing infection are similar, although different structures and adhesins are involved in binding bacteria to the uroepithelial cells. Flores-Mireles *et al.* (2015)[3] provide a description of such virulence factors for common uropathogens.

Diagnosis

Diagnosis of UTIs relies on assessment of clinical presentation and biological tests. The chance of cystitis in women who present with dysuria, increased urinary frequency or urgency, or suprapubic pain is 50%, and increases to 90% when dysuria and increased urinary frequency occur in the absence of vaginal discharge or irritation.[44] In men, dysuria, increased urinary urgency or frequency, and/or suprapubic pain suggest UTI.[45] Fever, flank pain and costovertebral angle tenderness are more indicative of upper UTI.[45]

Midstream urinalysis for pyuria (presence of white blood cells in urine) provides only a small increase in diagnostic accuracy when typical symptoms are present.[2] Urinalysis may assist in diagnosis when symptoms are not clear, and can be performed using a dipstick or by microscopy.[46] A result of greater than 10 leucocytes per microlitre is considered abnormal.[47] A midstream urine culture quantifies uropathogen colonisation, typically using a colony count criteria of $\geq 10^3$ colony forming units/millilitre.[45,46]

Clinical diagnosis of cystitis is made in women with typical signs and symptoms.[46] Diagnosis should be supported by urinalysis and urine culture for women with atypical symptoms.[46] Diagnosis of cystitis in men is made when symptoms are typical of cystitis, and when urinalysis and urine culture indicate pyuria and bacteriuria, respectively.[45]

When pyelonephritis is suspected based on symptoms, urinalysis and urine culture should be performed to confirm diagnosis.[48] Pyelonephritis may be present in adults with fever and flank pain, without typical symptoms of cystitis.[49] Physical examination should include assessment of costovertebral, suprapubic or abdominal tenderness.[49] Pelvic examination of sexually active women with less convincing symptoms of UTI may be performed to exclude pelvic inflammatory disease.[49] Rectal examination to exclude acute prostatitis may be warranted in men with pelvic or perineal pain.[49] Imaging studies are not usually required for diagnosis.[49]

In women with recurrent uncomplicated UTI, a physical examination should be performed, including pelvic examination, to exclude structural or functional abnormalities.[50] Imaging and cystoscopy are not necessary for diagnosis in all women, while postvoid residual and uroflowmetry may be used for postmenopausal women with recurrent UTI.[50] If abnormality is strongly suspected, computed tomography may be useful to aid diagnosis.[50]

Management

Management of UTI involves patient education and counselling, and pharmacological and non-pharmacological treatments. The clinical practice guidelines of the European Association of Urology (EAU),[2] Canadian Urological Association (CUA),[50] Society of Obstetricians and Gynaecologists of Canada (SOGC),[7,51] American College of Obstetricians and Gynecologists (ACOG),[8] Infectious Diseases Society of America and the European Society for Microbiology and Infectious Diseases (IDSA/ESCMID),[48] German Urological Society (Deutsche Gesellschaft fur Urologie, DGU),[17] National Institute for Health and Care Excellence (NICE),[52,53] Scottish Intercollegiate Guidelines Network (SIGN)[54] and the Korean guideline for UTI,[55] as well as the joint guideline of the American Urological Association (AUA), CUA and Society of Urodynamics, Female Pelvic Medicine & Urogenital Reconstruction (SUFU)[56] were reviewed to identify treatments for acute and recurrent UTI. While the list of guidelines consulted is not exhaustive, these were considered to be representative of management for UTI. Additional resources that can inform clinical practice include USA Choosing Wisely®;[57] the policy statement on antimicrobial stewardship by the Society for Healthcare Epidemiology of America, the Infectious Diseases Society of America and the Pediatric Infectious Diseases Society;[58] and the Japanese Society of Chemotherapy and Japanese Association for Infectious Diseases guideline for clinical research of antimicrobial agents on urogenital infections.[59]

Antibiotics are the mainstay of treatment. However, misuse and over-prescription have contributed to antibiotic resistance in uropathogenic bacteria.[2] Fluoroquinolones and trimethoprim/sulfamethoxazole have high resistance rates in some countries, while some of the older antibiotics, such as fosfomycin and nitrofurantoin, have continued to have high microbial activity against uropathogens.[4] Antimicrobial stewardship programmes have been developed that require adherence to guidelines in clinical care, as well as developing approaches to ensure adherence to such guidelines.[2] Such programmes have been effective in improving prescribing practices and reducing duration of antibiotic use.[60]

Acute Urinary Tract Infection

Antibiotics are an affordable and effective treatment for bacterial UTIs. Bacteriuria in the absence of symptoms does not require treatment in non-pregnant women.[54] For symptomatic women with uncomplicated cystitis, the choice of antibiotic should be made based on susceptibility of uropathogen, effectiveness, safety, cost, availability, allergy and prevalence of resistance in the local community.[2,48] The NICE guideline recommends offering women the option of immediate or back-up antibiotics, which can be used if symptoms don't improve within 48 hours or if symptoms worsen.[53]

Recommendations in clinical guidelines vary in terms of antibiotic, dose and duration of treatment. The treatment duration of antibiotics recommended as first-choice treatment for acute uncomplicated cystitis is summarised in Table 1.1. Not all guidelines indicated

Table 1.1. Guideline-recommended Treatment Duration for Acute Uncomplicated Cystitis

Antibiotic	ACOG[8]	DGU[17]	EAU[2]	IDSA/ ESCMID[48]	NICE[52,53]	SIGN[54]	Korea[55]
Fosfomycin	sd	sd	sd	sd	—	—	sd
Pivmecillinam	—	3 d	3–5 d	5 d	—	—	≥ 3 d
Nitrofurantoin	7 d	7 d/5 d (sr)	5 d	5 d	3 d ♀; 7 d ♂	3 d	≥ 5 d
Trimethoprim	3 d	—	5 d	—	3 d ♀; 7 d ♂	3 d	—
Trimethoprim/ Sulfamethoxazole	3 d	—	3 d ♀; 7 d ♂	—	3 d ♀; 7 d ♂	3 d	—
Ciprofloxacin	3 d	—	—	—	—	—	≥ 3 d

Table 1.1. (*Continued*)

Antibiotic	ACOG[8]	DGU[17]	EAU[2]	IDSA/ ESCMID[48]	NICE[52,53]	SIGN[54]	Korea[55]
Levofloxacin	3 d	—	—	—	—	—	—
Norfloxacin	3 d	—	—	—	—	—	—
Gatifloxacin	3 d	—	—	—	—	—	—
Nitroxoline	—	5 d	—	—	—	—	—
Beta-lactams	—	—	—	—	—	—	≥ 3 d

Guidelines: ACOG, American College of Obstetricians and Gynaecologists; DGU, German Urological Society (Deutsche Gesellschaft fur Urologie); EAU, European Association of Urology; IDSA/ESCMID, Infectious Diseases Society of America and the European Society for Microbiology and Infectious Diseases; NICE, National Institute for Health and Care Excellence; SIGN, Scottish Intercollegiate Guidelines Network.

Abbreviations: ♀, women; ♂, men; d, days; sd, single dose; sr, slow release.

first-choice treatments; where this information was not specified, all recommended antibiotics are listed. Readers are encouraged to review the guidelines to view second-choice treatments local to their region.

Differences in practice recommendations were noted, which may be due to local susceptibility and drug availability. For example, the Korean guideline recommended nitrofurantoin and pivmecillinam as first-choice treatment, despite these drugs not yet being available in Korea.[26] Nitrofurantoin was recommended as a first-choice antibiotic in all guidelines reviewed, while fosfomycin, trimethoprim and pivmecillinam were recommended as first-choice treatment in at least four guidelines. Most first-choice antibiotics should be used for three to five days.

People with pyelonephritis should be offered pain relief and an antibiotic, and be encouraged to maintain fluid intake to avoid dehydration.[52] Cases of acute pyelonephritis can be managed as outpatients or inpatients according to severity. Outpatient management using oral fluoroquinolones, cephalosporines,[2,48,52] or trimethoprim/sulfamethoxazole if the uropathogen is susceptible,[48] is appropriate. An initial intravenous dose of ciprofloxacin[48] or ceftriaxone[55] may be used.

Inpatient management of pyelonephritis typically involves intravenous administration of antibiotics for seven to 14 days. Antibiotics recommended in guidelines include fluoroquinolones, cephalosporin, aminoglycosides, penicillin or a carbapenem where urine culture has shown multidrug-resistant uropathogens.[2,17,48,52,55] Choice of antibiotic should be made based on known local residence data.[48] Co-amoxiclav is recommended in the NICE guideline based on urine culture.[52] Second-choice treatments vary, and can be found in the reviewed guidelines.

Recurrent Urinary Tract Infection

Conservative measures for people with recurrent UTI include education about avoidance of risk factors, use of alternatives to spermicides and diaphragms as contraception, and non-antimicrobial treatments.[2,51] Dason *et al.* (2011)[50] suggest that, despite a lack of evidence, voiding before and after sexual intercourse is unlikely to be harmful.

Antimicrobial prophylaxis should be offered after obtaining urine culture to confirm resolution[8,51,56] and based on patient preferences and history.[8] Continuous low-dose antibiotic therapy is recommended to prevent recurrent UTI.[50] Guidelines vary in their recommendation of treatment duration; the EAU recommends continuous low-dose treatment for three to six months,[2] while the SOGC[51] and ACOG[8] recommend treatment for six to 12 months.

Antibiotics for continuous use include once-daily nitrofurantoin, trimethoprim, trimethoprim/sulfamethoxazole,[2,17,50,51] cephalexin,[50,51] norfloxacin, ciprofloxacin,[8,17,50] cotrimoxazole[17] or a quinolone,[51] or fosfomycin every ten days.[2,17] While these may be offered, uptake of antibiotic prophylaxis was reported in less than 40% of people with recurrent UTI.[1]

Postcoital antibiotic therapy commenced within two hours of coitus is effective[2] and may be considered for women with recurrence associated with sexual activity.[8] Postcoital prophylaxis should be offered to women as an alternative to continuous therapy.[51] Antibiotics for postcoital prophylaxis include trimethoprim/sulfamethoxazole, ciprofloxacin, cephalexin, nitrofurantoin, norfloxacin and oflaxacin.[17,50] 'Self-start' antibiotic use for three days is an alternative option for women able to identify the symptoms of UTI.[50]

Non-antibiotic treatments exist for which there is varying evidence. Guidelines differ in their recommendations about oestrogen therapy for postmenopausal women. The SIGN guideline advises against oestrogens for routine prevention of recurrent UTI in postmenopausal women,[54] while guidelines of the CUA,[50] the SOGC[51] and the EAU[2] all support the use of vaginal oestrogens for postmenopausal women with recurrent UTI.

Other non-antibiotic treatments for recurrent UTI show varying results. Methenamine hippurate acts as a urinary alkaliser and has bactericidal actions against *E. coli*.[61] Methenamine shows promise in preventing UTI in people with no abnormalities of the renal tract.[54,62] Bacterial extracts can act as immune stimulants, and meta-analysis has shown one product, OM-89, which contains five serotypes of heat-killed *E. coli*, is more effective than placebo at preventing UTI recurrence[63] and is recommended in the EAU guidelines.[2] There is no evidence to support the use of urinary alkalisation in preventing UTI recurrence.[61]

Complementary and Alternative Medicine

Foxman, (2010),[14] notes that the problem of antibiotic resistance may signal a need to examine other options for UTI. Many women with bladder-related problems seek alternatives to antibiotics, including complementary and alternative medicines.[64] The guideline of the SOGC suggests that acupuncture may be considered for prevention of recurrent UTI in women who do not respond to, or are intolerant of, antibiotic treatment.[51] A recent systematic review of non-antibiotic treatments for prophylaxis of UTI found two studies that showed acupuncture was more effective than no treatment in preventing recurrence.[65]

Chinese herbal medicine (CHM) for UTI has been the subject of a Cochrane systematic review by Flower *et al.* (2015).[66] Seven small studies were included in this review that found CHM was effective when used alone, or combined with antibiotics in resolving acute infection, and may prevent recurrence for six months after treatment has ended. The authors were unable to make strong conclusions due to the small number of studies and suboptimal study quality.

Cranberry products have been recommended in several of the earlier guidelines;[7,54] however, more recent evidence has cast doubt over their effectiveness, particularly for women with recurrent UTI.[67] The CUA[50] and EAU[2] recommend against the use of cranberry products, while the guidelines of the SOGC continue to recommend their use.[51] The joint guideline of the AUA, CUA and SUFU suggests there is no apparent benefit or harm with cranberry product use.[56] Probiotics were found to be no better than placebo, or no treatment, in preventing recurrent UTI, with limited evidence for their effectiveness compared to antibiotics.[68]

Prognosis

Uncomplicated cystitis will usually resolve if untreated, although the recovery time is slower than when antibiotics are administered.[14] Untreated UTIs may lead to kidney damage, kidney failure or sepsis, so receiving appropriate treatment is important. Cystitis is responsive to appropriate antibiotic treatment, with relief of symptoms occurring within hours of the first dose.[45,46] When symptoms have resolved with a short course of treatment, there is no requirement for additional urine culture. Urinalysis should be repeated in patients who presented with haematuria initially.[46] Women whose symptoms persist after 48 hours, or recur within a few weeks of antibiotic treatment, should be evaluated to exclude other causes.[45,46] Urological evaluation in men with persistent symptoms should include assessment for prostatitis.[45]

Patients receiving outpatient antibiotic therapy for pyelonephritis should receive rapid relief from symptoms, and should be followed up within 48 hours.[49] Additional evaluation, including imaging, is required for patients who do not respond to treatment, whose symptoms worsen or who have symptoms of upper UTI such as pyelonephritis.[49] Urine culture should be repeated to allow appropriate selection of an antibiotic according to the susceptibility of the infective organism.[49]

Initial infection with UPEC increases the likelihood of recurrent infection.[16] Low-dose continuous therapy and postcoital therapy may reduce recurrence, but many people continue to experience recurrent infections despite their use.[3] New treatments targeting the initial stages of infection may provide alternative solutions to antibiotics in the future.[3]

References

1. Wagenlehner F, Wullt B, Ballarini S, *et al.* (2018) Social and economic burden of recurrent urinary tract infections and quality of life: A patient web-based study (GESPRIT). *Expert Rev Pharmacoecon Outcomes Res* **18**(1): 107–117.

2. Bonkat G, Pickard R, Bartoletti R, *et al.* (2018) EAU guidelines on urological infections 2018. European Association of Urology Guidelines 2018 Edition presented at the EAU Annual Congress, Copenhagen 2018. European Association of Urology Guidelines Office, Arnhem, the Netherlands.

3. Flores-Mireles AL, Walker JN, Caparon M, *et al.* (2015) Urinary tract infections: Epidemiology, mechanisms of infection and treatment options. *Nat Rev Microbiol* **13**(5): 269–284.

4. Concia E, Bragantini D, Mazzaferri F. (2017) Clinical evaluation of guidelines and therapeutic approaches in multi drug-resistant urinary tract infections. *J Chemother* **29**(Suppl 1): 19–28.

5. Nosseir SB, Lind LR, Winkler HA. (2012) Recurrent uncomplicated urinary tract infections in women: A review. *J Womens Health (Larchmt)* **21**(3): 347–354.

6. Kranz J, Schmidt S, Lebert C, *et al.* (2018) The 2017 update of the German clinical guideline on epidemiology, diagnostics, therapy, prevention, and management of uncomplicated urinary tract infections in adult patients: Part 1. *Urol Int* **100**(3): 263–270.

7. Epp A, Larochelle A, SOGC Urogynaecology Committee, *et al.* (2010) Recurrent urinary tract infection. SOGC Clinical Practice Guideline No. 250. *J Obstet Gynaecol Can* **32**(11): 1082–1090.

8. American College of Obstetricians and Gynecologists. (2008) ACOG Practice Bulletin No. 91: Treatment of urinary tract infections in non-pregnant women. *Obstet Gynecol* **111**(3): 785–794.

9. Hooton TM. (2001) Recurrent urinary tract infection in women. *Int J Antimicrob Agents* **17**(4): 259–268.

10. Hooton TM. (2012) Clinical practice: Uncomplicated urinary tract infection. *N Engl J Med* **366**(11): 1028–1037.

11. Stamm WE, Hooton TM. (1993) Management of urinary tract infections in adults. *N Engl J Med* **329**(18): 1328–1334.

12. Ramakrishnan K, Scheid DC. (2005) Diagnosis and management of acute pyelonephritis in adults. *Am Fam Physician* **71**(5): 933–942.

13. Ferry SA, Holm SE, Stenlund H, *et al.* (2007) Clinical and bacterio-logical outcome of different doses and duration of pivmecillinam compared with placebo therapy of uncomplicated lower urinary tract infection in women: The LUTIW project. *Scand J Prim Health Care* **25**(1): 49–57.

14. Foxman B. (2010) The epidemiology of urinary tract infection. *Nat Rev Urol* **7**(12): 653–660.

15. Kraft JK, Stamey TA. (1977) The natural history of symptomatic recurrent bacteriuria in women. *Medicine (Baltimore)* **56**(1): 55–60.

16. Foxman B, Gillespie B, Koopman J, *et al.* (2000) Risk factors for second urinary tract infection among college women. *Am J Epidemiol* **151**(12): 1194–1205.

17. Kranz J, Schmidt S, Lebert C, *et al.* (2017) Uncomplicated bacterial community acquired urinary tract infection in adults. *Dtsch Arztebl Int* **114**(50): 866–873.

18. Schappert SM, Rechtsteiner EA. (2011) Ambulatory medical care utili-zation estimates for 2007. *Vital Health Stat* **13**(169): 1–38.

19. Foxman B, Barlow R, D'Arcy H, *et al.* (2000) Urinary tract infection: Self-reported incidence and associated costs. *Ann Epidemiol* **10**(8): 509–515.

20. Ikaheimo R, Siitonen A, Heiskanen T, *et al.* (1996) Recurrence of urinary tract infection in a primary care setting: Analysis of a 1-year follow-up of 179 women. *Clin Infect Dis* **22**(1): 91–99.

21. Harding GK, Ronald AR. (1994) The management of urinary infections: What have we learned in the past decade? *Int J Antimicrob Agents* **4**(2): 83–88.

22. Taur Y, Smith MA. (2007) Adherence to the Infectious Diseases Society of America guidelines in the treatment of uncomplicated urinary tract infection. *Clin Infect Dis* **44**(6): 769–774.

23. Medina M, Castillo-Pino E. (2019) An introduction to the epidemiology and burden of urinary tract infections. *Ther Adv Urol* **11**: 175628721 9832172.

24. Foxman B. (1990) Recurring urinary tract infection: Incidence and risk factors. *Am J Public Health* **80**(3): 331–333.

25. Britt H, Miller G, Henderson J, *et al.* (2016) General practice activity in Australia 2015–2016. Sydney University Press, Sydney. Available from: purl.library.usyd.edu.au/sup/9781743325131.

26. Qiao LD, Chen S, Yang Y, *et al.* (2013) Characteristics of urinary tract infection pathogens and their in vitro susceptibility to antimicrobial agents in China: Data from a multicenter study. *BMJ Open* **3**(12): e004152.

27. Ling JM, Lam AW, Chan EW, *et al.* (2003) What have we learnt from community-acquired infections in Hong Kong? *J Antimicrob Chemother* **51**(4): 895–904.

28. Little P, Merriman R, Turner S, *et al.* (2010) Presentation, pattern, and natural course of severe symptoms, and role of antibiotics and antibiotic resistance among patients presenting with suspected uncomplicated urinary tract infection in primary care: Observational study. *BMJ* **340**: b5633.

29. Bermingham SL, Ashe JF. (2012) Systematic review of the impact of urinary tract infections on health-related quality of life. *BJU Int* **110**(11 Pt C): e830–e836.

30. Foxman B. (2014) Urinary tract infection syndromes: Occurrence, recurrence, bacteriology, risk factors, and disease burden. *Infect Dis Clin North Am* **28**(1): 1–13.

31. Ronald A. (2003) The etiology of urinary tract infection: Traditional and emerging pathogens. *Dis Mon* **49**(2): 71–82.

32. Stapleton AE. (2014) Urinary tract infection pathogenesis: Host factors. *Infect Dis Clin North Am* **28**(1): 149–159.

33. Madersbacher S, Thalhammer F, Marberger M. (2000) Pathogenesis and management of recurrent urinary tract infection in women. *Curr Opin Urol* **10**(1): 29–33.

34. Scholes D, Hooton TM, Roberts PL, *et al.* (2000) Risk factors for recurrent urinary tract infection in young women. *J Infect Dis* **182**(4): 1177–1182.

35. Laupland KB, Ross T, Pitout JD, *et al.* (2007) Community-onset urinary tract infections: A population-based assessment. *Infection* **35**(3): 150–153.

36. Chung A, Arianayagam M, Rashid P. (2010) Bacterial cystitis in women. *Aust Fam Physician* **39**(5): 295–298.

37. Goldstein I. (2010) Recognizing and treating urogenital atrophy in postmenopausal women. *J Womens Health (Larchmt)* **19**(3): 425–432.

38. Floyd KA, Moore JL, Eberly AR, *et al.* (2015) Adhesive fiber stratification in uropathogenic Escherichia coli biofilms unveils oxygen-mediated control of type 1 pili. *PLoS Pathog* **11**(3): e1004697.
39. Schaeffer A. (2010) Pathogeneis of urinary tract infections: Introduction. In: Naber K, Schaeffer A, Heyns C, *et al.* (eds), *Urogenital infections,* 2010 ed. The European Association of Urology, the Netherlands.
40. Mak RH, Kuo HJ. (2006) Pathogenesis of urinary tract infection: An update. *Curr Opin Pediatr* **18**(2): 148–152.
41. Song J, Bishop BL, Li G, *et al.* (2009) TLR4-mediated expulsion of bacteria from infected bladder epithelial cells. *Proc Natl Acad Sci U S A* **106**(35): 14966–14971.
42. Floyd KA, Meyer AE, Nelson G, *et al.* (2015) The yin-yang driving urinary tract infection and how proteomics can enhance research, diagnostics, and treatment. *Proteomics Clin Appl* **9**(11–12): 990–1002.
43. Blango MG, Ott EM, Erman A, *et al.* (2014) Forced resurgence and targeting of intracellular uropathogenic Escherichia coli reservoirs. *PLoS One* **9**(3): e93327.
44. Bent S, Nallamothu BK, Simel DL, *et al.* (2002) Does this woman have an acute uncomplicated urinary tract infection? *JAMA* **287**(20): 2701–2710.
45. Hooton TM. (2018) Acute simple cystitis in men. Available from: https://www.uptodate.com/contents/acute-simple-cystitis-in-men.
46. Hooton TM, Gupta K. (2019) Acute simple cystitis in women. Available from: https://www.uptodate.com/contents/acute-simple-cystitis-in-women.
47. Stamm WE. (1983) Measurement of pyuria and its relation to bacteriuria. *Am J Med* **75**(1b): 53–58.
48. Gupta K, Hooton TM, Naber KG, *et al.* (2011) International clinical practice guidelines for the treatment of acute uncomplicated cystitis and pyelonephritis in women: A 2010 update by the Infectious Diseases Society of America and the European Society for Microbiology and Infectious Diseases. *Clin Infect Dis* **52**(5): e103–e120.
49. Hooton TM, Gupta K. (2019) Acute complicated urinary tract infection (including pyelonephritis) in adults. Available from: https://www.uptodate.com/contents/acute-complicated-urinary-tract-infection-including-pyelonephritis-in-adults.
50. Dason S, Dason JT, Kapoor A. (2011) Guidelines for the diagnosis and management of recurrent urinary tract infection in women. *Can Urol Assoc J* **5**(5): 316–322.
51. Epp A, Larochelle A. (2017) No. 250-Recurrent urinary tract infection. *J Obstet Gynaecol Can* **39**(10): e422–e431.

52. National Institute for Health and Care Excellence. (2018) Pyelonephritis (acute): Antimicrobial prescribing – NICE guideline (NG 111). Available from: https://www.nice.org.uk/guidance/ng111.

53. National Institute for Health and Care Excellence. (2018) Urinary tract infection (lower): Antimicrobial prescribing – NICE guideline (NG109). Available from: https://www.nice.org.uk/guidance/ng109.

54. Scottish Intercollegiate Guidelines Network. (2012) SIGN 88: Management of suspected bacterial urinary tract infection in adults. Available from: https://www.sign.ac.uk/assets/sign88.pdf.

55. Kang CI, Kim J, Park DW, *et al.* (2018) Clinical practice guidelines for the antibiotic treatment of community-acquired urinary tract infections. *Infect Chemother* **50**(1): 67–100.

56. Anger J, Lee U, Ackerman AL, *et al.* (2019) Recurrent uncomplicated urinary tract infections in women: AUA/CUA/SUFU guideline. *J Urol* **202**(2): 282–289.

57. ABIM Foundation. (2019) Choosing wisely®: Promoting conversations between patients and clinicians. Available from: https://www.choosing-wisely.org/.

58. Society for Healthcare Epidemiology of America, Infectious Diseases Society of America, Pediatric Infectious Diseases Society. (2012) Policy statement on antimicrobial stewardship by the Society for Healthcare Epidemiology of America (SHEA), the Infectious Diseases Society of America (IDSA), and the Pediatric Infectious Diseases Society (PIDS). *Infect Control Hosp Epidemiol* **33**(4): 322–327.

59. Yasuda M, Muratani T, Ishikawa K, *et al.* (2016) Japanese guideline for clinical research of antimicrobial agents on urogenital infections: Second edition. *J Infect Chemother* **22**(10): 651–661.

60. Davey P, Marwick CA, Scott CL, *et al.* (2017) Interventions to improve antibiotic prescribing practices for hospital inpatients. *Cochrane Database Syst Rev* **2**: Cd003543.

61. Barclay J, Veeratterapillay R, Harding C. (2017) Non-antibiotic options for recurrent urinary tract infections in women. *BMJ* **359**: j5193.

62. Lee BS, Bhuta T, Simpson JM, *et al.* (2012) Methenamine hippurate for preventing urinary tract infections. *Cochrane Database Syst Rev* **10**: Cd003265.

63. Naber KG, Cho YH, Matsumoto T, *et al.* (2009) Immunoactive prophylaxis of recurrent urinary tract infections: A meta-analysis. *Int J Antimicrob Agents* **33**(2): 111–119.

64. Flower A, Bishop FL, Lewith G. (2014) How women manage recurrent urinary tract infections: An analysis of postings on a popular web forum. *BMC Fam Pract* **15**: 162.

65. Beerepoot MA, Geerlings SE, van Haarst EP, *et al.* (2013) Nonantibiotic prophylaxis for recurrent urinary tract infections: A systematic review and meta-analysis of randomized controlled trials. *J Urol* **190**(6): 1981–1999.

66. Flower A, Wang LQ, Lewith G, *et al.* (2015) Chinese herbal medicine for treating recurrent urinary tract infections in women. *Cochrane Database Syst Rev* (6): Cd010446.

67. Jepson RG, Williams G, Craig JC. (2012) Cranberries for preventing urinary tract infections. *Cochrane Database Syst Rev* **10**: Cd001321.

68. Schwenger EM, Tejani AM, Loewen PS. (2015) Probiotics for preventing urinary tract infections in adults and children. *Cochrane Database Syst Rev* (12): Cd008772.

2

Urinary Tract Infection in Chinese Medicine

OVERVIEW

Urinary tract infection is part of a group of symptoms that are referred to as *lin zheng* 淋证 (strangury syndrome). Urinary tract infection is caused by dampness-heat binding in the Lower Energiser and inhibited transformation of Kidney and Bladder *qi*. Acute urinary tract infection is considered to be an exterior excess pattern and the treatments will focus on clearing heat and draining dampness. Recurrent or chronic persistent urinary tract infection involves both exterior excess and interior deficiency patterns, and treatments aim to reinforce the healthy *qi*, clear heat and drain dampness. This chapter explains the terminology, aetiology, pathogenesis, Chinese medicine syndrome differentiation and treatments for urinary tract infection. Treatments include acupuncture, Chinese herbal medicine and other Chinese medicine therapies. The prevention and management of urinary tract infections are also discussed.

Introduction

The Chinese biomedical term for urinary disease, including urinary stones, prostatic hypertrophy and bladder cancer, is *mi niao xi tong ji bing* 泌尿系統疾病, while *mi niao xi tong gan ran* 泌尿系統感染 specifically refers to urinary tract infection (UTI). These terms are not used in Chinese medicine (CM), which uses the term *lin zheng* 淋证

(*lin* 淋 syndrome, which has a meaning similar to strangury) to encompass a range of urinary diseases, including UTI.

The term, *lin* 淋 syndrome, has been used in many of the classical CM texts, and continues to be used in contemporary CM literature. Urinary disease has also been referred to as *long* 癃 disease prior to the Han dynasty (206 BC to 220 AD), and the terms *lin* 淋 and *long* 癃 were considered to be synonyms.[1] When it re-emerged in texts from the Song and Jin dynasty, the meaning changed, instead referring to urinary retention (for more information see Chapter 3).

Contemporary texts attribute clinical symptoms, such as frequent urination, small urine volume with stabbing pain, dribbling or inhibited urination, and lower abdominal (or lower back) pain, to *lin* 淋 syndrome.[2] Other terms used to describe *lin* 淋 syndrome in classical literature include *lin bi* 淋闭, *lin mi* 淋秘, *lin sou* 淋溲 and *lin li* 淋沥. The terms *lin bi* 淋闭 and *lin mi* 淋秘 can be translated as strangury and/or urinary retention, while *lin sou* 淋溲 and *lin li* 淋沥 refer to dribbling urination.

Several well-known passages from classical CM texts have described *lin* 淋 syndrome. In the *Su Wen·Liu Yuan Zheng Ji Da Lun* 素问·六元正纪大论 (published during the Warring States period, 457–221 BC), *lin bi* 淋閟 was described as: 'if the internal heat [is] not clear … the frenetic movement of Blood due to heat will lead to *lin bi* 淋閟'. In *Jin Kui Yao Lue·Xiao Ke Xiao Bian Bu Li Lin Bing Mai Bing Zhi* 金匮要略·消渴小便不利淋病脉证并治 (c. 206 AD), *lin mi* 淋秘 was caused by heat in the Lower Energiser. The CM dictionary *Zhong Yi Da Ci Dian* 中医大词典 highlights painful or dribbling discharge of urine with inability to achieve a full stream as the key symptoms of *lin* 淋 syndrome.[3]

Six subtypes of *lin* 淋 syndrome have been described according to the aetiology, pathogenesis and clinical symptoms of UTI.[4] These include *re lin* 热淋 (heat *lin*), *shi lin* 石淋 (stone *lin*), *qi lin* 气淋, *lao lin* 劳淋 (fatigue *lin*), *gao lin* 膏淋 (paste *lin*) and *xue lin* 血淋 (Blood *lin*). Contemporary CM scholars generally agree that UTI can be categorised under *lin* 淋 syndrome. However, slight changes in meaning between classical and contemporary CM literature, as highlighted above, should be noted.

Aetiology and Pathogenesis

There are four main causes of UTI: (1) external pathogenic invasion of dampness-heat, (2) dietary irregularities, (3) disharmony of emotions, and (4) constitutional insufficiency or chronic/consumptive disease.[5] The locations of the disease are the Bladder and Kidney, with a close relationship to the Liver and Spleen. Dampness-heat binds in the Lower Energiser and inhibits transformation of Kidney and Bladder *qi*. The main pathological factor is dampness-heat. As stated in *Zhu Bing Yuan Hou Lun Lin Bing Zhu Hou* 诸病源候论·淋病诸候 (c. 610), 'all symptoms of *lin* 淋 are caused by Kidney deficiency and Bladder heat'.

Urinary tract infection can be either an excess pattern or a deficiency pattern, or a combination of both deficiency and excess. The excess pattern of UTI is normally due to acute contraction of dampness-heat without debilitation of the healthy (*zheng* 正) *qi*. When the disease lasts for a long time or continually recurs, dampness-heat will invade not only the *fu* 腑 organs, but also the *zang* 脏 organs. The disease will turn from excess of pathogenic *qi* into deficiency of healthy *qi*, so that dual deficiency of *zang fu* 脏腑 organs will be seen, especially relating to the Spleen and Kidney. If both excess of pathogenic *qi* and debilitation of healthy *qi* occur in the disease process, the deficiency-excess complex pattern will appear; for example *yin* deficiency with excess dampness-heat complication, or *qi* deficiency with excess water-dampness complication. In addition, excess of any of the seven emotions can lead to the failure of Liver function of free flow of *qi* and Blood, Liver *qi* stagnation and inhibited Bladder *qi* transformation.

Uncomplicated UTI generally has a favourable prognosis and few complications. With appropriate and timely treatment at the onset of the disease, the dampness-heat can be cleared. However, critical symptoms, such as high temperature and loss of consciousness, may occur if dampness-heat enters the Blood (*xue* 血). In infections with long duration, the dampness-heat will damage the healthy *qi* and cause chronic deficiency, with symptoms such as oedema, difficult urination or anuria, and vomiting.

Syndrome Differentiation and Treatments

Dampness-heat binding in the Lower Energiser is the basic CM pathogenesis of UTI. Acute UTI is normally an exterior excess pattern, and treatments will focus on clearing heat and draining dampness. Recurrent or chronic persistent UTI is usually considered to involve both exterior excess and interior deficiency patterns, and treatments will focus on reinforcing the healthy *qi*, clearing heat and draining dampness.

Oral Chinese Herbal Medicine Treatment Based on Syndrome Differentiation

This chapter refers to the following guidelines, expert consensus, textbooks or monographs: *Guidelines for the Diagnosis and Treatment of Common Diseases in Chinese Internal Medicine (Lin Zheng)* 中医内科常见病诊疗指南—中医病症部分 (淋证),[2] *Chinese Internal Medicine* 中医内科学,[5] *Chinese Medicine Clinical Diagnosis and Treatment of Urological Diseases* 中医临床诊治泌尿科专病,[6] *Clinical Practice Guidelines for Common Infectious Diseases Treated by Single Chinese Herbal Medicine/Combined Antibiotics – Uncomplicated Lower Urinary Tract Infection* 中医药单用/联合抗生素治疗常见感染性疾病临床实践指南—单纯性下尿路感染.[7] Treatments according to syndrome differentiation have been summarised in Table 2.1.

Dampness-heat in the Bladder 膀胱湿热

Clinical manifestations: Increased frequency of urination, burning and sharp pain when voiding urine, dark yellow and murky urine or with blood, distending pain in the lower abdomen, fever or chills, bitter taste in the mouth, nausea and vomiting, low back pain that is aggravated by pressure, and constipation. The tongue will have a yellow coating; the pulse will be soggy and rapid, or slippery and rapid.

Treatment principle: Clear heat, drain dampness and relieve strangury.

Oral formula: Modified *Ba zheng san* 八正散.[2,5–7]

Herbs: *Che qian zi* 车前子, *qu mai* 瞿麦, *bian xu* 萹蓄, *hua shi* 滑石, *zhi zi* 栀子, *gan cao* 甘草, *chuan mu tong* 川木通, *da huang* 大黄, *bai hua she she cao* 白花蛇舌草, *ji cai* 荠菜 and *mu xiang* 木香.

Main actions of herbs: *Che qian zi* 车前子, *qu mai* 瞿麦, *bian xu* 萹蓄, *hua shi* 滑石, *chuan mu tong* 川木通 and *ji cai* 荠菜 drain dampness and relieve strangury; *zhi zi* 栀子, *da huang* 大黄 and *bai hua she she cao* 白花蛇舌草 clear heat and drain dampness; *mu xiang* 木香 moves *qi* to relieve pain and protects the Spleen and Stomach; and *gan cao* 甘草 harmonises the actions of all herbs in the formula.

Modification: For constipation and abdominal distention, add extra *da huang* 大黄 and add *zhi shi* 枳实 and *hou pu* 厚朴 to regulate the bowels and discharge heat. If symptoms are accompanied with fever or chill, a bitter taste in the mouth, nausea and vomiting, use *Xiao chai hu tang* 小柴胡汤. For blood in the urine, use *dai ji* 大蓟, *xiao ji* 小蓟, *bai mao gen* 白茅根 and *zhen zhu cao* 珍珠草 to clear heat and stop bleeding.

Manufactured medicines: Products that can be used for the syndrome dampness-heat in the Bladder, particularly for symptoms of frequent, urgent or painful urination include *Ba zheng he ji* 八正合剂,[8] *San jin pian* 三金片,[8,9] *Niao gan ning ke li* 尿感宁颗粒,[8] *Re lin qing ke li* 热淋清颗粒[8,9] and *Shen shu ke li* 肾舒颗粒.[8,9]

Ba Zheng He Ji 八正合剂[6,8]

Herbs: *Chuan mu tong* 川木通, *che qian zi* 车前子, *bian xu* 萹蓄, *qu mai* 瞿麦, *hua shi* 滑石, *da huang* 大黄, *zhi zi* 栀子, *deng xin cao* 灯心草 and *gan cao* 甘草.

Main actions of the formula: Clears heat, increases urine excretion and relieves strangury.

Dosage: Take 15–20 mL every eight hours. Shake well before taking. A period of three to seven days constitutes one course of treatment.

San Jin Pian 三金片[6-9]

Herbs: *Jin ying gen* 金樱根, *ba qia* 菝葜, *yang kai kou* 羊开口, *jin sha teng* 金沙藤 and *ji xue cao* 积雪草.

Main actions of the formula: Detoxify and clear heat, drain dampness and relieve strangury, and tonify the Kidney.

Dosage: Take five small pills or three big pills every six to eight hours. A period of three to seven days constitutes one course of treatment.

Niao Gan Ning Ke Li 尿感宁颗粒[6,8]

Herbs: *Hai jin sha teng* 海金沙藤, *lian qian cao* 连钱草, *feng wei cao* 凤尾草, *zi hua di ding* 紫花地丁 and *lv cao* 葎草.

Main actions of the formula: Detoxify and clear heat, drain dampness and relieve strangury, and tonify the Kidney.

Dosage: Mix 15 grams of granules with boiled water and take every six to eight hours. A period of three to seven days constitutes one course of treatment.

Re Lin Qing Ke Li 热淋清颗粒[6-9]

Herbs: *Tou hua liao* 头花蓼.

Main actions of the formula: Detoxify and clear heat, drain dampness and relieve strangury, and tonify the Kidney.

Dosage: Mix one or two sachets with boiled water and take every eight hours. A period of three to seven days constitutes one course of treatment.

Shen Shu Ke Li 肾舒颗粒[7-9]

Herbs: *Bai hua she she cao* 白花蛇舌草, *hai jin sha teng* 海金沙藤, *qu mai* 瞿麦, *da qing ye* 大青叶, *huang bai* 黄柏, *dan zhu ye* 淡竹叶, *bian xu* 萹蓄, *fu ling* 茯苓, *di huang* 地黄 and *gan cao* 甘草.

Main actions of the formula: Detoxify and clear heat, drain dampness and relieve strangury, and tonify the Kidney.

Dosage: Mix 30 grams of granules with boiled water and take every eight hours. A period of three to seven days constitutes one course of treatment.

Yin Deficiency and Dampness-heat 阴虚湿热

Clinical manifestations: Increased frequency of urination, uneasy and painful voiding of urine, dizziness, soreness and weakness of the waist and knees, low grade fever in the afternoon, 'five hearts hot' (heat in the chest, palms and soles), and dry mouth or bitter taste in the mouth. The tongue will be red with a thin yellow coating, and the pulse will be fine and rapid.

Treatment principle: Nourish *yin* to clear heat, drain dampness and relieve strangury.

Oral formula: Modified *Zhi bai di huang tang* 知柏地黄汤.[6,7]

Herbs: *Zhi mu* 知母, *huang bai* 黄柏, *shu di huang* 熟地黄, *shan zhu yu* 山茱萸, *mu dan pi* 牡丹皮, *shan yao* 山药, *fu ling* 茯苓, *ze xie* 泽泻, *pu gong ying* 蒲公英, *shi wei* 石韦 and *gan cao* 甘草.

Main actions of herbs: *Zhi mu* 知母 and *huang bai* 黄柏 clear heat and purge fire; *shan zhu yu* 山茱萸, *shan yao* 山药 and *shu di huang* 熟地黄 nourish the Liver, Spleen and Kidney; *mu dan pi* 牡丹皮 clears heat and cools the Blood; *fu ling* 茯苓 induces diuresis and drains dampness; *shi wei* 石韦 and *ze xie* 泽泻 drain dampness and relieve strangury; *pu gong ying* 蒲公英 clears heat and detoxifies. The combination of all herbs nourishes *yin* to clear heat, drain dampness and relieve strangury; *gan cao* 甘草 harmonises the actions of all herbs in the formula.

Modification: For patients with 'steaming bone fever' (dry and intense sensation of heat with flushing and tidal fever), add *qing hao* 青蒿 and *bie jia* 鳖甲 to strengthen *yin* and clear heat. For patients with 'five hearts hot' (heat in the chest, palms and soles), add *bai mao gen* 白茅根 and *dan zhu ye* 淡竹叶 to clear Heart fire. For patients with dizziness, add *tian ma* 天麻 and *gou teng* 钩藤 to pacify the Liver and extinguish wind. For patients with significant soreness of the loins, add *nv zhen zi* 女贞子 and *sang ji sheng* 桑寄生 to tonify the Kidney.

Manufactured medicines: *Zhi bai di huang wan* 知柏地黄丸.[6,8,9]

Herbs: *Zhi mu* 知母, *huang bai* 黄柏, *shu di huang* 熟地黄, *shan zhu yu* 山茱萸, *mu dan pi* 牡丹皮, *shan yao* 山药, *fu ling* 茯苓 and *ze xie* 泽泻.

Main actions of the formula: Nourish *yin* and downbear fire. This formula can be used for the overt symptoms of soreness and weakness of the waist; heat in the chest, palms and soles; and reddish urine with scant amount.

Dosage: Take eight pills every eight hours. One course of treatment takes four weeks.

Dual Deficiency of Spleen and Kidney with Retention of Dampness-heat 脾肾两虚, 湿热内蕴

Clinical manifestations: Atypical reddish and difficult urination, paroxysmal dribbling discharge of urine, relapse due to over-fatigue, lack of strength, soreness and weakness of the waist and knees, distending pain in the lower abdomen, and loose stools. The tongue will be pale or enlarged with teeth marks, and the tongue coat will be thin and white. The pulse will be thready and deep, or thready and weak.

Treatment principle: Tonify Spleen and Kidney, clear heat and drain dampness.

Oral formula: Modified *Wu bi shan yao wan* 无比山药丸.[5,7]

Herbs: *Shan yao* 山药, *rou cong rong* 肉苁蓉, *shu di huang* 熟地黄, *shan zhu yu* 山茱萸, *du zhong* 杜仲, *tu si zi* 菟丝子, *fu ling* 茯苓, *ba ji tian* 巴戟天, *wu wei zi* 五味子, *chi shi zhi* 赤石脂, *niu xi* 牛膝, *yi yi ren* 薏苡仁, *ze xie* 泽泻, *shi wei* 石韦 and *gan cao* 甘草.

Main actions of herbs: *Shan yao* 山药, *fu ling* 茯苓 and *yi yi ren* 薏苡仁 fortify the Spleen and drain dampness; *rou cong rong* 肉苁蓉, *du zhong* 杜仲, *tu si zi* 菟丝子, *ba ji tian* 巴戟天 and *wu wei zi* 五味子

boost the Kidney, consolidate and astringe; *shu di huang* 熟地黄 and *shan zhu yu* 山茱萸 nourish *yin* and tonify the Kidney; *ze xie* 泽泻, *niu xi* 牛膝 and *shi wei* 石韦 drain dampness and relieve strangury; and *chi shi zhi* 赤石脂 stops bleeding. The combination of all herbs tonifies the Spleen and Kidney, clears heat and drains dampness; *gan cao* 甘草 harmonises the actions of all herbs in the formula.

Modification: For patients with the syndrome of Spleen deficiency and sinking of *qi* with a bearing-down sensation in the anal area, shortage of *qi* and no desire to speak, add *dang shen* 党参, *huang qi* 黄芪, *bai zhu* 白术, *sheng ma* 升麻 and *chai hu* 柴胡 to replenish and raise the middle *qi*. For patients with pale complexion, cold extremities and lack of strength in the waist and knees, add *shu fu zi* 熟附子, *rou gui* 肉桂 and *yin yang huo* 淫羊藿 to warm and tonify Kidney *yang*. For patients with Blood stasis, add *dan shen* 丹参, *pu huang* 蒲黄 and *liu ji nu* 刘寄奴 to activate Blood to stop bleeding. For patients with heavy dampness-heat, add *zhen zhu cao* 珍珠草, *tu fu ling* 土茯苓 and *pu gong ying* 蒲公英 to strengthen the action of clearing heat and draining damp.

Manufactured medicines: *Jin gui shen qi wan* 金匮肾气丸.[6,9]

Herbs: *Di huang* 地黄, *shan yao* 山药, *shan zhu yu* 山茱萸, *fu ling* 茯苓, *mu dan pi* 牡丹皮, *ze xie* 泽泻, *gui zhi* 桂枝, *fu zi* 附子, *niu xi* 牛膝 and *che qian zi* 车前子.

Main actions of the formula: Warm and tonify Kidney *yang*; resolve *qi* to move water. This formula can be used for the overt symptoms of soreness and weakness of the waist, inhibited urination and fear of cold with cold extremities.

Dosage: Take four to five grams every 12 hours. One course of treatment takes four weeks.

Liver Depression and *Qi* Stagnation 肝郁气滞

Clinical manifestations: Uneasy and dribbling discharge of urine and distending pain in the lower abdomen. The tongue will have a thin and white coat, and the pulse will be deep and wiry.

Treatment principle: Soothe the Liver and regulate *qi*, drain dampness and relieve strangury.

Oral formula: Modified *Chen xiang san* 沉香散.[2,5–7]

Herbs: *Chen xiang* 沉香, *ju pi* 橘皮, *bai shao* 白芍, *shi wei* 石韦, *hua shi* 滑石, *dong kui zi* 冬葵子, *wang bu liu xing* 王不留行 and *gan cao* 甘草.

Main actions of herbs: *Chen xiang* 沉香 and *ju pi* 橘皮 soothe the Liver and regulate *qi*; *bai shao* 白芍 calms the Liver and relaxes tension; *shi wei* 石韦, *hua shi* 滑石, *dong kui zi* 冬葵子 and *wang bu liu xing* 王不留行 drain dampness and relieve strangury. The combination of all herbs will soothe the Liver and regulate *qi*, drain dampness and relieve strangury, and *gan cao* 甘草 harmonises the actions of all herbs in the formula.

Modification: For patients with oppression in the chest and distention in the hypochondrium, add *qing pi* 青皮, *wu yao* 乌药 and *xiao hui xiang* 小茴香 to soothe the Liver and regulate *qi*. For patients with Blood stasis due to chronic *qi* stagnation, add *hong hua* 红花, *chi shao* 赤芍, *chuan niu xi* 川牛膝 and *liu ji nu* 刘寄奴 to activate Blood and dissipate Blood stasis.

Chinese Herbal Medicine Steam Wash

Chinese herbal medicine can be used as a steam wash for all *lin* 淋 syndromes.[6,7] The use of a Chinese herbal medicine (CHM) steam wash can prevent UTIs caused by gynaecological inflammation and may complement the actions of oral CHM. The principles of treatment with CHM steam wash are to clear heat and drain dampness. Herbs commonly used include *wa song* 瓦松, *huang bai* 黄柏, *ku shen* 苦参, *tu fu ling* 土茯苓 and *she chuang zi* 蛇床子. To use a CHM steam wash, first clean the genital area with warm water, then apply the steam wash for 10 to 20 minutes daily. This treatment can be used for two to four weeks, which constitutes one course of treatment. Chinese herbal medicine steam wash should not be used for menstruating women or men who are preparing for conception.

Acupuncture Therapies

Both body acupuncture and ear acupuncture can be used for all *lin* 淋 syndromes.

Acupuncture

Acupuncture points which directly address the four main syndromes of UTI are described in Table 2.1. The main acupuncture points are BL28 *Pangguangshu* 膀胱俞, CV3 *Zhongji* 中极, SP9 *Yinlingquan* 阴陵泉, BL39 *Weiyang* 委阳 and SP6 *Sanyinjiao* 三阴交.[2,6] These acupuncture points have actions that benefit the Lower Energiser.[10] Both BL28 *Pangguangshu* 膀胱俞 and CV3 *Zhongji* 中级 clear damp-heat

Table 2.1.   Summary of Main Treatments for Urinary Tract Infection

Syndrome	Treatment Principle	Oral Chinese Herbal Medicine	Acupuncture
Dampness-heat in Bladder	Clear heat, drain dampness and relieve strangury	Modified *Ba zheng san* 八正散	Main points: BL28 *Pangguangshu* 膀胱俞, CV3 *Zhongji* 中级, SP9 *Yinlingquan* 阴陵泉, BL39 *Weiyang* 委阳 and SP6 *Sanyinjiao* 三阴交
Yin deficiency and dampness-heat	Nourish *yin* to clear heat, drain dampness and relieve strangury	Modified *Zhi bai di huang tang* 知柏地黄汤	Not available
Dual deficiency of Spleen and Kidney, retention of dampness-heat	Tonify Spleen and Kidney, clear heat and drain dampness	Modified *Wu bi shan yao wan* 无比山药丸	The main points plus BL20 *Pishu* 脾俞, BL23 *Shenshu* 肾俞, CV4 *Guanyuan* 关元 and ST36 *Zusanli* 足三里
Liver depression and *qi* stagnation	Soothe the Liver and regulate *qi*, drain dampness and relieve strangury	Modified *Chen xiang san* 沉香散	The main points plus BL18 *Ganshu* 肝俞 and LR3 *Taichong* 太冲

from the Lower Energiser, clear stagnation and regulate the Bladder. The point CV3 *Zhongji* 中级 also regulates *qi* transformation and strengthens the Kidneys. The point SP9 *Yinlingquan* 阴陵泉 regulates the Spleen and water passages and resolves dampness. The point BL39 *Weiyang* 委阳 regulates urination and harmonises the Upper, Middle and Lower Energisers. The point SP6 *Sanyinjiao* 三阴交 tonifies the Stomach and Spleen, harmonises the Liver, toni-fies the Kidneys, regulates urination and resolves dampness.

Supplementary points can be selected according to syndrome differentiation.[2,6] For Liver depression and *qi* stagnation syndrome, add BL18 *Ganshu* 肝俞 and LR3 *Taichong* 太冲. For Spleen and Kidney deficiency syndromes, add BL20 *Pishu* 脾俞, BL23 *Shenshu* 肾俞, CV4 *Guanyuan* 关元 and ST36 *Zusanli* 足三里.

Supplementary points can also be selected based on accompany-ing symptoms.[2,6] When blood is present in the urine, add SP10 *Xuehai* 血海 and BL17 *Geshu* 膈俞. If the UTI is accompanied by lower abdominal distension, add LI11 *Quchi* 曲池, and if accompa-nied by high fever, add both LI11 *Quchi* 曲池 and LI4 *Hegu* 合谷. When patients report additional symptoms of oppression in the chest, distention in the hypochondrium and a bitter taste in the mouth, add LR2 *Xiangjian* 行间. BL32 *Ciliao* 次髎 and BL33 *Zhongliao* 中髎 can be used for difficult urination.

Twisting-rotating needle manipulation can be applied to all acu-puncture points.[2,6] Reducing techniques should be used for excess syndromes and reinforcing techniques used for deficiency syn-dromes. Acupuncture can work in parallel with CHM to improve patient outcomes and reduce recurrence.

Ear Acupuncture

Ear acupuncture can also be used in conjunction with CHM.[6] The main acupuncture points are CO10 Kidney (*Shen* 肝), CO9 Bladder (*Pangguang* 膀胱), CO17 Triple Energiser (*Sanjiao* 三焦), CO18 Endocrine (*Neifenmi* 内分泌) and TG2p Adrenal Gland (*Shenshengxian* 肾上腺). Supplementary points can be selected based on symptoms.

When UTI is accompanied by fever, the ear apex can be pricked (EX-HN6 *Erjian* 耳尖). For painful urination add CO9,10i Ureter (*Shuniaoguan* 输尿管) and HX3 Urethra (*Niaodao* 尿道). Needles should be retained for 20 to 30 minutes. Daily treatment for ten days constitutes one course of treatment. Ear studs or seeds can also be applied to these acupuncture points to allow the patient to stimulate points at home.

Ultrashort Wave Therapy

Ultrashort wave therapy is a technique that uses a specialised machine to deliver CHM to acupuncture points. Two pads (a positive and a negative) are placed on acupuncture points and electromagnetic energy is applied at short wave frequencies. This technique is purported to regulate the nervous, cardiovascular, endocrine and immune systems as well as promote kidney function. Ultrashort wave therapy is suitable for patients with acute pyelonephritis and those with strong signs of irritation of the bladder.[6] For acute pyelonephritis, place one electrode on the abdomen and the other on the lower back near the renal region (located in costovertebral angle, the acute angle formed on either side between the twelfth rib and the vertebral column). Treat with micro-heat level for 10 to 15 minutes, once daily for five to ten days (one course of treatment). For patients with strong signs of irritation of the bladder, place the two electrodes opposite each other in the bladder region of the lower abdomen. Alternatively, one electrode can be placed in the renal region and the other in the bladder region. Treat with micro-heat level for ten to 15 minutes, once daily for five to ten days (one course of treatment).

Other Management Strategies

Treatment should focus on prophylactic and/or preventative approaches that aim to eliminate the risk factors of external pathogens and internal dampness-heat.[2,5–7] Patients should be encouraged to drink plenty of water and to void urine regularly in order to lower the risk of a UTI. Maintaining good genital hygiene includes washing with warm water daily to avoid the entry of pathogens into the urinary tract. Washing the genital area before sexual intercourse and urinating after intercourse may reduce the risk of infections due to excessive sexual activity.

Maintaining a healthy lifestyle is also important. This includes regular exercise, engaging in recreational activities that foster a positive mindset, and ensuring adequate rest. Patients can participate in traditional Chinese health-promoting exercises such as *taichi* 太极 and *ba duan jin* 八段锦, which promote the flow of healthy *qi* and relaxation in the mind and body.

Patients should maintain a healthy and light diet, increase fruit and vegetable intake, and avoid cold, fried and spicy foods. Foods which detoxify, clear heat and relieve strangury include chrysanthemum (*ju hua* 菊花), leek (*ji cai* 荠菜), *ma lan tou* 马兰头 (a green vegetable) and winter gourd (*dong gua* 冬瓜). Patients may replace tea with boiled herb drinks such as dandelion (*pu gong ying* 蒲公英), bamboo leaves (*zhu ye* 竹叶), honeysuckle (*jin yin hua* 金银花), chrysanthemum (*ju hua* 菊花), plantain (*che qian cao* 车前草) and *jin qian cao* 金钱草. Alcohol intake should not be excessive.

References

1. Barrett P, Flower A, Lo V. (2015) What's past is prologue: Chinese medicine and the treatment of recurrent urinary tract infections. *J Ethnopharmacol* **167**: 86–96.
2. 中华中医药学会. (2008) 中医内科常见诊疗指南—中医病证部分. 北京: 中国中医药出版社, pp. 111–113.
3. 李经绅, 邓铁涛主编. (1995) 中医大词典. 北京: 人民卫生出版社.
4. 张天, 陈以平主编. (1990) 实用中医肾病学. 上海: 上海中医学院出版社, pp. 161–163.
5. 薛博瑜, 吴伟. (2016) 中医内科学 (第3版). 北京: 人民卫生出版社.
6. 杨霓芝, 刘旭生. (2013) 中医临床诊治泌尿科专病 (第3版). 北京: 人民卫生出版社.
7. 中华中医药学会. (2017) 中医药单用/联合抗生素治疗常见感染性疾病临床实践指南-单纯性下尿路感染 (中华中医药学会团体标准). 北京: 中国中医药出版社.

8. 国家药典委员会. (2015) 中华人民共和国药典. 北京: 中国医药科技出版社.

9. 国家药典委员会. (2008) 中华人民共和国卫生部药品标准—中药成方制剂. 中国: 卫生部药典委员会.

10. Deadman P, Al-Khafaji M, Baker K. (2000) *A Manual of Acupuncture*. Journal of Chinese Medicine Publications, East Sussex, England.

3

Classical Chinese Medicine Literature

OVERVIEW

Classical Chinese medicine literature has contributed a valuable resource to the prevention and management of various health conditions. As an important component of the 'whole-evidence' approach, this chapter systematically summarises and evaluates the classical Chinese medicine literature for urinary tract infection in *Zhong Hua Yi Dian* 中华医典, one of the most complete collections of classical Chinese medicine works. More than 500 citations were identified. Search terms, aetiology and Chinese medicine management, including herbal medicine, acupuncture and other therapies, for urinary tract infection are described and analysed.

Introduction

The earliest written records of Chinese medicine (CM) history date back to the Spring and Autumn (770–476 BC) and Warring States (474–221 BC) periods. Texts from these periods describe concepts such as *yin* and *yang*, as well as descriptions of herbal decoctions, acupuncture and moxibustion as ways to treat health complaints.[1] Some of the earliest references to the treatment of urinary diseases cited in contemporary textbooks are from these eras, found in the well-known book *Huang Di Nei Jing* 黄帝内经 (c. 474–221 BC).

In a review of the classical CM literature to inform a clinical trial intervention, Barrett *et al.* (2015),[2] identified references to urinary disease in medical manuscripts from the *Mawangdui* 马王堆 tombs (closed in 168 BC) and Wuwei 武威 tombs (closed in the first century AD). In these texts, urinary diseases were referred to as *lin zheng* 淋证 (*lin* 淋 syndrome) or *long zheng* 癃证 (*long* 癃 syndrome), which appear to be synonyms prior to the Han dynasty. Characteristic symptoms included dripping and inhibited urination, and four different types of *long* 癃 disease were presented: *shi long* 石癃 (stone *long*), *xue long* 血癃 (Blood *long*), *gao long* 膏癃 (paste *long*) and *gan long* 泔癃 ('dirty water' *long*) (Zhang and Zhu, 1996, cited in Barrett *et al.*, 2015).[2]

Later seminal texts provided more detailed descriptions of symptoms and further subtypes of *lin* 淋 syndrome. In *Jin Kui Yao Lue Xiao Ke Xiao Bian Bu Li Lin Bing Mai Bing Zhi* 金匮要略·消渴小便不利淋病脉证并治 (c. 206 AD), Zhang Zhongjing 张仲景 summarised the characteristic symptoms of *lin* 淋 syndrome: 'dripping' urine, feeling tense in the lower abdomen, and pain around navel'. He also emphasised that *lin* 淋 syndrome is characterised by frequent, urgent and painful urination, accompanied by change in urine and abdominal discomfort. This is similar to the contemporary biomedical understanding of urinary tract infection (UTI). In later eras, UTI symptoms were described using various terms such as *lin men* 淋闷(闷), *lin mi* 淋秘 and *lin li* 淋沥, with dysuria and dripping urination as the main symptoms of *lin* 淋 syndrome.

Due to the different terminologies used for urinary disease in classical CM literature, it is important to conduct a systematic analysis to identify instances of UTI in the classical and pre-modern medical literature. We conducted electronic searches of the *Zhong Hua Yi Dian* (ZHYD) 中华医典 *Encyclopaedia of Traditional Chinese Medicine*.[3] This digitalised collection of more than 1,100 medical books is the largest currently available and is representative of other large collections of the classical and pre-modern CM literature.[4,5]

Search Terms

In classical CM literature, symptoms typical of UTI were referred to using many different terms or diseases names. Terms containing the word *lin* 淋 have been used throughout CM history. Another term, *long* 癃, has also been used in past eras. This term was used to describe urinary disorders such as UTI, urinary retention, haematuria and urinary tract stones before the Han dynasty (202 BC–220 AD).[2] During the Han dynasty, the term *long* 癃 disappeared from textbooks due to a prohibition that prevented the use of characters from the name of a deceased Chinese emperor. From this period on, the term *lin* 淋 gained prominence in describing UTI symptoms. During the Song and Jin dynasties (961–1271), *long* 癃 reappeared in classical texts; however, this term was used only for urinary retention until modern times.

Considering only four classical literature books from before the Han dynasty are included in the ZHYD, a test search for the term *long* 癃 was conducted. The search produced few citations that were judged as irrelevant to UTI. Chinese medicine experts were consulted about this term, and the consensus was that it was not likely to be relevant for UTI. For these reasons, *long* 癃 was not included as a search term to identify citations related to UTI.

A list of search terms was developed after consulting authoritative sources, including the contemporary CM textbook *Zhong Yi Nei Ke Xue* 中医内科学 (周仲瑛主编),[6] *Guidelines for Diagnosis and Treatment of Common Internal Diseases in Chinese Medicine Symptoms in Chinese Medicine* 中医内科常见病诊疗指南 • 中医病证部分 (中华中医药学会),[7] *Zhong Yi Lin Chuang Zhen Zhi • Mi Niao Ke Zhuan Bing* (*Clinical Chinese Medicine Diagnosis and Management: Urologic Diseases*) 中医临床诊治 泌尿科专病 (杨霓芝, 刘旭生主编)[8] and the CM dictionary *Zhong Yi Da Ci Dian* 中医大词典.[9] The list of search terms was reviewed by CM specialists and experts, and a total of 13 search terms were selected (Table 3.1). The Chinese character *lin* 淋, which can be translated as 'strangury', is contained in all the search terms. For this reason, *lin* 淋 was considered to be the most representative term describing UTI.

Table 3.1. Terms Used to Identify Classical Literature Citations

Search Terms of Urinary Tract Infection in Pinyin	Search Terms of Urinary Tract Infection in Chinese	English Translation
Lin men	淋閟 (淋闷)	Strangury and/or urinary retention
Lin bi	淋闭	Strangury and/or urinary retention
Lin mi	淋秘	Strangury and/or urinary retention
Re lin	热淋	Heat strangury
Qi lin	气淋	*Qi* strangury
Lao lin	劳淋	Fatigue strangury
Xue lin	血淋	Haematuria
Lin zheng	淋证	Strangury
Lin sou	淋溲	The syndrome of dribbling urination
Lin li	淋沥	The syndrome of dribbling urination
Lin bing	淋病	Strangury disease, including urinary tract infection and other reproductive system diseases
Han lin	寒淋	Cold strangury
Leng lin	冷淋	Cold strangury

Procedures for Search

Included terms were entered into the ZHYD search fields individually. Both headings and full-text searches were conducted for each term, and the search results were exported to spreadsheets for cleaning and coding. A 'citation' was defined as a distinct passage of text referring to one, or more, of the search terms. Duplicate citations, which were identified by different search terms, were removed from the dataset after noting each term that identified the passage. Citations published after 1949 (the end of the Minguo/Republic of China period) were also excluded. The search procedure is presented in Fig. 3.1.

Search	Search *Zhong Hua Yi Dian* 中华医典, which contains over 1, 000 books
Collect	Collect citations that mention any of the search terms (Table 3.1)
Sort	Sort citations and remove those that are not relevant
Analyse	Analyse formula, herbs and acupuncture points
	Total treatment citations = 563

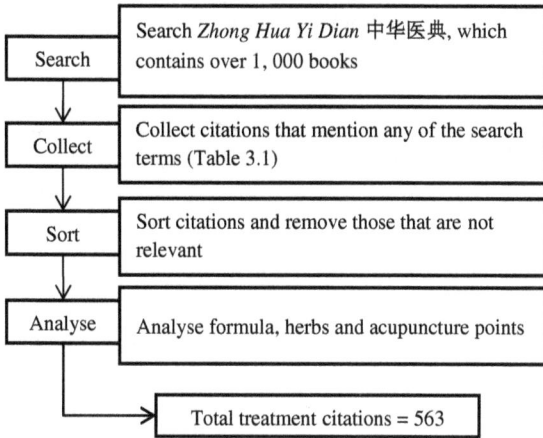

Fig. 3.1. Classical literature citations.

Data Coding and Data Analysis Procedures

After duplicate removal, citations were reviewed to identify signs and symptoms relevant to UTI. Citations that did not describe the treatment of UTI-like symptoms were excluded, as were citations describing UTI in children or pregnant women. Pharmacopaeia-style entries that described the indications of herbs were also excluded. Citations that described treatments for symptoms of urinary disease were included and were subject to further analysis.

Primary symptoms of UTI (Group A) included dysuria, burning sensation on urination, urinary frequency and urinary urgency (Table 3.2). Secondary symptoms of UTI (Group B) included symptoms that may or may not occur, and symptoms that could distinguish potential cases of cystitis from potential cases of pyelonephritis. An additional group of symptoms included symptoms and descriptions of medical history (Group C) to identify urinary symptoms that may be due to other causes such as vaginitis or diabetes. An exclusion criterion (C1: *Xing huo yue sheng huo shi* 性活跃生活史, translated as sexually active person) was used in an attempt to distinguish symptoms caused

Table 3.2. Symptom Categories for Rating Citations

Symptom Category	Descriptions	Possible Translation
Group A: Primary symptoms of UTI	A1: *Pai niao kun nan* 排尿困难	Dysuria
	A2: *Niao pin* 尿频	Urinary frequency
	A3: *Niao ji* 尿急	Urinary urgency
	A4: *Pai niao zhuo re* or *teng tong* 排尿灼热或疼痛	Urinary burning sensation or pain
Group B: Secondary symptoms of UTI	B1: *Xiao fu zhui zhang, ju ji* or *teng tong* 小腹坠胀, 拘急或疼痛	Suprapubic pain
	B2: *Yao bu teng tong* 腰部疼痛	Flank pain
	B3: *Xue niao* 血尿	Haematuria
	B4: *Niao ye hun zhuo* or even with *nong kuai* 尿液混浊, 甚至出现脓块	Cloudy urine
	B5: *Fa re* or *han zhan* 发热或寒战	Fever/chills
Group C: Symptoms/ medical history not related to UTI	C1: *Xing huo yue sheng huo shi* 性活跃生活史	Sexually active person
	C2: *Xing gong neng zhang ai zheng zhuang* 性功能障碍症状	Symptoms of sexual dysfunction
	C3: *Niao dao/yin dao fen mi wu zeng jia* 尿道/阴道分泌物增加	Urethral/vaginal discharge or odour
	C4: *Wai yin sao yang* 外阴瘙痒	Vaginal pruritus
	C5: *Hui yin bu teng tong* 会阴部疼痛	Perineal pain
	C6: *Jie he (lao) gan ran bing shi* 结核 (痨) 感染病史	Symptoms or history of tuberculosis infection
	C7: *Xiao bian pai chu sha shi* 小便排出砂石	Passing kidney stones
	C8: *Xiao bian shi hun zhuo cheng ru bai se* or *hun you xue se, dan wu niao tong* 小便时浑浊呈乳白色或混有血色, 但无尿痛	Chyluria
	C9: *Xue niao dan wu niao tong* 血尿, 但无尿痛	Haematuria without pain
	C10: *Yin yi sou yi* 饮一溲一	Profuse drink and profuse urine

Table 3.2. (*Continued*)

Symptom Category	Descriptions	Possible Translation
	C11: *Tian niao* 甜尿	Sweet urine
	C12: *Duo yin* 多饮	Increased thirst
	C13: *Duo shi* 多食	Increased hunger
	C14: *Xiao shou* 消瘦	Weight loss
	C15: *Shao niao* or *wu niao* 少尿或无尿	Oliguria/anuria
	C16: *Shui zhong* 水肿	Oedema
	C17: *Long bi* 癃闭	Urinary retention

Abbreviations: UTI, urinary tract infection.

by UTI from those caused by a sexually transmitted infection. None of the citations reported such information. Despite the term *long* 癃 being excluded from the search terms, citations were reviewed to identify any instances of this term which may have been written in traditional characters rather than simplified characters.

Criteria were developed to identify citations that were 'possibly' related to UTI and those that were 'most likely' describing UTI:

- Citations that contained two or more symptoms from Group A plus any sign or symptom from Group B were judged as 'most likely' UTI;
- Citations that contained two or more symptoms of Group A or contained one symptom from Group A and any sign or symptom from Group B were judged as 'possible' UTI.

Exclusion criteria were developed to identify citations with insufficient information and those that were judged as not UTI:

- Citations that contained one symptom from Group A, or any signs or symptoms from Group B, was considered to have insufficient information to make a judgment;
- Citations that contained any symptom from Group C (regardless of whether they contained symptoms from Groups A and B) were considered to be conditions other than UTI.

Citations that described multiple treatments were separated for analysis. In citations that did not describe herb ingredients for Chinese herbal medicine (CHM) formulas, these were sought from other mentions of the formula within the same book. If herb ingredients were not able to be identified from the same book, the data were marked as not available and were excluded from herb frequency analysis.

Treatments were analysed using descriptive statistics to identify the most frequently used CHM formulas, herb ingredients and acupuncture points in past eras. Formulas with the same name can vary in their ingredients, and the same combination of ingredients may have different names. For data analysis, formulas with the same name that have variations in a few ingredients were grouped together while those with large variations in ingredients were separated. Also, formulas with the same ingredients but different names have been grouped together. The results are presented for the total pool ('possible' UTI), and for a subset of the best citations ('most likely' UTI).

Search Results

The total number of instances (or hits) obtained by the 13 search terms was 6,423 (Table 3.3). The term *lin li* 淋沥, which can be translated as 'syndrome of dribbling urination', produced the largest number of instances (1,945 hits; 30.3%). Other terms that identified more than 10% of the total hits include *xue lin* 血淋 (Blood *lin*, 1,508 hits; 23.5%) and *re lin* 热淋 (heat *lin*, 829; 12.9%).

Citations Related to Urinary Tract Infection

A total of 563 treatment citations met the inclusion criteria and were judged as 'possible' UTI, and a subset of 181 of these described the typical symptoms of UTI ('most likely' UTI citations). All of the 563 citations contained CM treatment; 488 citations introduced CHM treatments, 51 citations described acupuncture and related therapies, and 24 citations mentioned other CM therapies such as diet therapy and *daoyin* 导引 (physical exercises).

Table 3.3.   Hit Frequency by Search Term

Pinyin	**Chinese Characters**	**Total Hit Frequency (*n*, %)**
Lin li	淋沥	1,945 (30.3)
Xue lin	血淋	1,508 (23.5)
Re lin	热淋	829 (12.9)
Lin bi	淋闭	483 (7.2)
Qi lin	气淋	461 (7.2)
Lin bing	淋病	253 (3.9)
Lao lin	劳淋	242 (3.8)
Lin zheng	淋证	178 (2.8)
Lin mi	淋秘	160 (2.5)
Leng lin	冷淋	160 (2.5)
Lin men	淋閦（淋闷）	101 (1.6)
Lin sou	淋溲	73 (1.1)
Han lin	寒淋	30 (0.5)

Descriptions of Urinary Tract Infection

In classical literature, urinary symptoms were described under the broad category of *lin* 淋 syndrome, which included different presentations of urinary symptoms. The Ming dynasty book *Jing Yue Quan Shu* 景岳全书 (c. 1624) by Zhang Jingyue 张景岳 described patients with *lin* 淋 syndrome as having symptoms of painful, dribbling and frequent urination (淋之为病, 小便痛涩滴沥, 欲去不去, 欲止不止者是也). This description is consistent with the contemporary clinical understanding of UTI.

Some of the best and most well-known descriptions of UTI came from other citations that did not describe treatment. In his book *Yan Shi Ji Sheng Fang* 严氏济生方 (c. 1253), Wei Yilin 危亦林 detailed the five different types of *lin* 淋: *qi lin* 气淋, *xue lin* 血淋 (Blood *lin*), *gao lin* 膏淋 (paste *lin*), *lao lin* 劳淋 (fatigue *lin*) and *shi lin* 石淋 (stone *lin*). He stated that *qi lin* 气淋 is a syndrome with difficult and dribbling urination as the main symptoms (气淋为病, 小便涩, 常有余沥). *Xue lin* 血淋 is a stranguria syndrome induced by a heat pathogen, manifesting in haematuria, yellow coloured nose and difficult urination (血淋为病, 热即发, 甚则尿血, 候其鼻头色黄者). *Gao lin* 膏淋 is a syndrome with fatty/creamy urine (膏淋为病, 尿似膏出), while *lao lin* 劳淋 is a stranguria syndrome with pain localised to the ST30 *Qichong* 气冲 point (at the superior border of the pubic symphysis), appearing when a person is fatigued (劳淋为病, 劳倦即发, 痛引气冲). Finally, *shi lin* 石淋 is characterised by penile pain and difficult urination (石淋为病, 茎中痛, 溺卒不得出). Note that *shi lin* 石淋 referred to urinary stone diseases in CM, and this was excluded from UTI search terms in this chapter. This categorisation of five subtypes of *lin* 淋 syndromes can be found in many contemporary CM textbooks.

Descriptions of the Aetiology of Urinary Tract Infection

As early as the Sui dynasty, Chao Yuanfang 巢元方 systematically summarised the aetiology and pathogenesis of *lin* 淋 syndrome in his book *Zhu Bing Yuan Hou Lun* 诸病源候论 (c. 610 AD). He postulated that the key mechanism of *lin* 淋 syndrome is Kidney deficiency and Bladder heat accumulation. Poor diet, uncontrolled emotions and unhealthy lifestyle are the main factors that generate the disharmony of *zang* 脏 and *fu* 腑 that could lead to Kidney deficiency and Bladder heat accumulation. In CM, the Bladder is responsible for storing and regulating the excretion of *jin* 津 (fluids). When heat accumulates in the Bladder, *jin* 津 flows into the testicles and blocks the waterways, leading to dysfunction of the transportation of water throughout the body. Kidney deficiency could result in frequent urination, while Bladder heat accumulation could induce dysuria. *Lin* 淋 is a disease manifesting with frequent urination, dysuria and dribbling urine (诸淋者, 由肾虚膀胱热故也…若饮食不节, 喜怒不时, 虚实不调, 则腑脏不和, 致肾虚而膀胱热也. 膀胱, 津液之府, 热则津液内溢而流于睾, 水道不通, 水不上不下, 停积于胞, 肾虚则小便数, 膀胱热则水下涩. 数而且涩, 则淋沥不宣, 故谓之为淋). The concept of lifestyle factors contributing to UTI persists in contemporary literature.

An additional passage of text from the same book described the subtypes of *lin* 淋 in greater detail. This passage of text did not describe treatment and thus was not included in the analyses of treatment presented below, but is worth highlighting due to the detailed description of the aetiology of each subtype and the addition of two further subtypes of *lin* 淋: *re lin* 热淋 (heat *lin*) and *han lin* 寒淋 (cold *lin*). He discussed their aetiology as follows:

- *Qi lin* 气淋 is caused by Kidney deficiency and Bladder heat accumulation, and *qi* distention. The Bladder and Kidney are related to exterior and interior *zang* 脏 and *fu* 腑. When heat accumulates in the Bladder, heat *qi* flows into the *bao* 胞 and induces interior excess syndrome. This could cause *qi* distention and fullness of the lower abdomen. Kidney deficiency could cause frequent urination and *lin* 淋 occurs (气淋者, 肾虚膀胱热, 气胀所为也. 膀胱合与肾为表里, 膀胱热, 热气流入于胞, 热则生实, 令胞纳气胀, 则小腹满, 肾虚不能制其小便, 故成淋). Note that in this book, the reference to *bao* 胞 does not appear to describe the contemporary understanding of *bao* 胞, which is generally considered to be the uterus. This book appears to suggest that the function of *bao* 胞 is to store urine;
- *Gao lin* 膏淋, a stranguria syndrome with oily and creamy urine, is also called *rou lin* 肉淋. This is caused by Kidney deficiency and dysfunction in control of fatty secretions. Fatty substance will be discharged with urine in this case (膏淋者, 淋而有肥, 状似膏, 故谓之膏淋, 亦曰肉淋. 此肾虚不能制于肥液, 故与小便俱出也);
- *Lao lin* 劳淋 is a stranguria syndrome that occurs when overstrain harms the Kidney *qi*. This could produce heat and induces *lin* 淋 (劳淋者, 谓劳伤肾气, 而生热成淋也);
- *Xue lin* 血淋, a severe case of *heat lin* 热淋, manifests with haematuria. The Heart governs Blood, which circulates around the body, flows through meridians and to the *zang fu* 脏腑. Excessive heat causes the Blood to escape the vessels and enter the Bladder, which results in *xue lin* 血淋 (血淋者, 是热淋之甚者, 则尿血, 谓之血淋. 心主血, 血之行身, 通遍经络, 循环脏腑. 其热甚者, 血则散失其常经, 溢渗入胞, 而成血淋也);
- *Re lin* 热淋 is generated by heat accumulating in the Triple Energiser. The heat pathogen overcomes *zheng qi* 正氣 in the Kidney, then flows into the Bladder and induces *lin* 淋. The symptoms of

re lin 热淋 include dark urine and dysuria. There is another type of chronic *lin* 淋 which is caused by heat pathogen, and it may manifest in haematuria when the heat is severe (热淋者, 三焦有热, 气博于肾, 流入于胞而成淋也. 其状: 小便赤涩. 亦有宿病淋, 今得热而发者, 其热甚则变尿血);

- *Han lin* 寒淋 usually manifests as chills and shivering before urination. It results from Kidney *qi* deficiency. Cold *qi* affects the Lower Energiser, and conflicts with healthy *qi* in the Bladder. Chills and shivering induce *lin* 淋 if cold *qi* predominates. When healthy *qi* predominates, cold is expelled and the urine is able to flow (寒淋者, 其病状, 先寒战, 然后尿是也. 由肾气虚弱, 下焦受于冷气, 入胞与正气交争, 寒气胜则战寒而成淋, 正气胜则战寒解, 故得小便也).

Several citations that did not include treatment information explained the dietary, emotional and lifestyle causes of urinary disease and are worth noting. In *San Yin Ji Yi Bing Zheng Fang Lun* 三因极一病证方论 (c. 1174), Chen Yan 陈言 suggested that cold, dampness and heat are the external pathogens that generate *lin* 淋. Emotions of fright, anxiety, fear and over-thinking (worry) contribute to *qi* stagnation in the Heart and Kidney. Dietary irregularities, excessive sexual activity, overexertion and fatigue, and not voiding regularly are additional causes (复有冷淋, 湿淋, 热淋等, 属外所因; 既言心肾气郁, 与夫惊忧恐思, 即内所因; 况饮啖冷热, 房室劳逸, 及乘急忍溺, 多致此病, 岂非不内外因). Further, Zhang Jingyue 张景岳 noted that *lin* 淋 is mainly generated by disharmony of the Heart and Kidney, heat toxin accumulation, sexual overindulgence after drinking wine, overeating dry and hot flavoured food, and stagnation of the seven emotions (*Jing Yue Quan Shu* 景岳全书 [c. 1624]: (大抵此证, 多由心肾不交, 积蕴热毒, 或酒后房劳, 服食燥热, 七情郁结所致).

Signs and Symptoms of Urinary Disease

The signs and symptoms described in included citations were reviewed. The most frequently described symptom in included citations was dysuria, mentioned in 451 of the 563 citations (80.1%) (Table 3.4). This was followed by burning sensation or pain, haematuria, suprapubic pain

Table 3.4. Frequency of Signs and Symptoms of Urinary Disease

Sign or Symptom	'Possible' UTI No. of Citations (%)	'Most Likely' UTI No. of Citations (%)
Dysuria (*pai niao kun nan* 排尿困难)	451 (80.1)	176 (97.2)
Urinary burning sensation or pain (*pai niao zhuo re* or *teng tong* 排尿灼热或疼痛)	407 (72.2)	146 (80.7)
Haematuria (*xue niao* 血尿)	212 (37.7)	93 (51.4)
Suprapubic pain (*xiao fu zhui zhang, ju ji* or *teng tong* 小腹坠胀, 拘急或疼痛)	171 (30.4)	78 (43.1)
Urinary frequency (*niao pin* 尿频)	93 (16.5)	55 (30.4)
Urinary urgency (*niao ji* 尿急)	36 (6.4)	14 (7.7)
Fever/chills (*fa re* or *han zhan* 发热或寒战)	29 (5.2)	20 (11.1)
Cloudy urine (*niao ye hun zhuo* 尿 液混浊), with or without pus (*nong kuai* 脓块)	24 (4.3)	17 (9.4)
Flank pain (*yao bu teng tong* 腰部疼痛)	9 (1.6)	0 (0)

Abbreviation: UTI, urinary tract infection.

and urinary frequency. The number of citations describing urinary urgency, fever and chills, and cloudy urine were similar. Flank pain, a symptom often reported in contemporary cases of pyelonephritis, was infrequently reported.

A similar pattern of signs and symptoms was seen in the best pool, that is, the 181 citations judged 'most likely' to be UTI. Again, dysuria was reported in all but five citations, and urinary burning or pain was frequently reported. None of the citations considered 'most likely' to be UTI described flank pain and only 20 citations described fever or chills. This may suggest that the included citations described lower urinary disease, as opposed to upper urinary infections.

Chinese Herbal Medicine

The 488 citations describing CHM management were obtained from 121 books. *Pu Ji Fang* 普济方 (c. 1406) was found to produce the largest number of citations. Other books yielding 15 citations or more included *Tai Ping Sheng Hui Fang* 太平圣惠方 (c. 992 AD; 40 citations), *Yi Xue Ru Men* 医学入门 (c. 1624; 20 citations), *Ben Cao Gang Mu* 本草纲目 (c. 1596; 15 citations) and *Ji Yang Gang Mu* 济阳纲目 (c. 1626; 15 citations). Twenty-four books contained five or more relevant citations describing CHM therapies. The vast majority of citations described CHM for oral use (480 citations), while topical treatments with CHM were discussed in eight citations.

Frequency of Treatment Citations by Dynasty

The included citations were obtained from books published from the Tang and Five dynasties (618–960 AD) through to the Minguo 民国/ Republic of China (1912–1949) (Table 3.5). Nineteen citations were found in Japanese books, two of which were published in the Song and Jin dynasties (961–1271) and 17 were from the Qing dynasty (1645–1911). The vast majority of citations were from the books published during the Ming and Qing dynasties (366 citations; 75%). More advanced printing techniques, and the duration of these two dynasties, are likely to have contributed to the larger number of citations from books from this period. A considerable number of citations were also found in the Song and Jin dynasties. Forty of the 88 citations identified from this period came from the book *Tai Ping Sheng*

Table 3.5. **Dynastic Distribution of Treatment Citations**

Dynasty	No. of Citations (*n*)
Tang and Five dynasties (618–960)	5
Song and Jin dynasties (961–1271)	88
Yuan dynasty (1272–1368)	5
Ming dynasty (1369–1644)	233
Qing dynasty (1645–1911)	133
Minguo/Republic of China (1912–1949)	5
Japan (Song and Jin dynasties)	2
Japan (Qing dynasty)	17
Total	488

Hui Fang 太平圣惠方, in which Wang Huaiyin 王怀隐 discussed various *lin* 淋 syndromes in detail.

The earliest included citation that described CHM treatment was from *Bei Ji Qian Jin Yao Fang* 备急千金要方 (c. 652 AD). In this citation, Sun Simiao 孙思邈 recommended an unnamed herbal formula to treat *han lin* 寒淋, *re lin* 热淋 and *lao lin* 劳淋, with some symptoms likely to be UTI, that is, having difficulty urinating, feeling fullness in abdomen and acute abdominal pain (治百种淋, 寒淋, 热淋, 劳淋, 小便涩, 胞中满, 腹急痛方: 通草 石苇 甘草 王不留行 [各二两] 冬葵子 滑石 瞿麦 白术 芍药 [各三两] 上九味). The most recent CHM citations were obtained from *Yi Xue Zhong Zhong Can Xi Lu* 医学衷中参西录 (c. 1934). Case reports of *lao lin* 劳淋 and *xue lin* 血淋 were described in this book. The author, Zhang Xichun 张锡纯, also detailed the aetiology and pathogenesis of *lao lin* 劳淋. He proposed that fatigue due to overexertion, sexual overindulgence or anxiety was the main factor causing *lao lin* 劳淋. These pathogens could induce internal heat, causing consumption of *yin*. Deficient *yin* and effulgent fire affected the patients' Bladder and caused *lin* 淋 syndrome (劳淋之证, 因劳而成. 其人或劳力过度, 或劳心过度, 或房劳过度, 皆能暗生内热, 耗散真阴. 阴亏热炽, 熏蒸膀胱, 久而成淋).

Treatment with Oral Chinese Herbal Medicine

In total, 480 citations described CHM treatments for oral use. Of these, a subset of 158 citations judged 'most likely' to relate to UTI described oral CHM formulas. Treatments used in these citations were analysed for the total pool and for the subset of 'most likely' UTI citations.

Most Frequent Oral Formulas in 'Possible' Urinary Tract Infection Citations

The earliest use of CHM in included citations came from the seventh century book *Bei Ji Qian Jin Yao Fang* 备急千金要方 (c. 652 AD). The unnamed formula included the herbs *tong cao* 通草, *shi wei* 石韦, *gan cao* 甘草, *wang bu liu xing* 王不留行, *dong kui zi* 冬葵子,

hua shi 滑石, *qu mai* 瞿麦, *bai zhu* 白术 and *bai shao* 白芍. Many formulas were not named (150 citations; 31.3%). These formulas were excluded from frequency analysis but the ingredients were included in herb frequency analysis.

One hundred and twenty-three different formulas were identified among the 480 citations. Formulas varied considerably in terms of the number of herb ingredients, ranging from one herb to 29 herbs. The median number of herbs in oral CHM formulas was six. The most frequently reported formulas and the ingredients are presented in Table 3.6. Formulas with different names, but similar ingredients, were pooled together for analysis. Herbal ingredients described in Table 3.6 were obtained from the earliest citation.

The most frequently reported formula was *Shi wei tang* (decoction)/*Shi wei san* (powder)/*Shi wei yin zi* (liquid) 石韦汤/石韦散/石韦饮子. The earliest citation of this formula was from *Wai Tai Mi Yao* 外台秘要 (c. 752 AD). The author, Wang Tao 王焘, wrote that '*Shi wei san* 石韦散 has been a popular formula to treat *shi lin* 石淋, *lao lin* 劳淋, and *re lin* 热淋 for many years including symptoms such as

Table 3.6. Most Frequent Formulas for Oral Use in 'Possible' Urinary Tract Infection Citations

Formula Name	Herb Ingredients	No. of Citations (*n*)
Shi wei tang/Shi wei san/Shi wei yin zi 石韦汤/石韦散/石韦饮子	*Tong cao* 通草, *shi wei* 石韦, *wang bu liu xing* 王不留行, *hua shi* 滑石, *zhi gan cao* 炙甘草, *dang gui* 当归, *bai zhu* 白术, *qu mai* 瞿麦, *bai shao* 白芍 and *kui zi* 葵子. (*Wai Tai Mi Yao* 外台秘要, c. 752)	24
Wu lin san 五淋散	*Fu ling* 茯苓, *dang gui* 当归, *gan cao* 甘草, *chi shao* 赤芍 and *zhi zi* 栀子. (*Tai Ping Hui Min He Ji Ju Fang* 太平惠民和剂局方, c. 1107)	18
Ba zheng san 八正散	*Che qian zi* 车前子, *qu mai* 瞿麦, *bian xu* 萹蓄, *hua shi* 滑石, *zhi zi* 栀子, *gan cao* 甘草, *mu tong* 木通, *da huang* 大黄 and *deng xin cao* 灯心草. (*Yu Ji Wei Yi* 玉机微义, c. 1396)	16

Table 3.6. (*Continued*)

Formula Name	Herb Ingredients	No. of Citations (n)
Cheng xiang san 沉香散	*Chen xiang* 沉香, *shi wei* 石韦, *hua shi* 滑石, *dang gui* 当归, *qu mai* 瞿麦, *bai zhu* 白术, *gan cao* 甘草, *kui zi* 葵子, *chi shao* 赤芍 and *wang bu liu xing* 王不留行. (*Tai Ping Sheng Hui Fang* 太平圣惠方, c. 992 AD)	12
Mu tong tang/san/ Mu tong yin zi 木通汤/散/饮子	*Mu tong* 木通, *ting li zi* 葶苈子 and *fu ling* 茯苓. (*Tai Ping Sheng Hui Fang* 太平圣惠方, c. 992 AD)	11
Dao chi san 导赤散	*Mu tong* 木通, *sheng di huang* 生地黄, *gan cao shao* 甘草梢 and *zhu ye* 竹叶. (*Mi Chuan Zheng Zhi Yao Jue Ji Lei Fang* 秘传证治要诀及类方, c. 1443)	10
Sheng fu tang/ Sheng fu san 生附汤/散	*Fu zi* 附子, *hua shi* 滑石, *qu mai* 瞿麦, *mu tong* 木通, *ban xia* 半夏, *sheng jiang* 生姜, *deng xin cao* 灯心草 and *mi* 蜜. (*Huo Ren Shi Zheng Fang Hou Ji* 活人事证方后集, c. 1216)	10
Wu ling tang/Wu ling san 五苓 汤/散	*Zhu ling* 猪苓, *fu ling* 茯苓, *bai zhu* 白术, *ze xie* 泽泻, *gui zhi* 桂枝 and *deng xin cao* 灯心草. (*Mi Chuan Zheng Zhi Yao Jue Ji Lei Fang* 秘传证治要诀及类方, c. 1443)	9
Qu mai tang 瞿麦汤	*Qu mai* 瞿麦, *sang gen bai pi* 桑根白皮, *hua shi* 滑石, *mu tong* 木通, *chi shao* 赤芍, *gan cao* 甘草, *yu bai pi* 榆白皮, *mang xiao* 芒硝 and *huang qin* 黄芩. (*Ji Feng Pu Ji Fang* 鸡峰普济方, c. 1133)	8
Si wu tang/Si wu tang jia wei 四物 汤/四物汤加味	*Shu di huang* 熟地黄, *dang gui* 当归, *bai shao* 白芍, *chuan xiong* 川芎 and *niu xi* 牛膝. (*Yi Xue Gang Mu* 医学纲目, c. 1565)	8
Tou ge san 1/Tou ge san 2/Xiao shi san 透膈散/透格 散/硝石散	*Xiao shi* 硝石, *kui zi* 葵子 and *mu tong* 木通 (*Zheng Lei Ben Cao* 证类本草, c. 1082)	8

The use of some herbs/ingredients may be restricted in some countries. For example, herbs *fu zi* 附子 and *mu tong* 木通 can be toxic. Readers are advised to comply with relevant regulations.

dysuria, tense abdomen, and pain localised at the navel' (古今录验疗石淋劳淋热淋, 小便不利, 胞中满急痛, 石苇散方). Ingredients in this formula have the function of clearing heat, inducing diuresis and relieving strangury.

Other common formulas, such as *Wu lin san* 五淋散, *Ba zheng san* 八正散, *Li xiao san* 立效散, *Qu mai tang* 瞿麦汤 and *Tou ge san 1/Tou ge san 2/Xiao shi san* 透膈散/透格散/硝石散 have similar actions of clearing heat, draining dampness and relieving strangury. In addition, each of these formulas treat specific syndromes. This is consistent with the current CM understanding from contemporary guidelines and textbooks, that dampness and heat are the main pathological factors of UTI (see Chapter 2).

Other common formulas had different actions. *Cheng xiang san* 沉香散 has actions of regulating *qi* and soothing the Liver, *Sheng fu tang/Sheng fu san* 生附汤/散 dissipates cold and dispels dampness, and *Si wu tang/Si wu tang jia wei* 四物汤/四物汤加味 activates Blood and resolves stasis. Both *Ba zheng san* 八正散 and *Cheng xiang san* 沉香散 are recommended in contemporary guidelines and textbooks for treating syndromes of dampness-heat in the Bladder and Liver depression and *qi* stagnation, respectively (see Chapter 2).

Most Frequent Herbs for Oral Use in 'Possible' Urinary Tract Infection Citations

A total of 340 herbs for oral use were extracted from the included citations. Six herbs were described in more than 100 formulas: *hua shi* 滑石, *mu tong* 木通, *gan cao* 甘草, *dang gui* 当归, *fu ling* 茯苓, and *qu mai* 瞿麦. The most frequently reported oral herbs are listed in Table 3.7. The key clinical function of these herbs is to drain dampness and relieve strangury. This was not surprising, as this was the function of the most common CHM formulas described above. Frequently used herbs had functions to do the following:

- Clear heat and induce diuresis to relieve strangury: *hua shi* 滑石, *mu tong* 木通, *zhi zi* 栀子, *ze xie* 泽泻, *che qian zi* 车前子, *huang qin* 黄芩 and *da huang* 大黄;

Table 3.7. Most Frequent Oral Herbs in 'Possible' Urinary Tract Infection Citations

Herb Name	Scientific Name	No. of Citations (*n*)
Hua shi 滑石	Hydrated magnesium silicate (talc)	170
Mu tong 木通	*Akebia* spp.	165
Gan cao 甘草	*Glycyrrhizae* spp.	119
Dang gui 当归	*Angelica sinensis* (Oliv.) Diels	108
Fu ling 茯苓	*Poria cocos* (Schw.) Wolf.	106
Qu mai 瞿麦	*Dianthus* spp.	102
Zhi zi 栀子	*Gardenia jasminoides* Ellis	87
Kui zi 葵子	*Abelmoschus manihot* (L.) Medic.	66
Sheng di huang 生地黄	*Rehmannia glutinosa* Libosch	66
Shi wei 石韦	*Pyrrosia* spp.	64
Ze xie 泽泻	*Alisma orientalis* (Sam.) Juzep.	64
Chi shao 赤芍	*Paeonia* spp.	60
Bai shao 白芍	*Paeonia lactiflora* Pall.	54
Che qian zi 车前子	*Plantago* spp.	54
Bai zhu 白术	*Atractylodes macrocephala* Koidz.	45
Mu xiang 木香	*Aucklandia lappa* Decne.	40
Huang qin 黄芩	*Scutellaria baicalensis* Georgi	39
Chen pi 陈皮	*Citrus reticulata* Blanco	36
Da huang 大黄	*Rheum palmatum* L.	35
Hu po 琥珀	Amber	35
Rou gui 肉桂	*Cinnamomum cassia* Presl	35

The use of some herbs, such as *mu tong* 木通, may be restricted in some countries. Readers are advised to comply with relevant regulations.

- Drain dampness and induce diuresis to relieve strangury: *fu ling* 茯苓, *qu mai* 瞿麦, *kui zi* 葵子 and *bai zhu* 白术;
- Activate Blood and resolve stasis to relieve strangury: *dang gui* 当归 and *hu po* 琥珀;
- Cool Blood and tonify *yin* to relieve strangury and/or stop bleeding: *sheng di huang* 生地黄, *shi wei* 石韦, *chi shao* 赤芍 and *bai shao* 白芍;
- Regulate *qi* and soothe the Liver to relieve strangury: *mu xiang* 木香;

- Dissipate cold, tonify *yang* and alleviate pain to relieve strangury: *rou gui* 肉桂.

Hua shi 滑石 was found to be the most frequently reported herb, identified in 170 formulas. *Hua shi* 滑石, is widely used for relieving stranguria and treating all kinds of *lin* 淋. Its frequent use, as well as its inclusion in guideline-recommended formulas *Ba zheng san* 八正散 and *Cheng xiang san* 沉香散, suggest it is an important herb for managing UTI.

Mu tong 木通 was the second most frequently reported herb (used in 165 citations). *Mu tong* 木通 can be sourced from various species and has been used for managing UTI symptoms throughout CM history. More recently, safety concerns have arisen about the use of this herb. In the 1990s, reports of nephrotoxicity due to aristolochic acid from the *Aristolochia* species (*guan mu tong* 关木通)[10–12] have resulted in prohibition of this herb in China and restricted use in other countries, including Australia.[13] The non-toxic *Clematis armandii* Franch. and *Clematis montana* Buch. Ham. species (*chuan mu tong* 川木通) are recommended in contemporary pharmacopoeia for CHM practice.[14]

Most Frequent Oral Formulas in 'Most Likely' Urinary Tract Infection Citations

Of the 480 citations that described oral CHM treatment, 158 were judged as 'most likely' to be UTI. Unnamed formulas were found in 37 citations, and 53 named formulas were described. Some formulas consisted of only one herb while others were more complex, involving up to 22 different ingredients. The median number of herbs in formulas for symptoms most likely to be UTI was six, which reflects the median number of herbs in formulas for the total pool. Ten formulas were documented in more than four citations (Table 3.8). Eight of these ten formulas were also found with high frequency in the total pool: *Shi wei tang/Shi wei san/Shi wei yin zi* 石韦汤/石韦散/石韦饮子, *Li xiao san* 立效散, *Sheng fu tang/Sheng fu san* 生附汤/生附散, *Wu lin san* 五淋散, *Ba zheng san* 八正散, *Qu mai tang* 瞿麦汤, *Tou*

Table 3.8. Most Frequent Oral Formulas in 'Most Likely' Urinary Tract Infection Citations

Formula Name	Herb Ingredients	No. of Citations (*n*)
Shi wei tang/Shi wei san/Shi wei yin zi 石韦汤/石韦散/石韦饮子	*Bai shao* 白芍, *bai zhu* 白术, *hua shi* 滑石, *kui zi* 葵子, *qu mai* 瞿麦, *shi wei* 石韦, *mu tong* 木通, *dang gui* 当归, *gan cao* 甘草 and *wang bu liu xing* 王不留行. (*Wei Sheng Bao Jian* 卫生宝鉴, c. 1343)	9
Li xiao san 立效散	*Qu mai* 瞿麦, *gan cao* 甘草, *zhi zi* 栀子, *cong gen* 葱根, *deng xin cao* 灯心草 and *sheng jiang* 生姜. (*Huo Ren Shi Zheng Fang Hou Ji* 活人事证方后集, c. 1216)	7
Sheng fu tang/ Sheng fu san 生附汤/生附散	*Fu zi* 附子, *hua shi* 滑石, *qu mai* 瞿麦, *mu tong* 木通, *ban xia* 半夏, *sheng jiang* 生姜, *deng xin cao* 灯心草 and *mi* 蜜. (*Huo Ren Shi Zheng Fang Hou Ji* 活人事证方后集, c. 1216)	7
Wu lin san 五淋散	*Fu ling* 茯苓, *dang gui* 当归, *gan cao* 甘草, *chi shao* 赤芍 and *zhi zi* 栀子. (*Tai Ping Hui Min He Ji Ju Fang* 太平惠民和剂局方, c. 1107)	7
Ba zheng san 八正散	*Che qian cao* 车前草, *qu mai* 瞿麦, *bian xu* 萹蓄, *hua shi* 滑石, *gan cao* 甘草, *zhi zi* 栀子, *mu tong* 木通, *da huang* 大黄 and *deng xin cao* 灯心草. (*Dan Xi Xin Fa* 丹溪心法, c. 1481)	5
Qu mai tang 瞿麦汤	*Qu mai* 瞿麦, *sang gen bai pi* 桑根白皮, *hua shi* 滑石, *mu tong* 木通, *chi shao* 赤芍, *gan cao* 甘草, *yu bai pi* 榆白皮, *mang xiao* 芒硝 and *huang qin* 黄芩. (*Ji Feng Pu Ji Fang* 鸡峰普济方, c. 1133)	5
Tou ge san 1/Tou ge san 2/Xiao shi san 透膈散/透格散/硝石散	*Xiao shi* 硝石, *kui zi* 葵子 and *mu tong* 木通. (*Zheng Lei Ben Cao* 证类本草, c. 1082)	5

(*Continued*)

Table 3.8. (*Continued*)

Formula Name	Herb Ingredients	No. of Citations (*n*)
Ze xie san 泽泻散	*Ze xie* 泽泻, *ji su* 鸡苏, *fu ling* 茯苓, *shi wei* 石韦, *dang gui* 当归, *rou gui* 肉桂, *bing lang* 槟榔, *sang piao qiao* 桑螵蛸, *zhi ke* 枳壳 and *hu po* 琥珀. (*Tai Ping Sheng Hui Fang* 太平圣惠方, c. 992)	5
Si wu tang/Si wu tang jia wei 四物汤/四物汤加味	*Shu di huang* 熟地黄, *dang gui* 当归, *bai shao* 白芍, *chuan xiong* 川芎, *niu xi* 牛膝, *hua shi* 滑石, *tao ren* 桃仁, *zhi shi* 枳实, *bei mu* 贝母, *zhi zi* 栀子 and *chai hu* 柴胡. (*Sun Shi Yi An* 孙氏医案, c. 1573)	4
Xi jiao di huang tang 犀角地黄汤	*Xi jiao* 犀角, *bai shao* 白芍, *mu dan pi* 牡丹皮 and *sheng di huang* 生地黄. (*Pu ji fang* 普济方, c. 1309)	4

The use of some herbs/ingredients may be restricted in some countries. For example, herbs such as *fu zi* 附子 and *mu tong* 木通 can be toxic; use of *xi jiao* 犀角 is prohibited under the Convention on International Trade in Endangered Species of Wild Fauna and Flora (CITES). Readers are advised to comply with relevant regulations.

ge san 1/Tou ge san 2/Xiao shi san 透膈散/透格散/硝石散, and *Si wu tang/Si wu tang jia wei* 四物汤/四物汤加味. This suggests a degree of consistency in managing urinary symptoms. The key clinical functions of the most frequently reported formulas were similar, including draining dampness and relieving strangury.

Of the remaining two formulas, both were found exclusively in citations judged 'most likely' to relate to UTI. *Ze xie san* 泽泻散 was first cited in the book *Tai Ping Sheng Hui Fang* 太平圣惠方 (c. 992 AD) to treat *leng lin* 冷淋 (cold strangury) with the symptoms of dysuria and tense lower abdomen. (治冷淋, 小便不通, 涩痛胀满, 泽泻散方) Herbs were formulated to regulate *qi* to induce diuresis, warm *yang* and drain dampness. The formula *Xi jiao di huang tang* 犀角地黄汤 has the clinical function of clearing heat, cooling Blood and resolving stasis. This formula was widely used for treating *xue lin* 血淋 (haematuria) historically.

Most Frequent Herbs for Oral Use in 'Most Likely' Urinary Tract Infection Citations

A total of 203 oral herbs were extracted from the 'most likely' UTI citations. The most frequently reported herbs are listed in Table 3.9. The most frequently cited herbs in the 'most likely' UTI citations were consistent with the herbs in the total pool, likely due to the large number of citations judged 'most likely' to be UTI. Thus, the best

Table 3.9. Most Frequent Oral Herbs in 'Most Likely' Urinary Tract Infection Citations

Herb Name	Scientific Name	No. of Citations (*n*)
Hua shi 滑石	Hydrated magnesium silicate (talc)	61
Mu tong 木通	*Akebia* spp.	53
Qu mai 瞿麦	*Dianthus superbus* L.	41
Gan cao 甘草	*Glycyrrhizae* spp.	40
Dang gui 当归	*Angelica sinensis* (Oliv.) Diels	38
Zhi zi 栀子	*Gardenia jasminoides* Ellis	37
Fu ling 茯苓	*Poria cocos* (Schw.) Wolf.	28
Shi wei 石韦	*Pyrrosia* spp.	23
Kui zi 葵子	*Abelmoschus manihot* (L.) Medic.	22
Chi shao 赤芍	*Paeonia* spp.	21
Sheng di huang 生地黄	*Rehmannia glutinosa* Libosch	21
Bai shao 白芍	*Paeonia lactiflora* Pall.	20
Bai mao gen 白茅根	*Imperata cylindrica* (L.) P. Beauv.	16
Mu xiang 木香	*Aucklandia lappa* Decne.	15
Rou gui 肉桂	*Cinnamomum cassia* Presl	15
Ze xie 泽泻	*Alisma orientalis* (Sam.) Juzep	15
Bai zhu 白术	*Atractylodes macrocephala* Koidz.	13
Da huang 大黄	*Rheum palmatum* L.	13

The use of some herbs/ingredients, such as *mu tong* 木通, may be restricted in some countries. Readers are advised to comply with relevant regulations.

pool is reflective of the total pool. Draining dampness and relieving strangury are the key clinical functions of these herbs that could be beneficial for treating *lin* 淋 syndrome.

Treatment with Topical Chinese Herbal Medicine

Topical CHM treatments were mentioned in eight 'possible' UTI citations, three of which were considered as 'most likely' UTI. These citations were obtained from seven classical literature texts published in the Ming and Qing dynasties (1369–1911). The limited number of citations suggests that topical CHM treatments were used less frequently than oral CHM treatments for UTI in past eras.

Application of topical CHM around the navel was described in five citations, including the three 'most likely' UTI citations. For example, in the book *Qi Xiao Liang Fang* 奇效良方 (c. 1470), Dong Suyuan 董宿原 described application of a powdered mixture of *hua shi* 滑石 and *che qian zi* 车前子 four *cun* 寸 (anatomical units) around the navel (车前子散, 治诸淋闭涩不通…车前子 滑石 [各一两] 上为细末, 一方涂脐四畔, 约四寸, 水和调服亦可). This treatment could be used for all kinds of *lin* 淋 syndromes. In *Mi Chuan Zheng Zhi Yao Jue Ji Lei Fang* 秘传证治要诀及类方 (c. 1443), *hu po* 琥珀 and salt were mentioned as the topical ingredients for treating *lin bi* 淋闭. Although the herbs/ingredients for topical applications varied among the included citations, the functions of these herbs/ingredients were similar, including inducing diuresis to relieve strangury.

Two citations reported another topical treatment for *re lin* 热淋 in men. These citations applied the herb *she xiang* 麝香 to the penis. This can have the action of cooling Blood and alleviating pain. One citation used *cong bai* 葱白 decoction as an enema for symptoms of frequent urination and penile pain (小便频数, 茎中切痛…外以葱汤频洗谷道, 则便数及痛自愈). *Cong bai* 葱白 has the function of relieving dysuria.

Discussion of Chinese Herbal Medicine for Urinary Tract Infection

The results of the analyses showed that CHM was an important treatment for UTI symptoms in past eras. In particular, classical texts emphasised use of herbal prescriptions for oral consumption. Diversity was seen amongst these formulas, with over 120 different named formulas identified. The diversity in formulas is reflected in the low number of citations for the most frequently used formula *Shi wei tang* (decoction)/*Shi wei san* (powder)/*Shi wei yin zi* (liquid) 石韦汤/石韦散/石韦饮子 (24 citations of the total of 480 oral CHM citations).

Oral CHM formulations varied in complexity, ranging from simple one- or two-herb formulas to more complex formulations involving up to 29 different herbs. This appears to be in contrast to findings from Barrett *et al.* (2015),[2] who described more simple treatments for urinary symptoms in their analysis of key classical literature. This difference may be influenced by the number of texts consulted; this analysis used a digitalised collection of more than 1,100 texts, while Barrett *et al.* (2015) selected a sample of 23 key texts dating back to the *Mawangdui* 马王堆 tomb medical manuscripts.

Among the ten most frequently cited formulas in the total pool, two formulas have demonstrated long history of use for urinary symptoms: *Ba zheng san* 八正散 and *Cheng xiang san* 沉香散. These formulas were found in citations judged 'most likely' to relate to UTI. Further, both formulas continue to be used in clinical practice and are recommended in contemporary textbooks and guidelines.[7,8,15,16] As highlighted above, *Ba zheng san* 八正散 has actions to clear heat, drain dampness and relieve strangury, while *Cheng xiang san* 沉香散 regulates *qi* and soothes the Liver.

Of note, formulas *Zhi bai di huang wan* 知柏地黄汤 and *Wu bi shan yao wan* 无比山药丸, which are both recommended in contemporary texts,[8,15,16] were not found in the included citations. The reasons for this are unclear but may relate to the criteria used for selecting citations. For example, if citations that described treatment of *lin* 淋 syndromes did not describe the symptoms used to select citations, or described urinary symptoms in children or pregnant women, they were excluded from further analysis. A second possible explanation for this finding may relate to the formula name; it is possible that the same set of herb ingredients were given different formula names in different books, or that the formula name changed over time. While efforts were made to identify CHM treatments which were composed of the same ingredients but with different names, it is possible that such instances were missed.

The most frequently used herbs in the total pool were *hua shi* 滑石, *mu tong* 木通, *gan cao* 甘草, *dang gui* 当归, *fu ling* 茯苓 and *qu mai* 瞿麦. *Hua shi* 滑石, *gan cao* 甘草, *fu ling* 茯苓 and *qu mai* 瞿麦 are all found in formulas recommended for contemporary practice (see Chapter 2). Despite being the fourth most cited herb, *dang gui* 当归 is not included in any of the formulas included in Chapter 2. It seems unusual to have a herb with high frequency in classical literature that is not an ingredient of formulas in contemporary texts. One possible explanation for this relates to syndromes. Blood stagnation is not described as a key syndrome in any of the texts reviewed for Chapter 2; however, contemporary textbooks and guidelines do describe modifications to formulas for patients with Blood stagnation. As detailed analysis of aetiology and CM syndromes was not undertaken as part of this review, it is unclear whether Blood stagnation was discussed in relation to UTI in classical texts. A second explanation for this is that other herbs with functions of activating Blood may be used in place of *dang gui* 当归 in contemporary texts. The herbs *dai ji* 大蓟, *xiao ji* 小蓟, *bai mao gen* 白茅根, *zhen zhu cao* 珍珠草, *hong hua* 红花, *chi shao* 赤芍 and *chuan niu xi* 川牛膝, all of which activate Blood, can be found in formulas described in Chapter 2.

Contemporary textbooks use *chuan mu tong* 川木通 in place of *mu tong* 木通 in the formula *Ba zheng san* 八正散 due to toxicity of *mu tong* 木通. In this way, advances in technology that allow evaluation of safety have changed practice of CM. Chinese medicine practice has also been changed by environmental factors. Some herbal products from animals, such as *xi jiao* 犀角 (rhinoceros skin or horn) that may have been abundant in past eras are now endangered or at risk of becoming endangered. Trade in such products is prohibited under the provisions of the Convention on International Trade in Endangered Species of Wild Fauna and Flora (CITES). Appropriate alternatives to such products are available.

The earliest oral CHM treatment among included citations came from *Bei Ji Qian Jin Yao Fang* 备急千金要方 dated 652 AD. The unnamed formula included herbs *hua shi* 滑石 and *qu mai* 瞿麦, among others. But the use of these herbs for urinary diseases appears to have a longer history, with both herbs being mentioned in relation to urinary symptoms in the Wuwei 武威 tomb medical manuscripts (first century AD).[2] These herbs were used in a recipe for *lin* 淋/*long* 癃 syndrome. Both herbs continue to be important for UTI in contemporary practice and are included in the formula *Ba zheng san* 八正散.

Topical CHM treatments were infrequently used for urinary symptoms. Treatment with topical CHM varied in terms of herbs used and techniques employed. Such methods were not found in contemporary texts, although the practice of using CHM as a topical wash is described in Chapter 2. In any case, treatment of urinary symptoms with CHM was predominantly with formulas for oral use.

Acupuncture and Related Therapies

A total of 51 citations describing acupuncture and related therapies were found in 19 books. Nine books provided two or more citations, and two books provided nine citations each: *Zhen Jiu Zi Sheng Jing* 针灸资生经 (c. 1220) and *Pu Ji Fang* 普济方 (c. 1390).

Frequency of Treatment Citations by Dynasty

Citations describing acupuncture therapies were also found in books from the Tang and Five dynasties (618–960 AD) through to the Minguo 民国/Republic of China (1912–1949) (Table 3.10). One citation was obtained from a Japanese book published in the Song dynasty (960–1279). No citations came from books produced during the Yuan dynasty, which was not surprising given the small number of CHM citations in books from this dynasty.

The earliest citations were obtained from *Bei Ji Qian Jin Fang* 备急千金方 (c. 652 AD). In this book, Sun Simiao 孙思邈 used moxibustion therapy for treating symptoms 'possibly' related to UTI. Moxibustion on the point *Niaobao* 尿胞 (CV2 *Qugu* 曲骨, one *cun* 寸 below the point, *Yuquan* 玉泉 [CV3 *Zhongji* 中极]) is recommended for sensations of fullness in the abdomen with frequent

Table 3.10. Dynastic Distribution of Treatment Citations

Dynasty	No. of Citations (*n*)
Tang and Five dynasties (618–960)	3
Song and Jin dynasties (961–1271)	15
Ming dynasty (1369–1644)	24
Qing dynasty (1645–1911)	6
Minguo/Republic of China (1912–1949)	2
Japan (Song and Jin dynasties)	1
Total	51

urination (腹中满小便数起, 灸玉泉下一寸, 名尿胞). Moxibustion to LR3 *Taichong* 太冲 is recommended for *lin* 淋 syndrome with dysuria and penile pain (淋病不得小便, 阴上痛, 灸足太冲五十壮). Sun Simiao 孙思邈 also suggested ST30 *Qichong* 气冲 could be used for treating feeling fullness and heat in the abdomen, strangury and urinary retention (气冲主腹中满热, 淋闭不得尿).

The most recent citation was obtained from the book *Jin Zhen Mi Chuan* 金针秘传 (1937). This citation recommended the combination of acupuncture and moxibustion to BL27 *Xiaochangshu* 小肠俞 for managing haematuria, dribbling urination and lower abdomen pain (小肠腧…治小便赤涩淋沥, 少腹·痛…针入三分, 留六呼, 可灸三壮).

Treatment with Acupuncture and Related Therapies

Of the included 51 citations, 20 described the combination of acupuncture and moxibustion therapies for managing UTI symptoms (39.2%), 14 recommended moxibustion individually as a treatment for UTI symptoms (27.5%), while four mentioned acupuncture alone (7.8%). Thirteen citations (25.5%) were entries describing the functions of points in relation to urinary symptoms or mentioned the use of certain points without specifying the acupuncture technique that could be employed. The result suggested that moxibustion might have been a popular therapy for managing UTI symptoms in dynastic China. Acupuncture points used in the included citations were analysed to identify those most frequently used.

Most Frequent Acupuncture Points in 'Possible' Urinary Tract Infection Citations

A total of 34 acupuncture points was used in the included citations. Ten acupuncture points were described in three or more citations (Table 3.11). Acupuncture points KI4 *Dazhong* 大钟, CV2 *Qugu* 曲骨, BL27 *Xiaochangshu* 小肠俞 and SP9 *Yinlingquan* 阴陵泉 were the four most cited acupuncture points, used in six citations each.

Approximately two-thirds of the acupuncture points used were on the Kidney, Bladder or Conception Vessel meridians (22 of the 34 acupuncture points; 64.7%). In CM, one function of the Kidney is to govern urinary function, while the Bladder stores and discharges urine. As the key syndromes of *lin* 淋 syndrome in classical texts were Kidney deficiency and Bladder heat accumulation (see 'Descriptions of the Aetiology of UTI' section), stimulating acupuncture points on the Kidney and Bladder meridians can tonify Kidney *qi* and clear Bladder heat. Most Conception Vessel points were between the pubic symphysis (CV2 *Qugu* 曲骨) and the navel (CV8 *Shenque* 神阙). These points have functions that benefit the Bladder, Kidney and the Lower Energiser, and drain dampness, hence their relevance for UTI.

Table 3.11. Most Frequent Acupuncture Points in 'Possible' Urinary Tract Infection Citations

Acupuncture Point	No. of Citations (*n*)
KI4 *Dazhong* 大钟	6
CV2 *Qugu* 曲骨	6
BL27 *Xiaochangshu* 小肠俞	6
SP9 *Yinlingquan* 阴陵泉	6
KI7 *Fuliu* 复溜	4
CV8 *Shenque* 神阙	4
LR3 *Taichong* 太冲	4
CV4 *Guanyuan* 关元	3
SP6 *Sanyinjiao* 三阴交	3
CV5 *Shimen* 石门	3

The acupuncture point BL27 *Xiaochangshu* 小肠俞 may be useful for urinary symptoms for several reasons. The point is located on the Bladder channel and is the back *shu* 俞 point of the Small Intestine. Both the Bladder and Small Intestine are *Taiyang* 太阳 meridians, the outermost pair of the six divisions, and are the body's first line of defence in external pathogenic attacks. The acupuncture point BL27 *Xiaochangshu* 小肠俞 drains dampness and clears damp-heat, and regulates Small Intestine *qi*. A key function of the Small Intestine is to separate clear and turbid fluids, hence stimulating this point can further contribute to draining dampness.

Two of the most frequently used points are on the Spleen meridian (SP9 *Yinlingquan* 阴陵泉 and SP6 *Sanyinjiao* 三阴交). Stimulating these points can promote the circulation of Spleen *qi* to enhance the transportation of fluids, which is beneficial for draining dampness and relieving strangury in *lin* 淋 syndrome.

Most Frequent Acupuncture Points in 'Most Likely' Urinary Tract Infection Citations

Seven citations describing acupuncture and/or moxibustion from the total pool were judged as 'most likely' UTI. Three citations referred to acupuncture points without specifying which acupuncture technique could be used; two citations described the actions of the *Yinqiao* 阴跷 meridians, and one citation used the acupuncture point KI6 *Zhaohai* 照海. Four citations described moxibustion as a treatment for *lin* 淋 syndrome, while one citation recommended a combination of acupuncture and moxibustion.

Moxibustion on CV8 *Shenque* 神阙 was mentioned in three citations for various *lin* 淋 syndromes. For example, in *Zhen Jiu Da Cheng* 针灸大成 (c. 1601), the author stated that *lin* 淋 syndrome manifesting with painful urination was induced by heat accumulating in Bladder that could not be expelled from the body. To treat the five *lin* 淋 syndromes, the practitioner can fill the patient's navel (the location of acupuncture point CV8 *Shenque* 神阙) with warm salt and apply moxibustion with seven *zhuang* 壮 (moxibustion cones). Alternatively, moxibustion could be applied to SP6 *Sanyinjiao*

三阴交 (淋, 小便涩痛也, 热客膀胱, 郁结不能渗泄故也. 以上五淋, 皆用盐炒热, 填满病人脐中, 却用筋头大艾, 灸七壮, 或灸三阴交即愈).

Acupuncture points CV4 *Guanyuan* 关元, BL27 *Xiaochangshu* 小肠俞 and SP6 *Sanyinjiao* 三阴交 were mentioned in one citation each. These points were also the most cited points in the 'possible' UTI citations pool. Stimulation of these points can regulate the function of the Bladder and Spleen.

Discussion of Acupuncture for Urinary Tract Infection

Acupuncture and moxibustion were not found as frequently in classical literature citations as CHM treatments; nevertheless, they provided another treatment option for cases of urinary symptoms. Over two-thirds of acupuncture points described in the 51 citations were on the Kidney, Bladder or Conception Vessel meridians, emphasising the importance of these organs and meridians in managing urinary symptoms. This aligns with the aetiology described in multiple citations, which attributed *lin* 淋 syndrome to deficiency of the Kidney and heat in the Bladder.

Moxibustion was used in 34 of the 51 citations, sometimes in combination with acupuncture. The focus on moxibustion seems surprising given that urinary symptoms were attributed, in part, to heat pathogens. However, in these citations, moxibustion appears to be used to provide dynamic *yang* when stimulating acupuncture points, rather than with the intention of introducing additional heat.

The earliest use of moxibustion identified in this review was in the seventh century book *Bei Ji Qian Jin Fang* 备急千金方. However, this does not appear to be the earliest description of using moxibustion for urinary symptoms. Moxibustion was described as a treatment for urological disease in a medical manuscript from the *Mawangdui* 马王堆 tombs in Changsha (Ma 1992, in Barrett *et al.*, 2015).[2] Despite not being recommended in leading contemporary CM textbooks and clinical guidelines reviewed in Chapter 2, it is likely that this technique continues to be used in clinical practice.

Three citations described using moxibustion to CV8 *Shenque* 神阙 for urinary symptoms. This point is traditionally recommended for moxibustion therapy and is contraindicated for needling in contemporary texts.[17] Applying moxibustion to this point can harmonise the *qi* and Blood in the Conception Vessel meridian, regulate functions of the Middle and Lower Energisers, and is used for various conditions caused by Kidney and Spleen deficiency. Thus, through these actions, moxibustion to CV8 *Shenque* 神阙 could be beneficial for managing *lin* 淋 syndromes.

Other Chinese Medicine Therapies

Other CM therapies were described in 24 citations. Most of the citations were from the Song and Jin dynasties (961–1271, 21 citations), likely due to 14 citations found in the book *Tai Ping Sheng Hui Fang* 太平圣惠方 (c. 992). Two citations came from books published during the Ming dynasty and one citation was from *Zhu Bing Yuan Hou Lun* 诸病源候论 (c. 610 AD), published before the Tang and Five dynasties. Three different types of therapies were cited; diet therapy (22 citations), *daoyin* 导引 (a style of *qigong* 气功 exercise, one citation), and external application of hot and cold items (one citation).

The citation that described *daoyin* 导引 was the earliest citation in the total pool. In *Zhu Bing Yuan Hou Lun* 诸病源候论 (c. 610 AD), Cao Yuanfang 巢元方 described the use of a *qigong* 气功 style exercise for managing *qi lin* 气淋: ask the patient to lie on his back, place his hands on his knees, move his heels under his hip, open his mouth and take a deep breath until the abdomen feels tense, then exhale via the nose. This exercise can treat *qi lin* 气淋, frequent urination, penile pain, wet perineum, lower abdomen pain and weak knees (气淋者, 肾虚膀胱热, 气胀所为也…偃卧, 以两手布膝头, 取踵置尻下, 以口纳气, 腹胀自极, 以鼻出气七息, 除气癃, 数小便, 茎中痛, 阴以下湿, 小腹痛, 膝不随也). This citation did not explain the cause of 'wet perineum'; this could be due to either post-void dribbling or sweat. This citation also described other types of treatment, including treatment with CHM. However, as the details of CHM treatment were not described (that is, the formula and herb ingredients were not named), this citation was not included in the CHM analysis.

One citation recommended external application of heat for symptoms of painful and dripping urination, and haematuria. The author described that placing hot and cold items on the lower abdomen could expel pathogenic heat *qi* which caused dysuria symptoms (淋沥尿血, 阴中疼, 此是热气所致, 熨之即愈, 熨法前以冷物熨少腹, 冷熨已, 又以热物熨前, 热熨之以后复冷熨).

Of the 22 diet therapy citations, 19 were named recipes while three were unnamed. *Pu tao jian* 葡萄煎 (grape soup/decoction), *Qing tou ya geng* 青头鸭羹 (duck soup) and *Yu pi suo bing* 榆皮索饼 (cake made with the bark of the elm tree) were obtained from multiple citations. Most citations described therapy with a Chinese herbal porridge (ten citations) or soup (nine citations). A total of 31 herbs/foods were cited in the included citations. Table 3.12 lists the herbs/foods that were cited in multiple citations. The most frequently cited herb was *cong bai* 葱白 (a type of onion), obtained from 11 citations.

Table 3.12. **Most Frequent Herbs and Foods Mentioned in Diet Therapy**

Herb Name	Scientific Name	No. of Citations (*n*)
Cong bai 葱白	*Allium fistulosum* L.	11
Jing mi 粳米	*Oryza sativa* L.	7
Qing liang mi 青粱米	*Setaria italica* (L.) Beauv	5
Feng mi 蜂蜜	Honey	5
Ou zhi 藕汁	*Nelumbo nucifera* Gaertn.	4
Sheng di huang 生地黄	*Rehmannia glutinosa* Libosch	4
Dan dou chi 淡豆豉	*Glycine max* (L.) Merr.	3
Dong gua 冬瓜	*Benincasa hispida* (Thunb.) Cogn.	3
Dong ma zi 冬麻子	*Cannabis sativa* L.	3
Che qian cao 车前草	*Plantago* spp.	2
Dong kui 冬葵	*Malva verticillata* L.	2
Jiang shui 浆水	*Oryza sativa* L.	2
Pu tao 葡萄	Grape (no species specified)	2
Qing tou ya 青头鸭	Duck	2
Yu bai pi 榆白皮	*Ulmus pumila* L.	2

It has the function of releasing the exterior and relieving dysuria. Other foods found in multiple citations were *jing mi* 粳米 (rice, seven citations), *qing liang mi* 青粱米 (millet, five citations) and *feng mi* 蜂蜜 (honey, five citations) which have the function to tonify Spleen and Kidney *qi*, draining dampness and relieving strangury, which are beneficial for treating *lin* 淋 syndrome.

Discussion of Other Chinese Medicine Therapies for Urinary Tract Infection

In addition to CHM and acupuncture, doctors and scholars in past eras considered dietary therapy as a valuable tool for urinary symptoms. Some of the herbs used in recipes may overlap with herbs used in CHM formulas, posing a challenge in terms of classifying treatments as CHM or other CM therapies. Citations presented in this section used the Chinese characters for dietary therapy (*shi zhi* 食治) to distinguish this treatment from CHM treatments.

The earliest use of dietary therapy in included citations was from the tenth century book *Tai Ping Sheng Hui Fang* 太平圣惠方. Similar to CHM and acupuncture, food as medicine for urinary symptoms pre-dates the earliest citations included in this review. Recipes for urinary disorders were found in the *Mawangdui* 马王堆 tomb manuscripts, showing the long history of dietary therapy.[2]

Daoyin 导引 exercises were found in just one included citation, which was the earliest citation included in the total pool. This citation from *Zhu Bing Yuan Hou Lun* 诸病源候论 describes *daoyin* 导引 as a treatment for *qi lin* 气淋. This is significant, as it provides an indication of early engagement of patients in their own health care.

Classical Literature in Perspective

Classical CM texts provide the basis for many treatments used in contemporary clinical practice. Chinese medicine practice is not static; it evolves and adapts to cultural and environmental changes as well as advances in knowledge. This analysis has identified several contemporary treatments which have their origins in early CM history, and highlights areas where practice has changed.

The patient's experience of UTI is one that does not appear to have changed over time. Dysuria and burning sensation or pain with urination were key symptoms in the included citations of *lin* 淋 syndrome and reflect the symptoms described in conventional biomedical textbooks. Flank pain, fever and chills are often seen in cases of pyelonephritis. Among the included citations, flank pain was found in only nine of the 563 included citations, while fever and/or chills were found in 29 of the included treatment citations.

Based on the frequently reported symptoms, it seems likely that cases of *lin* 淋 syndrome described in classical CM literature refer to acute lower UTI rather than upper UTI. Of course, such distinctions are modern disease classifications which would not be found in classical CM literature. Doctors in past eras would not have been able to distinguish between what is now considered as uncomplicated and complicated UTI cases, unless such cases were obviously more complex, for example UTI during pregnancy or when symptoms clearly refer to diabetes.

Similarly, few citations distinguished between sporadic UTI and recurrent infections. A small number of citations (fewer than 10 citations) mentioned chronicity (*su* 宿) in relation to UTI; these terms were found using the terms *lin zheng* 淋证, *xue lin* 血淋 and *re lin* 热淋. But these terms found many other possible cases of UTI that did not mention chronicity, so the terms alone are unlikely to directly relate to chronic or recurrent infections. A more detailed analysis of citations would be required to identify whether specific terms were used in cases of recurrent UTI.

Citations included in this review described multiple subtypes of *lin* 淋 syndrome. Research by Barrett *et al.* (2015)[2] highlighted variation among key texts, ranging from five to eight different subtypes. Five types of *lin* 淋 were among the most productive search terms that identified possible UTI citations: *xue lin* 血淋 (162 citations), *qi lin* 气淋 (72 citations), *re lin* 热淋 (65 citations), *lao lin* 劳淋 (34 citations) and *leng lin* 冷淋 (32 citations). Frequency of other subtypes of *lin* 淋, such as *shi lin* 石淋 and *gao lin* 膏淋, was not recorded as these subtypes were not included in the set of search terms. Despite this, we know that they were found in several of the included citations. It is possible that more subtypes of *lin* 淋 have been described in the classical literature, which may describe symptoms similar or different to those seen in UTI.

Oral CHM was the main treatment approach used in the included citations. Diversity was seen in formulas and herb ingredients used for urinary symptoms. The formula most often described was *Shi wei tang* 石韦汤, which was prepared as a decoction, powder (*san* 散) or liquid (*yin zi* 饮子) for oral consumption. The key ingredient, *shi wei* 石韦, has actions to relieve dysuria, clear heat and induce diuresis, and was among the ten most frequently used herbs in the included studies. While *Shi wei tang* 石韦汤 was not found in the references that informed Chapter 2, *shi wei* 石韦 is an ingredient of three of the four traditional formulas that are recommended for UTI. *Shi wei* 石韦 was an important herb for urinary symptoms in the past and continues to be important in contemporary clinical practice.

Two formulas that continue to be used in contemporary clinical practice were among the most frequently used in classical citations: *Ba zheng san* 八正散 and *Cheng xiang san* 沉香散. Both formulas were found with high frequency in the total pool, and were also found in the best citations, that is, those judged 'most likely' to relate to UTI. The longevity of these formulas highlights their importance for *lin* 淋 syndrome.

Acupuncture and moxibustion were additional treatments that could provide benefit in cases of *lin* 淋 syndrome. Acupuncture and moxibustion were frequently applied to points on the Bladder, Kidney and Conception Vessel meridians. Acupuncture points on the Bladder and Conception Vessel meridians are described in contemporary textbooks and clinical guidelines, but points on the Kidney meridian were noticeably absent. However, BL23 *Shenshu* 肾俞, the back *shu* 俞 point of the Kidney, is recommended in the textbooks and guidelines and this point can be used to tonify Kidney *qi*.

Dietary therapy was used less frequently than CHM, acupuncture or moxibustion. Recipes were simple and involved few ingredients that were probably readily available. Dietary therapy and recommendations for UTI continue to be described in contemporary textbooks and guidelines, although the food and herbs described in contemporary literature differ from those found in classical literature. Despite these differences, classical CM literature provided a model of treatment that allowed patients to participate in their own health care[2] that continues to be used in contemporary practice.

References

1. Needham J, Lu G, Sivin N. (2000) *Science and Civilisation in China. Volume 5, Part VI: Medicine.* Cambridge University Press, UK.
2. Barrett P, Flower A, Lo V. (2015) What's past is prologue: Chinese medicine and the treatment of recurrent urinary tract infections. *J Ethnopharmacol* **167**: 86–96.
3. Hu R, ed. (2000) *Encyclopedia of Traditional Chinese Medicine.* Hunan Electronic and Audio-Visual Publishing House, Changsha.
4. May B, Lu C, Xue C. (2012) Collections of traditional Chinese medical literature as resources for systematic searches. *J Altern Complement Med* **18**(12): 1101–1107.
5. May B, Lu Y, Lu C, *et al.* (2013) Systematic assessment of the representativeness of published collections of the traditional literature on Chinese medicine. *J Altern Complement Med* **19**(5): 403–409.
6. 周仲瑛. (2017) 中医内科学 (第 1 版). 北京: 中国中医药出版社.
7. 中华中医药学会. (2008) 中医内科常见诊疗指南—中医病证部分. 北京: 中国中医药出版社, pp. 111–113.
8. 杨霓芝, 刘旭生. (2013) 中医临床诊治泌尿科专病 (第 3 版). 北京: 人民卫生出版社.
9. 李经绅, 邓铁涛主编. (1995) 中医大词典. 北京: 人民卫生出版社.
10. Cheung TP, Xue C, Leung K, *et al.* (2006) Aristolochic acids detected in some raw Chinese medicinal herbs and manufactured herbal products: A consequence of inappropriate nomenclature and imprecise labelling? *Clin Toxicol* **44**(4): 371–378.
11. Shaw D. (2010) Toxicological risks of Chinese herbs. *Planta Medica* **76**(17): 2012–2018.
12. Zhao Z, Hu Y, Liang Z, *et al.* (2006) Authentication is fundamental for standardization of Chinese medicines. *Planta Medica* **72**(10): 865–874.

13. Department of Health. SUSMP NO. 24: Standard for the Uniform Scheduling of Medicines and Poisons No. 24 (2019) SUSMP Canberra: Australia Government Department of Health; 2019. Available from: https://www.legislation.gov.au/Details/F2019L00685.

14. 国家药典委员会. (2015) 中华人民共和国药典. 北京: 中国医药科技出版社.

15. 薛博瑜, 吴伟. (2016) 中医内科学 (第 3 版). 北京: 人民卫生出版社.

16. 中华中医药学会. (2017) 中医药单用/联合抗生素治疗常见感染性疾病临床实践指南-单纯性下尿路感染 (中华中医药学会团体标准). 北京: 中国中医药出版社.

17. Deadman P, Al-Khafaji M, Baker K. (2000) *A Manual of Acupuncture*. Journal of Chinese Medicine Publications, East Sussex, England.

4

Methods for Evaluating Clinical Evidence

OVERVIEW

Clinical studies of Chinese medicine interventions for uncomplicated urinary tract infection were identified through searching electronic databases. Studies were assessed against eligibility criteria, and a review was conducted using standardised methods. This chapter describes the methods used to evaluate the efficacy and safety of Chinese medicine treatments for urinary tract infection.

Introduction

The use of Chinese medicine (CM) for urinary tract infections (UTIs) has been described in the contemporary literature (Chapter 2) and in classical CM texts (Chapter 3). Several systematic reviews have been conducted to evaluate the efficacy and safety of CM treatment for the management of acute and recurrent UTIs. The evidence from controlled clinical trials (CCTs) was analysed using meta-analysis where possible, and details from non-controlled studies have been described. The findings of these analyses have been presented according to the type of intervention: Chinese herbal medicine (CHM; see Chapter 5), acupuncture and related therapies (see Chapter 7) and combinations of CM therapies such as CHM plus acupuncture, or acupuncture plus taichi 太极 (see Chapter 8).

This chapter describes the methods used to evaluate evidence from clinical studies. References to clinical trials were obtained and assessed by an expert group. Evidence from randomised controlled trials (RCTs), non-randomised CCTs, and non-controlled studies were evaluated separately. The same approach was used to evaluate RCTs and CCTs, which was to describe the characteristics of the studies and CM treatments, and to conduct meta-analyses using the approach outlined below. This approach was not suitable for non-controlled studies. Instead, a summary is provided of the characteristics of the studies, CM treatments and any adverse events reported.

References to included studies are indicated by a letter followed by a number. Studies of CHM are indicated by an 'H' (e.g., H1); studies of acupuncture and related therapies indicated by an 'A' (e.g., A1); and studies of combinations of CM therapies indicated by a 'C' (e.g., C1).

Search Strategy

A comprehensive search was conducted in English and Chinese language databases guided by the methods of the Cochrane Handbook of Systematic Reviews.[1] English language databases included PubMed, Excerpta Medica Database (Embase), Cumulative Index of Nursing and Allied Health Literature (CINAHL), Cochrane Central Register of Controlled Trials (CENTRAL) including the Cochrane Library, and Allied and Complementary Medicine Database (AMED). Chinese language databases included China BioMedical Literature (CBM), China National Knowledge Infrastructure (CNKI), Chongqing VIP (CQVIP) and Wanfang. Chinese language databases were searched from inception to March 2018, and English language databases were searched from inception to July 2018. No restrictions were applied. Search terms were mapped to controlled vocabulary (where applicable) in addition to being searched as keywords.

To conduct a comprehensive search of the literature, searches were run according to the study design (reviews, controlled trials and non-controlled studies). This was done for each of the three intervention types (CHM, acupuncture and related therapies, and other CM therapies) resulting in nine searches in each of the nine databases:

1. CHM — reviews;
2. CHM — controlled trials (randomised and non-randomised);
3. CHM — non-controlled studies;

4. Acupuncture and related therapies — reviews;
5. Acupuncture and related therapies — controlled trials (randomised and non-randomised);
6. Acupuncture and related therapies — non-controlled studies;
7. Other CM therapies — reviews;
8. Other CM therapies — controlled trials (randomised and non-randomised);
9. Other CM therapies — non-controlled studies.

Studies of combination CM therapies were identified through the above searches. In addition to electronic databases, reference lists of systematic reviews and included studies were searched for additional publications. Clinical trial registries were searched on 4 October 2018 to identify clinical trials that were ongoing or complete. The searched trial registries were the Australian New Zealand Clinical Trial Registry (ANZCTR), the Chinese Clinical Trial Registry (ChiCTR), the European Union Clinical Trials Register (EU-CTR) and the United States of America National Institutes of Health Register (ClinicalTrials.gov). If required, trial investigators were contacted to obtain further information. Trial investigators were contacted by email or telephone and were followed up after two weeks if no reply was received. Where no response was received after one month, any unknown information was marked as not available.

Inclusion Criteria

Eligible studies were those focusing on the treatment of acute, persistent or recurrent UTIs. Persistent UTI, also called chronic UTI, is not described in international guidelines, but is mentioned in Chinese guidelines.[1] Persistent UTI refers to infections that do not completely resolve with treatment. Studies that met the inclusion criteria for participants, interventions, comparators and outcome measures were included. Criteria were as follows:

- Participants: Adults (≥ 18 years) diagnosed with uncomplicated UTI, including cystitis, pyelonephritis or urethritis. Studies of patients with urethritis were included where evidence of infection was confirmed by urine culture;

- Interventions: CHM, acupuncture and related therapies, other CM therapies or combinations of CM therapies (Table 4.1);
- Comparators: No treatment/waitlist controls, placebo/sham, anti-microbials or other therapies recommended in clinical guidelines;
- Outcome measures: Studies reported at least one of the pre-specified outcome measures (Table 4.2).

Table 4.1.   Chinese Medicine Interventions Included in Clinical Evidence Evaluation

Category	Intervention
Chinese herbal medicine (CHM)	Oral or topical CHM
Acupuncture and related therapies	Acupuncture, acupressure, ear acupuncture, ear acupressure, electro acupuncture, laser acupuncture, moxibustion and transcutaneous electrical nerve stimulation (TENS)
Other Chinese medicine (CM) therapies	*Tuina* 推拿 (Chinese massage), cupping, CM diet therapy
Combination CM	Combination therapies are defined as two or more CM interventions from different categories administered together, for example, CHM plus acupuncture

Table 4.2.   Pre-specified Outcomes

Outcome Categories	Outcome Measures	Scoring
Cure	Composite cure	Number of cases; higher is better
	Clinical cure	Number of cases; higher is better
Recurrence	Recurrence	Number of cases; lower is better
Duration of symptoms	Urinary frequency, urinary urgency, dysuria, flank pain, suprapubic pain, haematuria, fever and global symptoms	Time; lower is better

Table 4.2. (*Continued*)

Outcome Categories	Outcome Measures	Scoring
Biological tests	Microbiologically positive result for urine culture	Number of cases; lower is better
	Urine culture count	Abnormal range $\geq 10^3$ CFU/ml[13]
	Presence of leucocyte esterase on urine dipstick	Number of cases; lower is better
	Leucocyte count	Abnormal range ≥ 10 erythrocyte/μL[14]
	SCr concentration	Normal range 62 to 115 μmol/L or 0.7 to 1.3 mg/dL[15]
	CrCl	Normal range ≥ 90 ml/min[15]
	GFR/eGFR	Normal range ≥ 90 ml/min/1.73cm^2 [15]
	Proteinuria	Normal range < 150 mg/24h[15]
	Urine β2-MG	Lower is better[16]
	Urine α1-MG	Lower is better[16]
Health-related quality of life	ACSS[7]	Variable for domains; lower is better
	AIA[8]	0–20 points; lower is better
	UTISA[9]	Variable; lower is better
	SF-36[11]	0–100 points; higher is better
	EQ-5D[12]	See text
Health care costs	Cost of health care utilisation	
Adverse events	Number and type of adverse events	

Changes in kidney function may vary depending on age, gender and race. The normal values referenced in this table are used as a guide only and may not be accurate depending on patient variables.

Abbreviations: α1-MG, alpha-1 microglobulin; β2-MG, beta-2 microglobulin; ACSS, Acute Cystitis Symptom Score; AER, albumin excretion rate; AIA, Activity Impairment Assessment; CFU, colony-forming units; cm, centimetre; CrCl, creatinine clearance; dL, decilitre; eGFR, estimated glomerular filtration rate; EQ-5D, EuroQoL Five Dimensions questionnaire; GFR, glomerular filtration rate; h, hours; L, litre; mg, milligrams; min, minute; mL, millilitres; SCr, serum creatinine; SF-36, Medical Outcome Study Short Form 36-item questionnaire; UTISA, Urinary Tract Infection Symptom Assessment.

Antimicrobials (antibiotics) are the first-line treatment of medical management,[2] and are an affordable and effective treatment for UTIs. As such, it was anticipated that few studies of acute UTIs would have used placebo, sham or no treatment controls. Placebo, sham and no treatment controls were considered more likely to be used in studies of recurrent UTIs. While there is little evidence for pre- and post-coital voiding and the use of spermicide and lactobacillus products as conservative measures for recurrent UTI,[3] these measures are unlikely to be harmful and may have been used as comparators.

For some interventions, such as those listed in the category 'other Chinese medicine therapies', no studies met the inclusion criteria.

Exclusion Criteria

Studies were excluded when:

- Participants had complicated UTIs, such as patients with structural and/or functional abnormalities of the urinary tract, patients with kidney disease or patients with comorbidities that could lead to more serious outcomes;
- Patients with asymptomatic UTIs;
- Urethritis showed a sexually transmitted infection on urine culture, or where urine culture was not conducted during patient eligibility screening;
- Participants were children or pregnant women.

Outcomes

The primary goal of treatment is resolution of symptoms and elimination of bacteria (where bacteria were cultured). Diagnosis of cure and failure has been poorly reported in the past[4] and efforts are underway to establish a core outcome set for clinical studies of acute or recurrent uncomplicated UTIs.[5] Outcomes selected for inclusion were agreed upon by consensus for studies of acute and recurrent UTIs (Table 4.2). Eligible studies reported at least one of the pre-specified outcomes. Outcome categories included composite/clinical cure rate, recurrence, duration of symptoms, biological tests, health-related quality of life, health resource utilisation and adverse events.

Cure

Studies published in Chinese language journals frequently report cure as part of a global assessment referred to as the 'therapeutic effective rate'. Treatment response is usually categorised into three categories: (1) 'ineffective' (typically described as no change or worsening of symptoms and/or signs); (2) 'improvement' (typically described as some improvement in symptoms, signs and/or biological tests); and (3) 'cure' (typically described as complete resolution of symptoms, signs and/or biological tests). Signs and symptoms include urinary frequency and urgency, dysuria and haematuria, while biological tests refer to urine dipstick test and bacterial culture. The term 'composite cure' is used in this book for resolution of symptoms/signs and biological tests, while the term 'clinical cure' refers to resolution of clinical symptoms/signs. Studies reported the number of people achieving a cure after treatment.

Recurrence

Recurrence is an important outcome for studies of both acute and recurrent UTI. Data were extracted where the number of people who experienced recurrence was reported, or as a frequency within a specified duration, for example, number of episodes within 12 months.

Duration of Symptoms

Duration of urinary frequency, urinary urgency, dysuria, flank pain, suprapubic pain, fever, all urinary symptoms and all general symptoms were extracted from eligible studies. All included studies that reported duration of symptoms measured duration in days.

Biological Tests

Biological tests included urine culture (culture count or microbiological cure rate), urine dipstick test for pyuria (leucocyte esterase in urine; number of positive cases), markers of kidney function and markers of kidney damage. Markers of kidney function included the concentration of creatinine in the blood (serum creatinine concentration, SCr), the rate at which creatinine is eliminated via urine in 24 hours (creatinine clearance rate, CrCl) and the actual or estimated glomerular filtration rate (GFR/eGFR). Other outcomes included markers of kidney damage, including proteinuria, urine β2 microglobulin (β2-MG) and urine α1 microglobulin (α1-MG).

Health-related Quality of Life

Despite being a common medical condition, few studies have examined the impact of UTIs on quality of life.[6] In their systematic review, Bermingham and Ashe (2012)[6] found most studies used generic well-being questionnaires to measure the impact of UTIs on health-related quality of life. Despite this, several disease-specific outcome tools have been developed. One such tool is the Acute Cystitis Symptom Score (ACSS),[7] an 18-item questionnaire that has been validated in female patients with acute uncomplicated UTI. The questionnaire includes six items related to typical symptoms ('Typical' subscale), four items related to differential diagnoses such as flank pain, fever or vaginal/urethral discharge ('Differential' subscale), three items on impact of UTI on quality of life ('QOL' subscale) and five items on additional conditions which may affect treatment, such as pregnancy or menopausal status ('Additional' subscale). Items for the Typical, Differential and QOL subscales are scored from zero to four, while Additional subscale items are answered as yes/no. Both total score and domain scores can be reported, and higher scores indicate worse severity.

The Activity Impairment Assessment (AIA),[8] which measures the amount of time that work or regular activities have been affected by UTI, has also been validated in uncomplicated UTI. The AIA is a self-reported, five-item scale. Responses are on a five-point Likert scale, with higher scores indicating greater impairment. The UTI Symptom Assessment questionnaire (UTISA)[9] is a 14-item self-administered questionnaire that measures levels of severity and bother from seven UTI symptoms: urgency, frequency, pain/burning on urination, incomplete voiding, pain in the pelvic area, pain in the lower back and blood in the urine. Items are scored on a four-point Likert scale, with higher scores indicating greater severity/bother. Additional questions relating to symptom changes are completed after the first visit. Scores are calculated for each of the four domains of 'urination regularity' (range 0 to 12), 'problems with urination' (range 0 to 12), 'pain associated with UTI' (range 0 to 12) and 'blood in the urine' (range 0 to 6). This questionnaire is also available in Chinese.[10]

Other general wellbeing questionnaires included the Medical Outcome Study Short Form 36-item questionnaire (SF-36)[11] and the EuroQoL Five Dimensions questionnaire (EQ-5D).[12] The SF-36 includes 36 items relating to eight domains: physical functioning, role functioning due to health problems, role functioning due to emotional problems, bodily pain, general health perceptions, vitality, social function and mental health. The EQ-5D includes five questions related to mobility, self-care, usual activities, pain or discomfort, and anxiety or depression. The EQ-5D also includes a 100-point visual analogue scale (VAS) to assess overall health status. Results can be presented in a variety of ways. For the five domains, a higher score indicates a greater level of perceived problems, while for the VAS component, a higher score indicates better health status.

Health Care Costs and Adverse Events

Information associated with health care/service utilisation was collected where reported. Adverse event information included the nature and number of events by group allocation.

Risk of Bias Assessment

Risk of bias was assessed for RCTs using the Cochrane Collaboration's tool.[17] In clinical trials, bias can be categorised as selection bias, performance bias, detection bias, attrition bias and reporting bias. Each domain is assessed to determine whether the bias is at 'low', 'high' or 'unclear' risk. 'Low' risk of bias indicates that bias is unlikely, 'high' risk indicates plausible bias that seriously weakens confidence in the results, and 'unclear' bias indicates lack of information or uncertainty over potential bias and raises some doubt about the results. Risk of bias assessment was verified by two people and disagreement was resolved by discussion or consultation with a third person.

Risk of bias is categorised using the following six domains:

- Sequence generation: The method used to generate the allocation sequence is given in sufficient detail to allow an assessment of whether it should produce comparable groups. 'Low' risk of bias refers to the use of appropriate methods, such as a random number table or computer random generator. 'High' risk of bias includes studies that describe a non-random sequence generation such as odd or even date of birth or date of admission;
- Allocation concealment: The method used to conceal the allocation sequence is given in enough detail to determine whether intervention allocations could have been foreseen before or during enrolment. Examples of 'low' risk of bias include central randomisation or sealed envelopes, and examples of 'high' risk of bias includes open random sequence;
- Blinding of participants and personnel: Measures used to describe whether the study participants and personnel are blind to the intervention received. In addition, information relating to whether the blinding was effective is also assessed. Studies that ensure blinding of participants and personnel are at 'low' risk of bias. If the study is not blind, or incompletely blind, it is at 'high' risk of bias;
- Blinding of outcome assessors: Measures used to describe whether the outcome assessors are blind to knowledge of which intervention a participant received. In addition, information relating to whether the blinding was effective is also assessed. Studies that ensure blinding of outcome assessors are at 'low' risk of bias. If the study is not blind, or incompletely blind, it is at 'high' risk of bias;

- Incomplete outcome data: Completeness of outcome data for each main outcome, including drop-outs, exclusions from the analysis with numbers missing in each group and reasons for drop-out or exclusions. Studies with 'low' risk of bias would include all outcome data or if there is missing data, it is unlikely to relate to the true outcome or is balanced between groups. Studies at 'high' risk of bias would have unexplained missing data;
- Selective reporting: The study protocol is available and the pre-specified outcomes are included in the report. Studies with a published protocol and which include all pre-specified outcomes in their report would be at 'low' risk of bias. Studies at 'high' risk of bias would not include all pre-specified outcomes or the outcome data may be reported incompletely.

Statistical Analyses

Studies of acute uncomplicated UTI were reported separate to those of persistent and recurrent UTI. Frequency of CM syndromes, CHM formulas, herbs and acupuncture points reported in included studies are presented using descriptive statistics. Chinese medicine syndromes reported in two or more studies were presented. The ten most frequently reported CHM formulas and 20 most frequently reported herbs were presented when used in at least two studies, although for CHM formulas this was not always possible. The top ten acupuncture points used in two or more studies are presented, or as available. Where data were limited, reports of single CM syndromes or acupuncture points were provided as a guide for the reader.

Definitions of statistical tests and results are described in the glossary. Dichotomous data are reported as a risk ratio (RR) with 95% confidence intervals (CI), and continuous data are reported as mean difference (MD) or standardised mean difference (SMD) with 95% CI. For dichotomous data, when the RR is greater than one and the upper and lower values of the 95% CI are both greater than one, this indicates we can be 95% certain that there is a difference between the groups and that the true effect lies within these CIs. The same is true for values less than one. In such cases, we say there is a 'significant difference' between the groups. For continuous data, when the MD is greater than zero and both the upper and lower values of the 95% CI are greater than zero, we say there is a 'significant difference' between the groups. The same is true on the negative side of the scale.[17] For all analyses, RR or MD and 95% CI were reported, together with a formal test for heterogeneity using the I^2 statistic. An I^2 score greater than 50% was considered to indicate substantial heterogeneity.[17]

Sensitivity analyses were undertaken to explore potential sources of heterogeneity, based on 'low' risk of bias for one of the risk of bias domains, sequence generation. Where possible and appropriate, planned subgroup analyses included location of UTI (upper, lower, both upper and lower, and not specified), gender (females, both females and males, and gender not specified), CM syndromes, CM formula, duration of treatment and comparator type. Available case analysis with a random effects model was used in all analyses. The random effects model was used to take into account the clinical heterogeneity likely to be encountered within, and between, included studies, and the variation in treatment effects between included studies.

Assessment Using Grading of Recommendations Assessment, Development and Evaluation

The Grading of Recommendations Assessment, Development and Evaluation (GRADE) approach was used.[18,19] The GRADE approach summarises and rates the strength and quality ('certainty') of evidence in systematic reviews using a structured process for presenting evidence summaries. The results are presented in summary of findings tables. The results provide an important overview for UTI outcomes.

A panel of experts was established to evaluate the certainty of evidence. The panel included the systematic review team, CM practitioners, integrative medicine experts, research methodologists and conventional medicine physicians. The experts were asked to rate the clinical importance of key interventions from CHM and acupuncture therapies, as well as comparators and outcomes. Results were collated and, based on the rating scores and subsequent discussion, a consensus on the content for the summary of findings tables was achieved.

The quality of evidence for each outcome was rated according to five factors outlined in the GRADE approach. The certainty of evidence may be rated based on:

- Limitations in study design (risk of bias);
- Inconsistency of results (unexplained heterogeneity);
- Indirectness of evidence (interventions, populations, and outcomes important to the patients with the condition);
- Imprecision (uncertainty about the results);
- Publication bias (selective publication of studies).

These five factors are additive and a reduction in one factor, or more than one factor, will reduce the certainty of the evidence for that outcome. The GRADE approach also includes methods for assessing observational studies. GRADE summaries in this book only include RCTs.

Treatment recommendations can also be assessed using the GRADE approach, but due to the diverse nature of CM practice, treatment recommendations were not included with the summary of findings. Therefore, the reader should interpret the evidence with reference to the local practice environment. It should also be noted that the GRADE approach requires judgments about the strength and quality of evidence, and some subjective assessment. However, the experience of the panel members suggests the judgments are reliable and transparent representations of the certainty of evidence.

The GRADE levels of evidence are grouped into four categories:

1. 'High' certainty: We are very confident that the true effect lies close to that of the estimate of the effect;
2. 'Moderate' certainty: We are moderately confident in the effect estimate: the true effect is likely to be close to the estimate of the effect, but there is a possibility that it is substantially different;

3. 'Low' certainty: Our confidence in the effect estimate is limited. The true effect may be substantially different from the estimate of the effect;

4. 'Very low' certainty: We have very little confidence in the effect estimate. The true effect is likely to be substantially different from the estimate of effect.

References

1. 第 2 届肾脏病学术会议组. (1985) 尿路感染的诊断治疗标准. 中华肾脏病杂志 **1**(4): 13.

2. Gupta K, Hooton TM, Naber KG, *et al.* (2011) International clinical practice guidelines for the treatment of acute uncomplicated cystitis and pyelonephritis in women: A 2010 update by the Infectious Diseases Society of America and the European Society for Microbiology and Infectious Diseases. *Clin Infect Dis* **52**(5): e103–e120.

3. Dason S, Dason JT, Kapoor A. (2011) Guidelines for the diagnosis and management of recurrent urinary tract infection in women. *Can Urol Assoc J* **5**(5): 316–322.

4. Fihn SD, Stamm WE. (1985) Interpretation and comparison of treatment studies for uncomplicated urinary tract infections in women. *Rev Infect Dis* **7**(4): 468–478.

5. Duane S, Vellinga A, Murphy AW, *et al.* (2019) COSUTI: A protocol for the development of a core outcome set (COS) for interventions for the treatment of uncomplicated urinary tract infection (UTI) in adults. *Trials* **20**(1): 106.

6. Bermingham SL, Ashe JF. (2012) Systematic review of the impact of urinary tract infections on health-related quality of life. *BJU Int* **110**(11 Pt C): e830–e836.

7. Alidjanov JF, Abdufattaev UA, Makhsudov SA, *et al.* (2014) New self-reporting questionnaire to assess urinary tract infections and differential diagnosis: Acute cystitis symptom score. *Urol Int* **92**(2): 230–236.

8. Wild DJ, Clayson DJ, Keating K, *et al.* (2005) Validation of a patient-administered questionnaire to measure the activity impairment experienced by women with uncomplicated urinary tract infection: The Activity Impairment Assessment (AIA). *Health Qual Life Outcomes* **3**: 42.

9. Clayson D, Wild D, Doll H, *et al.* (2005) Validation of a patient-administered questionnaire to measure the severity and bothersomeness of lower urinary tract symptoms in uncomplicated urinary tract infection (UTI): The UTI Symptom Assessment questionnaire. *BJU Int* **96**(3): 350–359.

10. Chang SJ, Lin CD, Hsieh CH, *et al.* (2015) Reliability and validity of a Chinese version of Urinary Tract Infection Symptom Assessment questionnaire. *Int Braz J Urol* **41**(4): 729–738.

11. Ware JJ, Sherbourne C. (1992) The MOS 36-item short-form health survey (SF-36). I. Conceptual framework and item selection. *Med Care* 30: 473–483.

12. Rabin R, de Charro F. (2001) EQ-5D: A measure of health status from the EuroQol Group. *Ann Med* **33:** 337–343.

13. Hooton TM, Roberts PL, Cox ME, *et al.* (2013) Voided midstream urine culture and acute cystitis in premenopausal women. *N Engl J Med* **369**(20): 1883–1891.

14. Stamm WE. (1983) Measurement of pyuria and its relation to bacteriuria. *Am J Med* **75**(1b): 53–58.

15. Stevens PE, Levin A. (2013) Evaluation and management of chronic kidney disease: Synopsis of the kidney disease: Improving global outcomes 2012 clinical practice guideline. *Ann Intern Med* **158**(11): 825–830.

16. Carter JL, Tomson CR, Stevens PE, *et al.* (2006) Does urinary tract infection cause proteinuria or microalbuminuria? A systematic review. *Nephrol Dial Transplant* **21**(11): 3031–3037.

17. Higgins JPT, Green S, eds. (2011) Cochrane handbook for systematic reviews of interventions version 5.1.0 [updated March 2011]. The Cochrane Collaboration. Available from www.cochrane-handbook.org2011.

18. Schunemann H, Brozek J, Guyatt G, Oxman A, eds. (2013) GRADE handbook for grading quality of evidence and strength of recommendations. The GRADE Working Group. Available from: http://www.guidelinedevelopment.org/handbook/.

19. Schunemann H, Higgins J, Vist G, *et al.* (2019) Chapter 14: Completing 'Summary of findings' tables and grading the certainty of the evidence. In: Higgins JPT, Thomas J, Chandler J, *et al.* (eds), *Cochrane Handbook for Systematic Reviews of Interventions* version 6.0 (updated July 2019). Available from: www.training.cochrane.org/handbook.

5

Clinical Evidence for Chinese Herbal Medicine

OVERVIEW

Clinical studies have evaluated Chinese herbal medicine in people with acute, persistent and recurrent urinary tract infections. This chapter reviews the Chinese medicine syndromes described, treatments tested, and efficacy and safety of Chinese herbal medicine in 188 clinical studies published in scientific journals. Oral Chinese herbal medicine was the main treatment tested, and has shown some benefit in improving the number of people achieving a cure.

Introduction

Chinese medicine (CM) includes a variety of interventions, among which Chinese herbal medicine (CHM) is one of the most frequently used. Chinese herbal medicine is prescribed according to CM syndrome differentiation in contemporary clinical guidelines and textbooks (Chapter 2). Analysis of classical literature shows CHM was a key treatment option in past eras (Chapter 3). Clinical studies have evaluated the effectiveness of CHM, and the results have been published in English and Chinese language biomedical journals. This chapter reviews the available evidence for clinical studies of CHM for people with urinary tract infection (UTI).

Randomised controlled trials (RCTs), controlled clinical trials (CCTs) and non-controlled studies have been selected for further analysis. Findings have been presented according to three categories: (1) acute UTI; (2) persistent UTI (infections that do not resolve after

7–14 days of antibiotic treatment); and (3) recurrent UTI (two or more infections within six months, or three or more within 12 months). Results for each category are presented according to the route of administration of CHM.

Previous Systematic Reviews

Six published systematic reviews that assessed the efficacy and safety of oral CHM for UTIs were identified. One systematic review included participants with complicated UTIs,[1] and one systematic review included studies with inappropriate comparisons, such as CM therapies as a control group.[2] Therefore, four published systematic reviews were consistent with the inclusion criteria, and the results are highlighted below.[3-6]

A 2015 Cochrane systematic review of CHM for women with recurrent UTIs included seven RCTs with 542 women.[6] Five of the included RCTs recruited exclusively postmenopausal women. Meta-analysis showed CHM to have a higher rate of effectiveness (partial or total improvement in signs, symptoms and biological tests) than antibiotics (selected according to microbial sensitivity) when used during an acute UTI (risk ratio (RR) 1.21 [1.11, 1.33]). Chinese herbal medicine also reduced the rate of recurrence compared to antibiotics (RR 0.28 [0.09, 0.82]; 'very low' certainty evidence). When CHM was used in combination with antibiotics, the effective rate during acute UTI was greater than antibiotics alone (RR 1.24 [1.04, 1.47]), and the rate of recurrence was lower (RR 0.53 [0.35, 0.80]). Two studies reported on safety, with no adverse events occurring during the trials.

Pu *et al.* (2016)[4] reported the efficacy and safety of a manufactured product, *San jin pian* 三金片, alone or combined with antibiotics for treating acute uncomplicated UTIs in adults. The primary outcome of this review was effectiveness rate, defined as a partial or total improvement of symptoms, physical signs and biological tests (including urine culture and pyuria on dipstick test). Other outcomes included microbiological cure rate, change in urine white blood cells from baseline to end of treatment, and recurrence.

The review included three RCTs with 260 participants. The results showed that oral *San jin pian* 三金片 combined with antibiotics was superior to antibiotics alone in improving the effectiveness rate and microbiological cure rate, while oral *San jin pian* 三金片 alone was not significantly different to antibiotic. One RCT reported four adverse events in the treatment group (two cases of nausea or indigestion, two of diarrhoea) and eight adverse events in the control group (five cases of indigestion, three cases of loss of appetite). However, the risk of bias in the original studies was generally 'high'. The unclear allocation concealment, lack of blinding, and other potential risks of bias, such as incomplete outcome data and selective reporting, may limit confidence in the results.

One 2010 systematic review reported the efficacy and safety of a manufactured product, *Re lin qing* 热淋清, alone or combined with antibiotics, for treating acute uncomplicated UTIs in adults.[3] The key outcomes were effective rate, microbiological cure rate, change in urinary white blood cells and recurrence. Five RCTs with 471 participants were included. Compared with antibiotics alone, oral *Re lin qing* 热淋清 combined with antibiotics improved both the effective rate and microbiological cure rate, and reduced recurrence (defined as the proportion of people who experienced recurrence within the follow-up period). When used alone, oral *Re lin qing* 热淋清 was not significantly different to antibiotics in improving the effective rate and microbiological cure rate. Three of the included studies reported adverse events, including indigestion and nausea. The methodological quality of the included studies was generally 'low'. The methods for sequence generation and allocation concealment were unclear, and a lack of blinding may have introduced bias.

Zhang *et al.* (2010),[3] examined the efficacy and safety of oral CHM formulas with the CM actions of clearing heat and draining dampness. Such formulas were used alone or in combination with antibiotics for treating UTIs. The review lacked detail about UTI diagnosis. Eighteen RCTs with 1,828 participants were included. The effective rate and recurrence were the primary outcomes. The results showed that oral CHM formulas alone and combined with antibiotics were superior to antibiotics alone in improving the effectiveness rate and reducing recurrence. Five of the included studies reported adverse events, with no adverse events occurring in three studies. Five adverse events were reported in two studies, and included bad breath, menorrhagia and indigestion. The quality of original studies was generally 'low', because of unclear allocation concealment, lack of blinding and other potential risks of bias.

Identification of Clinical Studies

After searching nine databases (see Chapter 4), more than 22,000 records were identified (Fig. 5.1). Duplicates were removed, and the titles and abstracts of 11,171 citations were reviewed for relevance. The full text was retrieved for 1,953 articles, and these were assessed against the inclusion criteria. In total, 189 articles were selected for further analysis. One hundred and forty-six were RCTs, 20 were CCTs and 21 were non-controlled studies. Two studies investigated an intervention not commonly practised outside of China (intravenous administration of CHM),[7,8] but they will not be presented here. The findings of 187 studies are described in this chapter. Included studies are referred to in text by an 'H' followed by a number, for example, 'H1'. The reference list for included studies can be found at the end of this chapter.

Acute Urinary Tract Infection

Sixty-seven studies tested CHM in 6,424 people with acute UTI (H1–H67). All studies used oral CHM as the intervention.

Randomised Controlled Trials of Oral Chinese Herbal Medicine for Acute Urinary Tract Infection

Sixty RCTs (H1–H60) tested the effectiveness of oral CHM in 5,825 people with acute UTI. Five studies included three groups, four of which included one treatment group of oral CHM alone and one treatment group of oral CHM used as integrative medicine with antibiotics (H41, H57, H59, H60). One study (H58) used a 'double

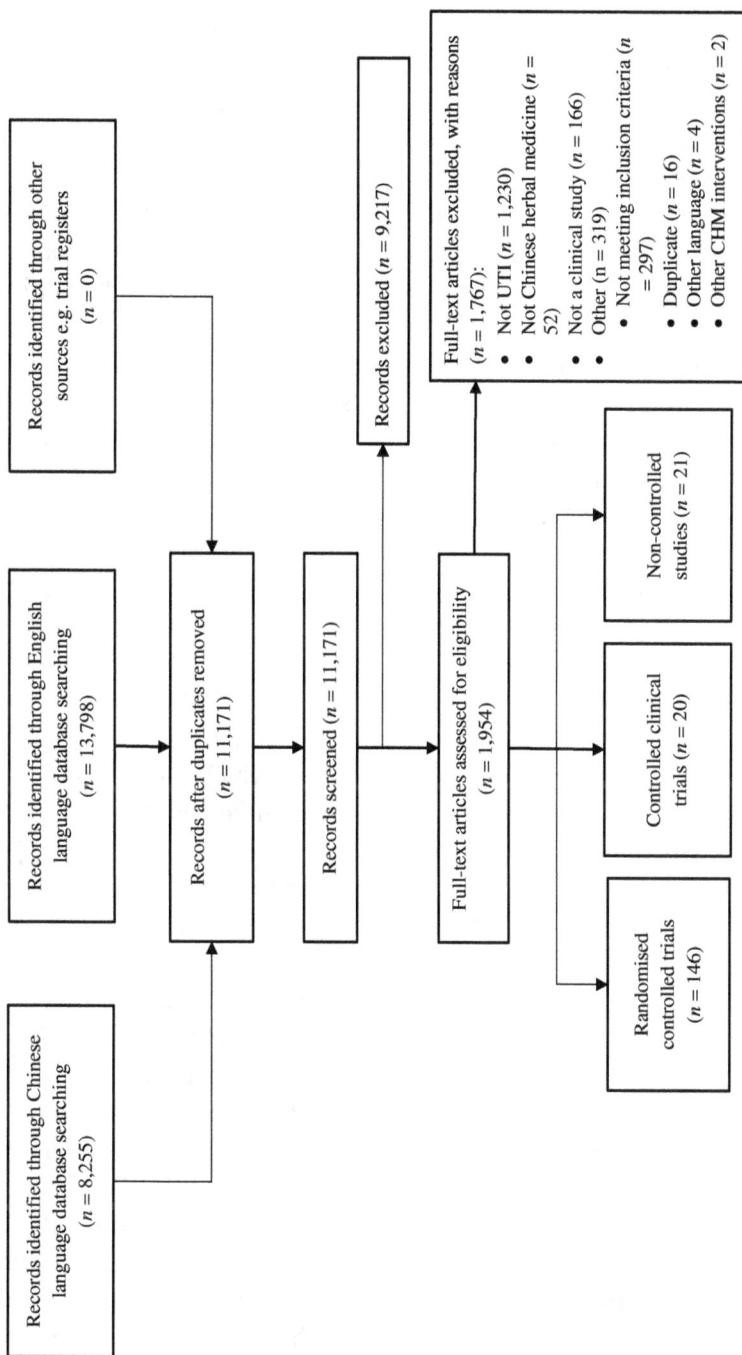

Fig. 5.1. Flowchart of study selection process: Chinese herbal medicine.

Records identified through Chinese language database searching (*n* = 8,255)

Records identified through English language database searching (*n* = 13,798)

Records identified through other sources e.g. trial registers (*n* = 0)

Records after duplicates removed (*n* = 11,171)

Records screened (*n* = 11,171)

Records excluded (*n* = 9,217)

Full-text articles assessed for eligibility (*n* = 1,954)

Full-text articles excluded, with reasons (*n* = 1,767):
- Not UTI (*n* = 1,230)
- Not Chinese herbal medicine (*n* = 52)
- Not a clinical study (*n* = 166)
- Other (*n* = 319)
  - Not meeting inclusion criteria (*n* = 297)
  - Duplicate (*n* = 16)
  - Other language (*n* = 4)
  - Other CHM interventions (*n* = 2)

Randomised controlled trials (*n* = 146)

Controlled clinical trials (*n* = 20)

Non-controlled studies (*n* = 21)

dummy' design. In this study, one group received oral CHM alone plus a placebo tablet designed to look like levofloxacin, one group received oral CHM and levofloxacin, and the control group received levofloxacin and a placebo tablet designed to look like the herbal product *San jin pian* 三金片.

All studies were conducted in China. In studies that reported participant recruitment, patients were recruited from hospital outpatient, inpatient or emergency departments, or community clinics. Fourteen studies (H2, H3, H5, H10–H13, H15, H17, H33, H41, H44, H50, H56) included only women. Six studies (H1, H7, H20, H30, H37, H52) included participants with upper UTI, 17 studies (H10, H11, H13, H15, H19, H28, H31, H35, H39, H42, H46, H47, H49, H50, H55, H58, H59) included participants with lower UTI, 14 studies (H9, H17, H18, H21, H24–H27, H33, H36, H40, H43, H48, H53) included participants with either upper or lower UTI and the remaining studies did not specify the location of infection.

Treatment duration ranged from three days (H19, H47) to nine weeks (H20), with the median duration of treatment being two weeks. Twenty-four studies (H3, H6, H8, H12, H14, H17, H25, H26, H29, H30, H31, H34, H35, H39, H44, H45, H50–H56, H59) conducted follow-up assessment after treatment ceased, which ranged from two weeks (H6, H39) to one year (H50). Three studies (H10, H58, H59) reported withdrawals, with 46 participants lost to follow-up.

Chinese medicine syndrome differentiation was used as an inclusion criterion or to guide treatment in 27 studies (H1, H3, H6, H7, H10, H14, H17, H19–H21, H27, H31–H34, H38, H40, H42, H45, H47, H48, H50–H52, H54, H55, H60). The most frequently reported syndrome was Lower Energiser dampness-heat (ten studies). Other syndromes reported in multiple studies include heat strangury (*re lin* 热淋, four studies), Bladder dampness-heat (three studies), *yin* deficiency and dampness-heat (three studies), dampness-heat syndrome (two studies) and fatigue strangury (*lao lin* 劳淋, two studies).

Thirty different CHM formulas were used among the 60 RCTs. Three studies used investigator-developed formulas, and these were excluded from formula frequency analysis. Formulas tested in multiple studies are described in Table 5.1. The most frequently tested

Table 5.1. Frequently Reported Oral Formulas in Randomised Controlled Trials for Acute Urinary Tract Infection

Most Common Formulas	No. of Studies	Ingredients
Ba zheng san 八正散	8	*Che qian zi* 车前子, *qu mai* 瞿麦, *bian xu* 萹蓄, *hua shi* 滑石, *zhi zi* 栀子, *gan cao* 甘草, *mu tong* 木通 and *da huang* 大黄
San jin pian 三金片	6	*Jin ying gen* 金樱根, *ba qia* 菝葜, *yang kai kou* 羊开口, *jin sha teng* 金沙藤 and *ji xue cao* 积雪草 (H12, H17, H41, H56, H58, H59)
Re lin qing ke li/pian 热淋清颗粒/片	4	*Tou hua liao* 头花蓼 (H9, H18, H27, H53)
Yin hua mi yan ling pian 银花泌炎灵片	4	*Jin yin hua* 金银花, *ban zhi lian* 半枝莲, *bian xu* 萹蓄, *qu mai* 瞿麦, *shi wei* 石韦, *chuan mu tong* 川木通, *che qian zi* 车前子, *dan zhu ye* 淡竹叶, *sang ji sheng* 桑寄生 and *deng xin cao* 灯心草 (H13, H29, H50, H55)
Jin qian cao ke li 金钱草颗粒	3	Variant 1: *Jin qian cao* 金钱草, *che qian cao* 车前草, *shi wei* 石韦 and *yu mi xu* 玉米须 (H24, H28) Variant 2: *Jin qian cao* 金钱草 (H39)
Bi xie fen qing wan/yin 萆薢分清丸/饮	2	*Bi xie* 萆薢, *huang bai* 黄柏, *shi chang pu* 石菖蒲, *fu ling* 茯苓, *bai zhu* 白术, *lian zi xin* 莲子心, *dan shen* 丹参 and *che qian zi* 车前子
Fu zheng qu shi fang 扶正祛湿方	2	*Di fu zi* 地肤子, *dang gui* 当归, *ku shen* 苦参, *chai hu* 柴胡, *zhi shi* 枳实, *huang bai* 黄柏, *chi shao* 赤芍 and *bei mu* 贝母 (H16, H45)
Long qing pian 癃清片	2	*Ze xie* 泽泻, *che qian zi* 车前子, *bai jiang cao* 败酱草, *jin yin hua* 金银花, *mu dan pi* 牡丹皮, *bai hua she she cao* 白花蛇舌草, *chi shao* 赤芍, *xian he cao* 仙鹤草, *huang lian* 黄连 and *huang bai* 黄柏 (H11, H60)
Ning mi tai jiao nang 宁泌泰胶囊	2	*Si ji hong* 四季红, *bai mao gen* 白茅根, *da feng teng* 大风藤, *san ke zhen* 三颗针, *xian he cao* 仙鹤草, *fu rong ye* 芙蓉叶 and *lian qiao* 连翘 (H21, H30)
Qing re li shi fang/tang 清热利湿方/汤	2	Variant 1: *Ma chi xian* 马齿苋, *huang qi* 黄芪, *mu tong* 木通, *hong hua* 红花, *che qian cao* 车前草, *huang qin* 黄芩, *mu dan pi* 牡丹皮, *shi wei* 石韦, *sheng di huang* 生地黄, *gan cao* 甘草, *huang bai* 黄柏 and *bai hua she she cao* 白花蛇舌草 (H8)

(*Continued*)

Table 5.1. (*Continued*)

Most Common Formulas	No. of Studies	Ingredients
		Variant 2: *Zhi mu* 知母, *huang bai* 黄柏, *qu mai* 瞿麦, *che qian cao* 车前草, *pu gong ying* 蒲公英, *shi wei* 石苇, *ze xie* 泽泻, *sheng di huang* 生地黄 and *gan cao* 甘草 (H48)
Xie re san yu tong ling tang 泻热散瘀通淋汤	2	Variant 1: *Che qian zi* 车前子, *shi wei* 石苇, *hua shi* 滑石, *da huang* 大黄, *huai niu xi* 怀牛膝, *bian xu* 萹蓄, *fu ling* 茯苓, *jin yin hua* 金银花, *lian qiao* 连翘 and *jin qian cao* 金钱草 (H1)
		Variant 2: *Da huang* 大黄, *huang bai* 黄柏, *pu gong ying* 蒲公英, *sheng gan cao* 生甘草, *zhi zi* 栀子, *mu dan pi* 牡丹皮, *chi shao* 赤芍, *jin qian cao* 金钱草, *che qian zi* 车前子 and *hua shi* 滑石 (H7)

Ingredients are referenced to the original studies where possible. If herb ingredients varied across studies, the herb ingredients were sourced from *Zhong Yi Fang Ji Da Ci Dian* 中医方剂大辞典.

The use of some herbs may be restricted in some countries. Readers are advised to comply with relevant regulations.

CHM formulas were *Ba zheng san* 八正散 (used in eight studies) and *San jin pian* 三金片 (used in six studies). Several of the frequently reported formulas in RCTs of acute UTI are commercially manufactured products, which may explain their higher frequency compared to traditional formulas. There was great variety in the herb ingredients used across the studies, with 115 individual herbs described. The most frequently used herbs for acute UTI were *che qian zi* 车前子, *bian xu* 萹蓄, *qu mai* 瞿麦 and *gan cao* 甘草 (Table 5.2).

Oral CHM was compared with antibiotic therapy in 18 studies (H5, H8, H10, H11, H14, H17, H28, H33, H34, H39, H40, H41, H49, H56–H60) and was combined with antibiotic therapy in 47 studies (H1–H4, H6, H7, H9, H12, H13, H15, H16, H18–H27, H29–H32, H35–H38, H41–H48, H50–H55, H57–H60). All studies used antibiotics in the control group. Two studies (H14, H43) added sodium bicarbonate tablets to antibiotics, and one study (H58) provided a CHM placebo, as well as antibiotics, to the control group.

Table 5.2. Frequently Reported Orally Used Herbs in Randomised Controlled Trials for Acute Urinary Tract Infection

Most Common Herbs	Scientific Name	Frequency of Use
Che qian zi 车前子	*Plantago* spp.	24
Bian xu 萹蓄	*Polygonum aviculare* L.	21
Qu mai 瞿麦	*Dianthus* spp.	21
Gan cao 甘草	*Glycyrrhiza* spp.	20
Huang bai 黄柏	*Phellodendron chinense* Schneid.	18
Shi wei 石韦	*Pyrrosia* spp.	18
Hua shi 滑石	Hydrated magnesium silicate	17
Mu tong 木通	*Akebia* spp.	14
Zhi zi 栀子	*Gardenia jasminoides* Ellis	14
Da huang 大黄	*Rheum* spp.	12
Fu ling 茯苓	*Poria cocos* (Schw.) Wolf	11
Jin yin hua 金银花	*Lonicera japonica* Thunb.	11
Jin qian cao 金钱草	*Lysimachia christinae* Hance	10
Che qian cao 车前草	*Plantago* spp.	8
Deng xin cao 灯心草	*Juncus effusus* L.	8
Huang qi 黄芪	*Astragalus membranaceus* (Fisch.) Bge.	8
Niu xi 牛膝	*Achyranthes bidentata* Bl.	8
Dan zhu ye 淡竹叶	*Lophatherum gracile* Brongn.	7
Ji xue cao 积雪草	*Centella asiatica* (L.) Urb.	7
Sheng di huang 生地黄	*Rehmannia glutinosa* Libosch.	7

The use of some herbs, such as *mu tong* 木通, may be restricted in some countries. Readers are advised to comply with relevant regulations.

Risk of Bias

None of the studies were free from bias (Table 5.3). Fourteen studies (H1–H3, H13, H16, H30, H31, H33, H37, H38, H43, H48, H51, H54) used a random number table or block randomisation to allocate participants to groups and were judged as 'low' risk of bias. None of the studies reported the method for concealing group allocation, and all were assessed as 'unclear' risk. One study reported that both participants and personnel were blind and was judged 'low' risk (H58); all

Table 5.3. Risk of Bias of Randomised Controlled Trials for Acute Urinary Tract Infection: Oral Chinese Herbal Medicine

Risk of Bias Domain	Low Risk *n* (%)	Unclear Risk *n* (%)	High Risk *n* (%)
Sequence generation	14 (23.3)	42 (70.0)	4 (6.7)
Allocation concealment	0 (0)	60 (100)	0 (0)
Blinding of participants	1 (1.7)	0 (0)	59 (98.3)
Blinding of personnel	1 (1.7)	0 (0)	59 (98.3)
Blinding of outcome assessors	0 (0)	60 (100)	0 (0)
Incomplete outcome data	58 (96.7)	1 (1.7)	1 (1.7)
Selective outcome reporting	0 (0)	59 (98.3)	1 (1.7)

other studies were judged to pose 'high' risk of bias. None of the studies reported whether outcome assessors were blind to group allocation. The majority of studies (58 RCTs; 96.7%) had no missing data, while one study (H10) did not report the reasons for missing data and one study (H59) had a high proportion of drop-outs. These studies were judged as 'unclear' and 'high' risk, respectively. One study (H4) was judged 'high' risk for selective outcome reporting due to differences in the outcomes specified in the methods section and those described in the results. No trial protocols or trial registrations were able to be identified for the remaining studies, which were judged to be at 'unclear' risk of bias.

Outcomes

All studies reported the number of people who achieved a cure. Ten studies assessed recurrence and four of these studies assessed recurrence in people who achieved a cure at the end of treatment. Results for these four studies were analysed, as these were considered to be true cases of recurrence. Twenty-one studies reported duration of symptoms, which included duration of all urinary symptoms, as well as duration of specific symptoms such as dysuria. Nine studies reported the number of people with a positive microbiological urine culture at the end of treatment and four studies reported pyuria. Biological tests included serum creatinine (one study) and beta-2 microglobulin (β2-MG) (three studies). One study reported health care costs. Safety was reported in 32 studies. Some studies reported results in a way that did not allow for re-analysis. The findings presented below are for results that were able to be analysed.

Composite Cure

All studies reported the number of people who achieved a cure. Seventeen studies (H5, H8, H10, H11, H14, H17, H28, H33, H34, H39–H41, H49, H56, H57, H59, H60) compared oral CHM with antibiotic therapy, 46 studies (H1–H4, H6, H7, H9, H12, H13, H15, H16, H18, H19, H20–H27, H29–H32, H35–H38, H41–H48, H50–H55, H57, H59, H60) compared the combination of oral CHM and antibiotic therapy with antibiotic therapy alone, one study (H58) compared oral CHM plus placebo with antibiotics plus placebo, and the same study compared oral CHM plus antibiotics with antibiotics plus placebo. Results are presented according to these comparisons.

Oral Chinese herbal medicine plus placebo versus antibiotics plus placebo

Among 141 participants, those who received oral CHM plus placebo were not more likely to achieve a composite cure based on resolution of symptoms than people who received antibiotics plus placebo (RR 0.94 [0.71, 1.25]; H58).

Oral Chinese herbal medicine plus antibiotics versus antibiotics plus placebo

When oral CHM was combined with antibiotics, there was no difference in the number of people achieving a composite cure compared to antibiotics plus placebo (RR 1.15 [0.90, 1.48]; H58).

Oral Chinese herbal medicine versus pharmacotherapy

More than 1,000 people were included in meta-analyses of the effects of oral CHM compared to antibiotic-based therapy for short-term cure

(Table 5.4). Meta-analysis showed people who received oral CHM were more likely to achieve a cure in the short term (six weeks or less), compared to people who received antibiotic-based therapy (1,146 participants, RR 1.39 [1.18, 1.65], I^2 = 44%). Subgroup analyses were conducted to examine the effects on specific subpopulations. Oral CHM was superior to antibiotic-based therapy regardless of the site of infection (Table 5.4). In studies that included both males and females, oral CHM was more effective at producing a cure than antibiotic therapy (532 participants, RR 1.53 [1.13, 2.08], I^2 = 67%), while no such benefit was seen in studies that only included women (361 women,

Table 5.4. Oral Chinese Herbal Medicine versus Pharmacotherapy for Acute Urinary Tract Infection: Short-term Cure

Assessment	No. of Studies (Participants)	Effect Size (RR [95% CI], I^2)	Included Studies
All studies	13 (1,146)	1.39 [1.18, 1.65]*, 44%	H10, H11, H14, H28, H33, H34, H39–H41, H49, H56, H57, H59
Subgroup analyses			
Upper UTI	6 (460)	1.40 [1.03, 1.91]*, 65%	H10, H11, H28, H39, H49, H59
Both upper and lower UTI	2 (206)	1.40 [1.08, 1.81]*, 0%	H33, H40
Infection site NS	5 (480)	1.45 [1.05, 2.01]*, 47%	H14, H34, H41, H56, H57
Females	5 (361)	1.26 [0.97, 1.65], 38%	H10, H11, H33, H41, H56
Both females and males	6 (532)	1.53 [1.13, 2.08]*, 67%	H14, H28, H34, H39, H49, H59
Gender NS	2 (253)	1.45 [1.00, 2.10]#, 0%	H40, H57
Jin qian cao ke li 金钱草颗粒	2 (190)	1.57 [1.17, 2.10]*, 0%	H28, H39
San jian pian 三金片	3 (250)	0.99 [0.81, 1.22], 0%	H41, H56, H59

*Statistically significant, #p = 0.05, see Chapter 4.
Abbreviations: CI, confidence interval; NS, not specified; RR, risk ratio; UTI, urinary tract infection.

RR 1.26 [0.97, 1.65], I^2 = 38%). Two CHM formulas were tested in two or more studies: *Jin qian cao ke li* 金钱草颗粒 and *San jian pian* 三金片. *Jin qian cao ke li* 金钱草颗粒 was more effective than antibiotics in achieving a composite cure (190 participants, RR 1.57 [1.17, 2.10], I^2 = 0%), while no benefit over antibiotics was seen with *San jian pian* 三金片 (250 participants, RR 0.99 [0.81, 1.22], I^2 = 0%).

One study (H8) reported medium-term cure, assessed between six weeks and six months in people with acute UTI. There was a trend towards statistical significance favouring oral CHM over antibiotics (80 participants, RR 1.75 [1.00, 3.06], p = 0.05).

Long-term cure, measured at least six months after the end of treatment, was assessed in three studies (H5, H17, H60). Two hundred and sixty-three participants were included in the meta-analysis, which favoured oral CHM over antibiotic-based therapy (RR 1.60 [1.16, 2.20], I^2 = 0%; Table 5.5). Subgroup analyses according to infection site showed no difference between oral CHM and antibiotics in long-term composite cure when the infection site was not specified (163 participants, RR 1.34 [0.86, 2.08], I^2 = 0%).

Oral Chinese herbal medicine plus pharmacotherapy versus pharmacotherapy alone

The effect of the combination of oral CHM plus pharmacotherapy on short-term cure was assessed in 46 studies. Overall, the combination

Table 5.5. Oral Chinese Herbal Medicine versus Pharmacotherapy for Acute Urinary Tract Infection: Long-term Cure

Assessment	No. of Studies (Participants)	Effect Size (RR [95% CI], I^2)	Included Studies
All studies	3 (263)	1.60 [1.16, 2.20]*, 0%	H5, H17, H60
Subgroup analyses			
Both upper and lower UTI	1 (100)	1.94 [1.22, 3.06]*, NA	H17
Infection site NS	2 (163)	1.34 [0.86, 2.08], 0%	H5, H60

*Statistically significant, see Chapter 4.
Abbreviations: CI, confidence interval; NA, not applicable; NS, not specified; RR, risk ratio; UTI, urinary tract infection.

of oral CHM with pharmacotherapy improved the rate of short-term cure (3,302 participants, RR 1.37 [1.27, 1.47], I^2 = 29%; Table 5.6). Subgroup analyses were conducted for important clinical features and with studies that used the same CHM formula. Oral CHM as integrative medicine with antibiotic-based therapy was superior to antibiotic therapy alone regardless of the site of infection or gender

Table 5.6. Oral Chinese Herbal Medicine plus Pharmacotherapy versus Pharmacotherapy Alone for Acute Urinary Tract Infection: Short-term Cure

Assessment	No. of Studies (Participants)	Effect Size (RR [95% CI], I^2)	Included Studies
All studies	37 (3,302)	1.37 [1.27, 1.47]*, 29%	H2–H4, H6, H7, H9, H12, H13, H15, H18, H19, H21–H27, H29, H30, H32, H36–H38, H41–H43, H46, H47, H50–H55, H57, H59
Subgroup analyses			
Upper UTI	4 (304)	1.46 [1.22, 1.76]*, 0%	H7, H30, H37, H52
Lower UTI	9 (843)	1.29 [1.14, 1.47]*, 0%	H13, H15, H19, H42, H46, H47, H50, H55, H59
Both upper and lower UTI	10 (1,005)	1.38 [1.17, 1.62]*, 69%	H9, H18, H21, H24–H27, H36, H43, H53
Infection site NS	14 (1,150)	1.39 [1.24, 1.55]*, 0%	H2–H4, H6, H12, H22, H23, H29, H32, H38, H41, H51, H54, H57
Females	7 (720)	1.35 [1.17, 1.55]*, 0%	H2, H3, H12, H13, H15, H41, H50
Both females and males	23 (2,458)	1.37 [1.26, 1.49]*, 39%	H4, H6, H7, H9, H18, H19, H21–H27, H29, H30, H32, H36–H38, H42, H43, H46, H47, H51–H55, H59
Gender NS	1 (124)	2.29 [1.15, 4.57]*, NA	H57
Ba zheng san 八正散	4 (268)	1.32 [1.12, 1.55]*, 0%	H22, H47, H52, H54
Ning mi tai jiao nang 宁泌泰胶囊	2 (210)	1.55 [1.15, 2.10]*, 0%	H21, H30
Re lin qing ke li/pian 热淋清颗粒/片	4 (238)	1.41 [1.21, 1.64]*, 0%	H9, H18, H27, H53

Table 5.6. (*Continued*)

Assessment	No. of Studies (Participants)	Effect Size (RR [95% CI], I²)	Included Studies
San jin pian 三金片	3 (244)	1.24 [1.06, 1.44]*, 0%	H12, H41, H59
Yin hua mi yan ling pian 银花泌炎灵片	4 (436)	1.38 [1.12, 1.70]*, 0%	H13, H29, H50, H55

*Statistically significant, see Chapter 4.
Abbreviations: CI, confidence interval; NA, not applicable; NS, not specified; RR, risk ratio; UTI, urinary tract infection.

(Table 5.6). The formulas *Ba zheng san* 八正散, *Ning mi tai jiao nang* 宁泌泰胶囊, *Re lin qing ke li/pian* 热淋清颗粒/片, *San jin pian* 三金片 and *Yin hua mi yan ling pian* 银花泌炎灵片 were tested in two or more studies. Analysis of these oral CHM formulas showed benefits of adding CHM to antibiotic-based therapy, with treatment effects similar to results seen for the total pool of studies (Table 5.6).

Two studies (H31, H35) evaluated the effects of oral CHM plus antibiotics on cure between six weeks and six months after the end of treatment. Adding oral CHM to antibiotics increased the chances of achieving a medium-term cure (392 participants, RR 1.50 [1.27, 1.79], I² = 0%).

Cure at six months or beyond (long-term cure) was evaluated in seven studies (H1, H16, H20, H44, H45, H48, H60) involving 606 participants. The combination of oral CHM and antibiotics resulted in a higher number of people achieving a long-term cure than antibiotics alone (606 participants, RR 1.64 [1.36, 1.98], I² = 14%; Table 5.7). The treatment effect was higher in individual studies that included people with both upper and lower UTI (98 participants, RR 2.49 [1.56, 3.95]) and females (50 participants, RR 2.35 [1.06, 5.18]), although the variance in these studies limits confidence in the result.

Recurrence

Recurrence among people who achieved a cure at the end of treatment was assessed in four studies (H3, H8, H41, H52). Diversity was seen

Table 5.7. Oral Chinese Herbal Medicine plus Antibiotics versus Antibiotics Alone for Acute Urinary Tract Infection: Long-term Cure

Assessment	No. of Studies (Participants)	Effect Size (RR [95% CI], I²)	Included Studies
All studies	7 (606)	1.64 [1.36, 1.98]*, 14%	H1, H16, H20, H44, H45, H48, H60
Subgroup analyses			
Upper UTI	2 (198)	1.36 [1.03, 1.81]*, 0%	H1, H20
Both upper and lower UTI	1 (98)	2.49 [1.56, 3.95]*, NA	H48
Infection site NS	4 (310)	1.66 [1.30, 2.11]*, 0%	H16, H44, H45, H60
Females	1 (50)	2.35 [1.06, 5.18]*, NA	H44
Both females and males	6 (556)	1.61 [1.32, 1.96]*, 17%	H1, H16, H20, H45, H48, H60

*Statistically significant, see Chapter 4.
Abbreviations: CI, confidence interval; NA, not applicable; NS, not specified; RR, risk ratio; UTI, urinary tract infection.

in the time at which recurrence was assessed, and meta-analysis was not possible. Results are reported for individual studies.

Oral Chinese herbal medicine versus antibiotics

Two studies (H8, H41) that compared oral CHM with antibiotics assessed recurrence. No benefit of oral CHM over antibiotics was seen when recurrence was assessed at three months (33 participants, RR 0.38 [0.13, 1.09]; H8) or at an unspecified time point (58 participants, RR 0.54 [0.21, 1.37]; H41).

Oral Chinese herbal medicine plus antibiotics versus antibiotics alone

Three studies (H52, H3, H41) tested the combination of oral CHM plus antibiotics on recurrence. When recurrence was assessed one month after the end of treatment, there was no statistical difference between people who received oral CHM plus antibiotics and those who received antibiotics alone (108 participants, RR 0.47 [0.21, 1.05]; H52). The same result was seen when recurrence was assessed after six months (60 women, RR 1.00 [0.43, 2.31]; H3). One study that did not specify when recurrence was assessed showed benefit of oral CHM plus antibiotics (124 women, RR 0.20 [0.05, 0.88]; H41). However, the meaning of the results is unclear due to the lack of information about assessment of recurrence.

Duration of Symptoms

Seventeen studies (H2, H7, H13, H15, H23, H24, H27, H33, H35, H36, H37, H42, H43, H46, H48, H50, H53) reported the duration of all urinary or general symptoms of acute UTI, as well as duration of specific symptoms such as dysuria and urinary frequency. All but one of the studies (H33) that reported duration of symptoms compared oral CHM plus pharmacotherapy with pharmacotherapy alone. Results are presented according to comparisons.

Oral Chinese herbal medicine versus antibiotics

One study of 81 women (H33) that compared oral CHM with antibiotics assessed duration of symptoms. After two weeks of treatment, the formula *Gua lou xie bai ban xia tang* 瓜蒌薤白半夏汤 reduced the duration of all urinary symptoms by 0.8 days ([–1.05, –0.55]), reduced the duration of flank pain by 0.89 days ([–1.13, –0.65]) and reduced the duration of all general symptoms by 0.96 days ([–1.25, –0.67]) compared to antibiotics.

Oral Chinese herbal medicine plus pharmacotherapy versus pharmacotherapy alone

Studies that compared oral CHM plus antibiotic-based therapy reported duration of all urinary symptoms, urinary frequency, urinary urgency, dysuria, fevere, flank pain, suprapubic pain and haematuria. Meta-analysis of results for studies that reported duration of all urinary symptoms showed a shorter duration of urinary symptoms by two days (1,138 participants, [−2.68, −1.32], I^2 = 96%; Table 5.8). However, considerable statistical heterogeneity was detected. Subgroup analysis for studies that included people with upper UTI (112 participants, mean difference [MD] −2.41 days, [−3.65, −1.16], I^2 = 44%) and people with an upper or lower UTI (204 participants, MD −1.30 days, [−1.60, −1.00], I^2 = 33%) produced more homogenous results. Subgroup analyses according to gender also showed results that favoured the combination of oral CHM plus antibiotics; however, the considerable statistical heterogeneity reduces confidence in the results.

Table 5.8. Oral Chinese Herbal Medicine plus Antibiotics versus Antibiotics Alone for Acute Urinary Tract Infection: Duration of All Urinary Symptoms

Assessment	No. of Studies (Participants)	Effect Size (MD [95% CI], I^2)	Included Studies
All studies	11 (1,138)	−2.00 [−2.68, −1.32]*, 96%	H7, H13, H15, H23, H24, H35, H37, H42, H46, H48, H50
Subgroup analyses			
Upper UTI	2 (112)	−2.41 [−3.65, −1.16]*, 44%	H7, H37
Lower UTI	6 (622)	−2.41 [−3.46, −1.35]*, 96%	H13, H15, H35, H42, H46, H50
Both upper and lower UTI	2 (204)	−1.30 [−1.60, −1.00]*, 33%	H48, H24
Infection site NS	1 (200)	−0.60 [−0.81, −0.39]*, NA	H23
Females	3 (386)	−2.66 [−4.38, −0.95]*, 93%	H13, H15, H50
Both females and males	8 (752)	−1.77 [−2.58, −0.97]*, 97%	H7, H23, H24, H35, H37, H42, H46, H48

*Statistically significant, see Chapter 4.
Abbreviations: CI, confidence interval; MD, mean difference; NA, not applicable; NS, not specified; UTI, urinary tract infection.

Table 5.9. Oral Chinese Herbal Medicine plus Antibiotics versus Antibiotics Alone for Acute Urinary Tract Infection: Duration of Urinary Frequency

Assessment	No. of Studies (Participants)	Effect Size (MD [95% CI], I^2)	Included Studies
All studies	4 (397)	−2.16 [−2.62, −1.69]*, 71%	H2, H27, H36, H53
Subgroup analyses			
Both upper and lower UTI	3 (297)	−2.22 [−2.83, −1.61]*, 78%	H27, H36, H53
Infection site NS	1 (100)	−1.95 [−2.48, −1.42]*, NA	H2
Re lin qing ke li/pian 热淋清颗粒/片	2 (228)	−2.36 [−3.24, −1.47]*, 86%	H27, H53

*Statistically significant, see Chapter 4.

Abbreviations: CI, confidence interval; MD, mean difference; NA, not applicable; NS, not specified; UTI, urinary tract infection.

Duration of urinary frequency was 2.2 days less in people who received oral CHM plus antibiotics than in people who received antibiotics alone (397 participants, [−2.62, −1.69], I^2 = 71%; Table 5.9). Statistical heterogeneity seen in the overall and subgroup analyses lowers confidence in the results.

Studies that reported duration of urinary frequency also reported duration of urinary urgency (H2, H27, H36, H53). The duration of urinary urgency was reduced by 2.4 days in people who received oral CHM plus antibiotics (397 participants, [−3.15, −1.60], I^2 = 85%; Table 5.10). The potential reasons for statistical heterogeneity were not able to be identified through subgroup analyses according to infection site. Statistical heterogeneity persisted in two studies that used the formula *Re lin qing ke li/pian* 热淋清颗粒/片 with antibiotics (228 participants, MD −2.92 days [−4.98, −0.86], I^2 = 94%; Table 5.10).

Studies that reported urinary frequency and urgency also reported duration of dysuria. Results for meta-analysis of duration of dysuria were more homogenous than those seen for duration of urinary frequency and urgency. Duration of dysuria was 1.8 days less in people who received oral CHM plus antibiotics compared to antibiotics alone (397 participants, [−1.95, −1.56], I^2 = 0%; Table 5.11). Benefits

Table 5.10. Oral Chinese Herbal Medicine plus Antibiotics versus Antibiotics Alone for Acute Urinary Tract Infection: Duration of Urinary Urgency

Assessment	No. of Studies (Participants)	Effect Size (MD [95% CI], I^2)	Included Studies
All studies	4 (397)	−2.37 [−3.15, −1.60]*, 85%	H2, H27, H36, H53
Subgroup analyses			
Both upper and lower UTI	3 (297)	−2.55 [−3.67, −1.43]*, 90%	H27, H36, H53
Infection site NS	1 (100)	−1.95 [−2.48, −1.42]*, NA	H2
Re lin qing ke li/pian 热淋清颗粒/片	2 (228)	−2.92 [−4.98, −0.86]*, 94%	H27, H53

*Statistically significant, see Chapter 4.
Abbreviations: CI, confidence interval; MD, mean difference; NA, not applicable; NS, not specified; UTI, urinary tract infection.

Table 5.11. Oral Chinese Herbal Medicine plus Antibiotics versus Antibiotics Alone for Acute Urinary Tract Infection: Duration of Dysuria

Assessment	No. of Studies (Participants)	Effect Size (MD [95% CI], I^2)	Included Studies
All studies	4 (397)	−1.76 [−1.95, −1.56]*, 0%	H2, H27, H36, H53
Subgroup analyses			
Both upper and lower UTI	3 (297)	−1.70 [−1.92, −1.49]*, 0%	H27, H36, H53
Infection site NS	1 (100)	−1.94 [−2.34, −1.54]*, NA	H2
Re lin qing ke li/pian 热淋清颗粒/片	2 (228)	−1.69 [−1.94, −1.45]*, 0%	H27, H53

*Statistically significant, see Chapter 4.
Abbreviations: CI, confidence interval; MD, mean difference; NA, not applicable; NS, not specified; UTI, urinary tract infection.

Table 5.12 Oral Chinese Herbal Medicine plus Pharmacotherapy versus Pharmacotherapy Alone for Acute Urinary Tract Infection: Duration of Fever

Assessment	No. of Studies (Participants)	Effect Size (MD [95% CI], I²)	Included Studies
All studies	7 (613)	−1.75 [−2.25, −1.24]*, 85%	H7, H24, H27, H36 H37, H43, H53
Subgroup analyses			
Upper UTI	2 (112)	−1.81 [−2.74, −0.88]*, 71%	H7, H37
Both upper and lower UTI	5 (501)	−1.72 [−2.34, −1.11]*, 89%	H24, H27, H36, H43, H53
Re lin qing ke li/pian 热淋清颗粒/片	2 (228)	−2.00 [−2.40, −1.61]*, 10%	H27, H53

*Statistically significant, see Chapter 4.
Abbreviations: CI, confidence interval; MD, mean difference; UTI, urinary tract infection.

were seen regardless of the location of infection and in two studies that tested the formula *Re lin qing ke li/pian* 热淋清颗粒/片.

Oral CHM plus antibiotic-based therapy reduced the duration of fever by 1.8 days (613 participants, [−2.25, −1.24], I² = 85%; Table 5.12). Results for studies that tested the formula *Re lin qing ke li/pian* 热淋清颗粒/片 showed a slightly greater reduction in duration of fever, with little statistical heterogeneity. Other subgroup analyses according to location of infection did not account for the statistical heterogeneity seen in the overall analysis.

Analysis of studies that reported duration of suprapubic pain and haematuria in people with a lower UTI showed no statistical heterogeneity. Oral CHM combined with antibiotics reduced the duration of suprapubic pain (274 participants, MD −2.16 days [−2.60, −1.72], I² = 0%; Table 5.13) and duration of haematuria (274 participants, MD −0.98 days [−1.24, −0.72], I² = 0%, Table 5.14). These benefits did not appear to relate to participant gender.

One study (H37) reported duration of flank pain in people with an upper UTI. Duration of flank pain was 2.6 days less in people who

Table 5.13. Oral Chinese Herbal Medicine plus Antibiotics versus Antibiotics Alone for Acute Urinary Tract Infection: Duration of Suprapubic Pain

Assessment	No. of Studies (Participants)	Effect Size (MD [95% CI], I²)	Included Studies
All studies	3 (274)	−2.16 [−2.60, −1.72]*, 0%	H15, H35, H42
Subgroup analyses			
Females	1 (108)	−2.00 [−2.81, −1.19]*, NA	H15
Both females and males	2 (166)	−2.23 [−2.75, −1.70]*, 0%	H35, H42

*Statistically significant, see Chapter 4.
Abbreviations: CI, confidence interval; MD, mean difference; NA, not applicable.

Table 5.14. Oral Chinese Herbal Medicine plus Antibiotics versus Antibiotics Alone for Acute Urinary Tract Infection: Duration of Haematuria

Assessment	No. of Studies (Participants)	Effect Size (MD [95% CI], I²)	Included Studies
All studies	3 (274)	−0.98 [−1.24, −0.72]*, 0%	H15, H35, H42
Subgroup analyses			
Females	1 (108)	−0.90 [−1.36, −0.44]*, NA	H15
Both females and males	2 (166)	−1.01 [−1.32, −0.70]*, 0%	H35, H42

*Statistically significant, see Chapter 4.
Abbreviations: CI, confidence interval; MD, mean difference; NA, not applicable.

received *Jian pi yi shen qing re li shi fang* 健脾益肾清热利湿方 compared to quinolone ([−4.14, −1.16]).

Microbiologically Positive Urine Culture

Data were analysed for nine studies (H3, H9, H11, H17, H18, H21, H48, H58, H60) that reported the number of people with a positive urine culture at the end of treatment.

Oral Chinese herbal medicine plus placebo versus antibiotics plus placebo

Results from one RCT showed the number of people with a positive urine culture was not statistically different between oral CHM plus placebo and antibiotics plus placebo (141 participants, RR 0.65 [0.27, 1.57]; H58).

Oral Chinese herbal medicine plus antibiotics versus antibiotics plus placebo

Oral CHM plus antibiotics was compared with antibiotics plus placebo in one study of 141 participants (H58). Oral CHM plus antibiotics was not more likely to reduce the number of people with a positive urine culture than antibiotics plus placebo (RR 0.45 [0.16, 1.22]).

Oral Chinese herbal medicine versus antibiotics

Meta-analysis of three studies (203 participants) showed no difference between oral CHM and antibiotics in the number of people with a positive urine culture at the end of treatment (RR 0.92 [0.23, 3.73], $I^2 = 67\%$; H11, H17, H60). Subgroup analyses found similar results for two studies that only included women (140 women, RR 1.83 [0.72, 4.68], $I^2 = 0\%$; H11, H17) and studies that tested *Long qing pian* 癃清片 (103 participants, RR 0.64 [0.07, 5.75], $I^2 = 76\%$; H11, H60). One study (H17) described the bacteria detected on urine culture: *Escherichia coli, Proteus, Klebsiella, Aeronomas, Serratia* and *Streptococcus faecalis*. The frequencies of each organism were not reported.

Oral Chinese herbal medicine plus antibiotics versus antibiotics alone

Six studies (H3, H9, H18, H21, H48, H60) that tested the combination of oral CHM plus antibiotics reported on microbiologically positive urine culture at the end of treatment. There was no statistical difference between groups in the number of people with a positive

Table 5.15. Oral Chinese Herbal Medicine plus Antibiotics versus Antibiotics Alone for Acute Urinary Tract Infection: Microbiologically Positive Urine Culture

Assessment	No. of Studies (Participants)	Effect Size (MD [95% CI], I^2)	Included Studies
All studies	6 (458)	0.67 [0.37, 1.22], 57%	H3, H9, H18, H21, H48, H60
Subgroup analyses			
Both upper and lower UTI	4 (334)	0.76 [0.39, 1.48], 55%	H9, H18, H21, H48
Infection site NS	2 (124)	0.36 [0.04, 3.25], 76%	H3, H60
Females	1 (60)	0.88 [0.36, 2.11], NA	H3
Both females and males	5 (398)	0.59 [0.27, 1.28], 66%	H9, H18, H21, H48, H60
Re lin qing ke li/pian 热淋清颗粒/片	2 (110)	0.31 [0.12, 0.80]*, 0%	H9, H18

*Statistically significant, see Chapter 4.
Abbreviations: CI, confidence interval; NA, not applicable; NS, not specified; RR, risk ratio; UTI, urinary tract infection.

urine culture at the end of treatment (458 participants, RR 0.67 [0.37, 1.22], I^2 = 57%; Table 5.15). Results of subgroup analyses also showed no difference between groups regardless of the location of infection or gender. However, analysis of two studies that combined *Re lin qing ke li/pian* 热淋清颗粒/片 with antibiotics found fewer positive urine cultures in the treatment group, compared with the antibiotics group (110 participants, RR 0.31 [0.12, 0.80], I^2 = 0%).

Pyuria

Pyuria (presence of white blood cells in urine) was reported in four studies (H3, H17, H19, H24).

Oral Chinese herbal medicine versus antibiotics

One study (H17) compared *San jin pian* 三金片 with levofloxacin for the effects on pyuria. There was no statistical difference between groups in the number of people with pyuria (100 participants, RR 1.04 [0.71, 1.53]).

Oral Chinese herbal medicine plus antibiotics versus antibiotics alone

Meta-analysis was possible with three studies that tested the combination of oral CHM plus antibiotics. Among the 256 participants, there were fewer people with pyuria in those who received the combination of oral CHM plus antibiotics than in those who received antibiotics alone (RR 0.37 [0.18, 0.75], I^2 = 0%; H3, H19, H24).

Serum Creatinine

One study, with 84 participants, reported that the levels of serum creatinine were 11.74 μmol/L lower in people who received *Ning mi tai jiao nang* 宁泌泰胶囊 plus the antibiotics cefoperazone and sulbactam compared to cefoperazone and sulbactam alone ([−15.49, −7.99]; H30).

Urinary Beta-2 Microglobulin

Three studies reported urinary β2-MG. One study (H17) compared oral CHM with antibiotics and two studies (H1, H48) compared the combination of oral CHM plus antibiotics with antibiotics alone.

Oral Chinese herbal medicine versus antibiotics

The mean urinary β2-MG was lower at the end of treatment in people who received oral CHM than in people who received antibiotics (100 participants, MD −0.27 mg/L, [−0.36, −0.18]; H17). The mean values at the end of treatment for both groups were above the reference range for this outcome (oral CHM mean: 0.44 mg/L; antibiotics mean: 0.71 mg/L).

Oral Chinese herbal medicine plus antibiotics versus antibiotics alone

Of the two studies that reported urinary β2-MG, one study (H1) reported the results in mg/L, while the other study (H48) didn't report the units. Meta-analysis was conducted using standardised mean difference (SMD) due to these differences. There was no difference between oral CHM plus antibiotics with antibiotics alone in the level of urinary β2-MG at the end of treatment (222 participants, SMD −3.16 [−8.95, 2.62], I^2 = 99%).

Health Care Costs

One study (H31) reported on health care costs associated with lower UTI. The cost-effectiveness ratio was calculated by dividing the total cost of treatment divided by the reduction in score of clinical symptoms. The study authors reported that there were no statistical differences between groups in the cost-effectiveness ratio.

Assessment Using Grading of Recommendations Assessment, Development and Evaluation

Results for important clinical questions were summarised using the Grading of Recommendations Assessment, Development and Evaluation (GRADE) approach. Consensus on items for inclusion in GRADE tables was reached using the process outlined in Chapter 4. Outcomes that were considered important were cure, recurrence, duration of urinary symptoms, health-related quality of life, health care costs and adverse events.

Selected interventions were oral CHM used alone or in combination with antibiotics, and the formulas *Ba zheng san* 八正散 and *San jin pian* 三金片 used alone or as integrative medicine with antibiotics. The selected comparator was antibiotics. This resulted in six GRADE tables being prepared to summarise the strength and quality ('certainty') of the evidence for acute UTI:

- Oral CHM versus antibiotics for acute UTI;
- Oral CHM plus antibiotics versus antibiotics alone for acute UTI;

- *Ba zheng san* 八正散 versus antibiotics for acute UTI;
- *Ba zheng san* 八正散 plus antibiotics versus antibiotics alone for acute UTI;
- *San jin pian* 三金片 versus antibiotics for acute UTI;
- *San jin pian* 三金片 plus antibiotics versus antibiotics alone for acute UTI.

Oral Chinese Herbal Medicine versus Antibiotics for Acute Urinary Tract Infection

Sixteen studies (H5, H8, H10, H11, H17, H28, H33, H34, H39, H40, H41, H49, H56, H57, H59, H60) that compared oral CHM with antibiotics reported on the selected outcomes. The certainty of the evidence for oral CHM versus antibiotics for acute UTI was assessed as 'low' to 'very low' (Table 5.16). Whether oral CHM increases the

Table 5.16. GRADE: Oral Chinese Herbal Medicine versus Antibiotics for Acute Urinary Tract Infection

Outcome	Absolute Effect		Relative Effect (95% CI) No. of Participants (Studies)	Certainty of the Evidence (GRADE)
	With Oral CHM	With Antibiotics		
Short-term cure, treatment duration: 7 d to 4 w	**53 per 100** Difference: 15 more per 100 patients (95% CI: 6 to 26 more per 100 patients)	**38 per 100**	**RR 1.40*** (1.16 to 1.68) 1,044 (12 RCTs)	⊕◯◯◯ VERY LOW[a,b,c]
Medium-term cure, treatment duration: 56 d	**53 per 100** Difference: 23 more per 100 patients (95% CI: 0 to 62 more per 100 patients)	**30 per 100**	**RR 1.75** (1.00 to 3.06) 80 (1 RCT)	⊕⊕◯◯ LOW[a,b]
Long-term cure, treatment duration: 1 w to 28 d	**48 per 100** Difference: 18 more per 100 patients (95% CI: 5 to 36 more per 100 patients)	**30 per 100**	**RR 1.60*** (1.16 to 2.20) 263 (3 RCTs)	⊕⊕◯◯ LOW[a,b]

(Continued)

Table 5.16. (*Continued*)

Outcome	Absolute Effect		Relative Effect (95% CI) No. of Participants (Studies)	Certainty of the Evidence (GRADE)
	With Oral CHM	With Antibiotics		
Recurrence at 3 m, treatment duration: 56 d	**19 per 100** Difference: 31 fewer per 100 patients (95% CI: 44 fewer to 5 more per 100 patients)	**50 per 100**	**RR 0.38** (0.13 to 1.09) 33 (1 RCT)	⊕⊕◯◯ LOW[a,b]
Duration of urinary symptoms, treatment duration: 2 w	**3.24 days** Average difference: 0.8 days lower (95% CI: 1.05 to 0.55 days lower)	**4.04 days**	**MD –0.80*** (–1.05 to –0.55) 81 (1 RCT)	⊕⊕◯◯ LOW[a,b]

*Statistically significant result.

Abbreviations: CHM, Chinese herbal medicine; CI, confidence interval; d, days; GRADE, Grading of Recommendations Assessment, Development and Evaluation; m, months; MD, mean difference; RCT, randomised controlled trial; RR, risk ratio; w, weeks.

Notes
[a]High risk of bias due to lack of blinding of participants and personnel.
[b]Small sample size.
[c]Publication bias suspected.

Study references
Short-term cure: H10, H11, H28, H33, H34, H39–H41, H49, H56, H57, H59.
Medium-term cure: H8.
Long-term cure: H5, H17, H60.
Recurrence: H8.

number of people achieving a short-term cure is unclear ('very low' certainty evidence). However, oral CHM may improve long-term cure ('low' certainty evidence). Oral CHM may lead to little, or no difference, in medium-term cure rate ('low' certainty evidence) or recurrence at three months ('low' certainty evidence). Oral CHM may slightly reduce the duration of urinary symptoms ('low' certainty evidence). Safety was reported in five RCTs (H8, H49, H57, H59, H60). Reported adverse events with oral CHM were two cases of constipation, two cases of vomiting and nausea, and one case of gastrointestinal discomfort. Adverse events with antibiotics were five cases of nausea, four cases of gastrointestinal discomfort and nausea, two cases of rash and two cases of gastrointestinal discomfort.

Oral Chinese Herbal Medicine plus Antibiotics versus Antibiotics Alone for Acute Urinary Tract Infection

Forty-five studies (H1–H4, H6, H7, H9, H12, H13, H15, H16, H18–H27, H29–H32, H35–H38, H41, H42, H44–H48, H50–H55, H57, H59, H60) that compared oral CHM plus antibiotics with antibiotics alone for acute UTI reported on the outcomes selected by group consensus. The certainty of evidence was 'moderate' to 'low' (Table 5.17). Oral CHM plus antibiotics is likely to increase the number of people achieving a short- or long-term cure ('moderate' certainty evidence) and may increase the number of people achieving a medium-term cure ('low' certainty evidence). Oral

Table 5.17. GRADE: Oral Chinese Herbal Medicine plus Antibiotics versus Antibiotics Alone for Acute Urinary Tract Infection

	Absolute Effect		Relative Effect (95% CI) No. of Participants (Studies)	Certainty of the Evidence (GRADE)
Outcome	With Oral CHM IM	With Antibiotics		
Short-term cure, treatment duration: 3 d to 15 d	**63 per 100** Difference: 17 more per 100 patients (95% CI: 12 to 21 more per 100 patients)	**46 per 100**	**RR 1.36*** (1.27 to 1.46) 3,204 (36 RCTs)	⊕⊕⊕◯ MODERATE[a]
Medium-term cure, treatment duration: 7 d to 14 d	**71 per 100** Difference: 24 more per 100 patients (95% CI: 13 to 37 more per 100 patients)	**47 per 100**	**RR 1.50*** (1.27 to 1.79) 392 (2 RCTs)	⊕⊕◯◯ LOW[a,b]
Long-term cure, treatment duration: 7 d to 9 w	**59 per 100** Difference: 23 more per 100 patients (95% CI: 13 to 35 more per 100 patients)	**36 per 100**	**RR 1.64*** (1.36 to 1.98) 606 (7 RCTs)	⊕⊕⊕◯ MODERATE[a]
Recurrence at 6 m, treatment duration: 2 w	**27 per 100** Difference: 0 fewer per 100 patients (95% CI: 15 fewer to 35 more per 100 patients)	**27 per 100**	**RR 1.00** (0.43 to 2.31) 60 (1 RCT)	⊕⊕◯◯ LOW[a,b]

(Continued)

Table 5.17. (*Continued*)

Outcome	Absolute Effect		Relative Effect (95% CI) No. of Participants (Studies)	Certainty of the Evidence (GRADE)
	With Oral CHM IM	With Antibiotics		
Recurrence at 1 m, treatment duration: 2 w	**13 per 100**	**28 per 100**	**RR 0.47**	⊕⊕○○ LOW[a,b]
	Difference: 15 fewer per 100 patients (95% CI: 22 fewer to 1 more per 100 patients)		(0.21 to 1.05) 108 (1 RCT)	
Duration of urinary symptoms, treatment duration: 4 w to 2 m	**4.13 days**	**6.13 days**	**MD –2.00***	⊕⊕○○ LOW[a,c]
	Average difference: 2 days lower (95% CI: 2.68 to 1.32 days lower)		(–2.68 to –1.32) 1,138 (11 RCTs)	

*Statistically significant result.

Abbreviations: CHM, Chinese herbal medicine; CI, confidence interval; d, days; GRADE, Grading of Recommendations Assessment, Development and Evaluation; IM, integrative medicine; m, months; MD, mean difference; RCT, randomised controlled trial; RR, risk ratio; w, weeks.

Notes
[a]High risk of bias due to lack of blinding of participants and personnel.
[b]Small sample size.
[c]High heterogeneity and wide variance in effect estimates.

Study references
Short-term cure: H2–H4, H6, H7, H9, H12, H13, H15, H18, H19, H21–H27, H29, H30, H32, H36–H38, H41, H42, H46, H47, H50–H55, H57, H59.
Medium-term cure: H31, H35.
Long-term cure: H1, H16, H20, H44, H45, H48, H60.
Recurrence at 6 months: H3.
Recurrence at 1 month: H52.
Duration of urinary symptoms: H7, H13, H15, H23, H24, H35, H37, H42, H46, H48, H50.

CHM combined with antibiotics may make little or no difference, in terms of recurrence one, or six, months after the end of treatment ('low' certainty evidence) but may reduce the duration of urinary symptoms ('low' certainty evidence). Evidence from one study showed oral CHM plus antibiotics may make little or no difference, in cost-effectiveness ('low' certainty evidence).

Adverse events were reported in 27 RCTS, nine of which reported no adverse events occurring (H1, H2, H19, H22, H35, H37, H47,

H48, H52). Adverse events were reported in the remaining 18 RCTs (H9, H15, H18, H21, H24, H26, H30, H31, H36, H42, H46, H50, H51, H53, H55, H57, H59, H60). Adverse events among people who received oral CHM plus antibiotics were 18 cases of gastrointestinal discomfort, nine cases of mild diarrhoea, five cases of nausea and stomach upset, four cases of nausea and loss of appetite, four cases of nausea, three cases of loss of appetite, three cases of rash, two cases of mild nausea and diarrhoea, two cases of nausea and vomiting, two cases of vomiting and one case each of dizziness and headache. Adverse events among people who received antibiotics were 21 cases of gastrointestinal discomfort, 12 cases of nausea, 11 cases of diarrhoea, ten cases of vomiting, seven cases of nausea and stomach upset, four cases of loss of appetite, two cases of mild dizziness and headache, two cases of nausea and vomiting, and one case each of stomachache and diarrhoea, allergy and mild dizziness.

Ba Zheng San 八正散 *versus Antibiotics for Acute Urinary Tract Infection*

Two studies (H5, H34) that compared *Ba zheng san* 八正散 with antibiotics reported the pre-specified outcomes. *Ba zheng san* 八正散 may increase the number of people achieving a short-term cure, compared to antibiotics ('low' certainty evidence), but may make little, or no difference, in the chance of achieving a long-term cure ('low' certainty evidence; Table 5.18). Neither study reported on the safety of *Ba zheng san* 八正散.

Ba Zheng San 八正散 *plus Antibiotics versus Antibiotics Alone for Acute Urinary Tract Infection*

Five studies (H22, H35, H47, H52, H54) that tested *Ba zheng san* 八正散 as integrative medicine with antibiotics reported on relevant outcomes. When combined with antibiotics, *Ba zheng san* 八正散 may improve the chance of a short- or medium-term cure, compared with antibiotics alone ('low' certainty evidence) (Table 5.19). *Ba zheng san* 八正散 as integrative medicine may have little, or no,

Table 5.18. GRADE: *Ba Zheng San* 八正散 **versus Antibiotics for Acute Urinary Tract Infection**

Outcome	Absolute Effect		Relative Effect (95% CI) No. of Participants (Studies)	Certainty of the Evidence (GRADE)
	With *Ba Zheng San* 八正散	With Antibiotics		
Short-term cure, treatment duration: 2 w	**64 per 100**	**29 per 100**	**RR 2.20***	⊕⊕○○ LOW[a,b]
	Difference: 35 more per 100 patients (95% CI: 7 to 84 more per 100 patients)		(1.23 to 3.94) 70 (1 RCT)	
Long-term cure, treatment duration: 1 w	**42 per 100**	**28 per 100**	**RR 1.50**	⊕⊕○○ LOW[a,b]
	Difference: 14 more per 100 patients (95% CI: 4 fewer to 45 more per 100 patients)		(0.86 to 2.60) 100 (1 RCT)	

*Statistically significant result.

Abbreviations: CI, confidence interval; d, days; GRADE, Grading of Recommendations Assessment, Development and Evaluation; m, months; RCT, randomised controlled trial; RR, risk ratio; w, weeks.

Notes
[a]High risk of bias due to lack of blinding of participants and personnel.
[b]Small sample size.

Study references
Short-term cure: H34.
Long-term cure: H5.

effect in reducing recurrence ('low' certainty evidence). Four studies (H22, H47, H52, H54) reported on safety, with no adverse events occurring.

San Jin Pian 三金片 *versus Antibiotics for Acute Urinary Tract Infection*

Evidence from four studies (H17, H41, H56, H59) for the commercial product *San jin pian* 三金片 compared to antibiotics was judged to be of 'low' certainty. Used alone, *San jin pian* 三金片 may have little, or no, effect in improving the number of people achieving a short-term cure,

Table 5.19. GRADE: *Ba Zheng San* 八正散 **plus Antibiotics versus Antibiotics Alone for Acute Urinary Tract Infection**

Outcome	Absolute Effect		Relative Effect (95% CI) No. of Participants (Studies)	Certainty of the Evidence (GRADE)
	With *Ba Zheng San* 八正散 IM	With Antibiotics		
Short-term cure, treatment duration: range 3 to 14 d	**75 per 100** Difference: 18 more per 100 patients (95% CI: 7 to 32 more per 100 patients)	**57 per 100**	**RR 1.32*** (1.12 to 1.55) 268 (4 RCTs)	⊕⊕○○ LOW[a,b]
Medium-term cure, treatment duration: 14 d	**67 per 100** Difference: 24 more per 100 patients (95% CI: 2 to 56 more per 100 patients)	**43 per 100**	**RR 1.55*** (1.05 to 2.28) 92 (1 RCT)	⊕⊕○○ LOW[a,b]
Recurrence at 1 m, treatment duration: 14 d	**13 per 100** Difference: 15 fewer per 100 patients (95% CI: 22 fewer to 1 more per 100 patients)	**28 per 100**	**RR 0.47** (0.21 to 1.05) 108 (1 RCT)	⊕⊕○○ LOW[a,b]

*Statistically significant result.

Abbreviations: CI, confidence interval; d, days; GRADE, Grading of Recommendations Assessment, Development and Evaluation; IM, integrative medicine; m, months; RCT, randomised controlled trial; RR, risk ratio.

Notes
[a]High risk of bias due to lack of blinding of participants and personnel.
[b]Small sample size.

Study references
Short-term cure: H22, H47, H52, H54.
Medium-term cure: H35.
Recurrence at one month: H52.

or in reducing UTI recurrence ('low' certainty evidence; Table 5.20). However, *San jin pian* 三金片 may result in a greater increase in the number of people achieving a long-term cure than antibiotics ('low' certainty evidence). Adverse events in one study (H59) included one case of gastric discomfort with *San jin pian* 三金片 and two cases of gastric discomfort with levofloxacin.

Table 5.20.   GRADE: *San Jin Pian* 三金片 **versus Antibiotics for Acute Urinary Tract Infection**

Outcome	Absolute Effect		Relative Effect (95% CI) No. of Participants (Studies)	Certainty of the Evidence (GRADE)
	With *San Jin Pian* 三金片	With Antibiotics		
Short-term cure, treatment duration: 7 d to 4 w	**51 per 100**	**52 per 100**	**RR 0.99**	⊕⊕〇〇
	Difference: 1 fewer per 100 patients (95% CI: 10 fewer to 11 more per 100 patients)		(0.81 to 1.22) 250 (3 RCTs)	LOW[a,b]
Long-term cure, treatment duration: 28 d	**62 per 100**	**32 per 100**	**RR 1.94***	⊕⊕〇〇
	Difference: 30 more per 100 patients (95% CI: 7 to 66 more per 100 patients)		(1.22 to 3.06) 100 (1 RCT)	LOW[a,b]
Recurrence (time NS), treatment duration: mean 11 d	**18 per 100**	**33 per 100**	**RR 0.54**	⊕⊕〇〇
	Difference: 15 fewer per 100 patients (95% CI: 26 fewer to 12 more per 100 patients)		(0.21 to 1.37) 58 (1 RCT)	LOW[a,b]

*Statistically significant result.

Abbreviations: CI, confidence interval; d, days; GRADE, Grading of Recommendations Assessment, Development and Evaluation; NS, not specified; RCT, randomised controlled trial; RR, risk ratio.

Notes

[a]High risk of bias due to lack of blinding of participants and personnel.
[b]Small sample size.

Study references
Short-term cure: H41, H56, H59.
Long-term cure: H17.
Recurrence: H41.

San Jin Pian 三金片 *plus Antibiotics versus Antibiotics for Acute Urinary Tract Infection*

Three studies (H12, H41, H59) reporting on pre-specified outcomes compared *San jin pian* 三金片 plus antibiotics with antibiotics alone. Results showed that adding *San jin pian* 三金片 to antibiotics may increase the number of people achieving a short-term cure ('low'

Table 5.21. **GRADE:** *San Jin Pian* 三金片 **plus Antibiotics versus Antibiotics for Acute Urinary Tract Infection**

Outcome	Absolute Effect		Relative Effect (95% CI) No. of Participants (Studies)	Certainty of the Evidence (GRADE)
	With *San Jin Pian* 三金片 IM	With Antibiotics		
Short-term cure, treatment duration: 7 to 14 d	76 per 100	61 per 100	RR 1.24*	⊕⊕○○
	Difference: 15 more per 100 patients (95% CI: 4 to 27 more per 100 patients)		(1.06 to 1.44) 244 (3 RCTs)	LOW^[a,b]
Recurrence (time NS), treatment duration: mean 11 d	3 per 100	16 per 100	RR 0.20*	⊕⊕○○
	Difference: 13 fewer per 100 patients (95% CI: 15 to 2 fewer per 100 patients)		(0.05 to 0.88) 124 (1 RCT)	LOW^[a,b]

*Statistically significant result.

Abbreviations: CI, confidence interval; d, days; GRADE, Grading of Recommendations Assessment, Development and Evaluation; IM, integrative medicine; NS, not specified; RCT, randomised controlled trial; RR, risk ratio.

Notes
[a]High risk of bias due to lack of blinding of participants and personnel.
[b]Small sample size.

Study references
Short-term cure: H12, H41, H59.
Recurrence: H41.

certainty evidence; Table 5.21) and may reduce the rate of recurrence at an unspecified time point ('low' certainty evidence). Adverse events reported in one study (H59) included three cases of gastric discomfort and one case of rash with *San jin pian* 三金片 plus antibiotics, and two cases of gastric discomfort with levofloxacin.

Randomised Controlled Trial Evidence for Individual Oral Formulas

Several oral CHM formulas and manufactured products were evaluated in multiple RCTs (see Table 5.1). Meta-analysis was possible for several formulas and outcomes: *Ba zheng san* 八正散, *Jin qian cao ke li* 金钱草颗粒, *Long qing pian* 癃清片, *Ning mi tai jiao nang* 宁泌泰胶囊, *Re lin qing ke li/pian* 热淋清颗粒/片, *San jian pian* 三金片 and *Yin hua mi yan ling pian* 银花泌炎灵片. Oral CHM formulas used alone showed that the benefit with *Jin qian cao ke li* 金钱草颗粒 was greater than that with antibiotics, in terms of short-term cure (190 participants, RR 1.57 [1.17, 2.10], I^2 = 0%; H28, H39). *San jian pian* 三金片 was not superior to antibiotics in increasing chances of achieving a short-term cure (250 participants, RR 0.99 [0.81, 1.22], I^2 = 0%; H41, H56, H59), nor was *Long qing pian* 癃清片 more effective than antibiotics in reducing the number of people with a positive urine culture (103 participants, RR 0.64 [0.07, 5.75], I^2 = 76%; H11, H60).

Due to the larger number of studies that tested oral CHM as integrative medicine with antibiotic-based therapy, it was possible to conduct several meta-analyses for different oral CHM formulas. *Ba zheng san* 八正散 was shown to increase chances of achieving a short-term cure when combined with antibiotics (268 participants, RR 1.32 [1.12, 1.55], I^2 = 0%; H22, H47, H52, H54). Similar findings were seen with *Ning mi tai jiao nang* 宁泌泰胶囊 as integrative medicine (210 participants, RR 1.55 [1.15, 2.10], I^2 = 0%; H21, H30), *San jian pian* 三金片 as integrative medicine (244 participants, RR 1.24 [1.06, 1.44], I^2 = 0%; H12, H41, H59) and *Yin hua mi yan ling pian* 银花泌炎灵片 as integrative medicine (436 participants, RR 1.38 [1.12, 1.70], I^2 = 0%; H13, H29, H50, H55).

Meta-analyses of results for several outcomes were possible with studies that tested *Re lin qing ke li/pian* 热淋清颗粒/片 as integrative medicine with antibiotics. The combination:

- Increased the chances of achieving a short-term cure (238 participants, RR 1.41 [1.21, 1.64], I^2 = 0%; H9, H18, H27, H53);
- Reduced the duration of urinary frequency (228 participants, MD −2.36 days [−3.24, −1.47], I^2 = 86%; H27, H53);
- Reduced the duration of urinary urgency (228 participants, MD −2.92 days [−4.98, −0.86], I^2 = 94%; H27, H53);
- Reduced the duration of dysuria (228 participants, MD −1.69 days [−1.94, −1.45], I^2 = 0%; H27, H53);

- Reduced the duration of fever (228 participants, MD –2.00 days [–2.40, –1.61], I² = 10%; H27, H53);
- Reduced the chance of a positive urine culture at the end of treatment (110 participants, RR 0.31 [0.12, 0.80], I² = 0%; H9, H18).

Frequently Reported Orally Used Herbs in Meta-analyses Showing Favourable Effect

Several of the meta-analyses of oral CHM for acute UTI have shown benefit in achieving a composite cure, reducing the duration of symptoms and improving results of some biological tests. The herb ingredients of studies that were included in these meta-analyses were reviewed to identify the frequently used herbs that may be contributing to the treatment effect (Table 5.22).

Table 5.22. Frequently Reported Orally Used Herbs in Meta-analyses Showing Favourable Effect for Acute Urinary Tract Infection

Herbs	Scientific Name	Frequency of Use
Composite cure: five meta-analyses, 52 studies		
Che qian zi 车前子	*Plantago* spp.	24
Bian xu 萹蓄	*Polygonum aviculare* L.	21
Qu mai 瞿麦	*Dianthus* spp.	21
Gan cao 甘草	*Glycyrrhiza* spp.	19
Hua shi 滑石	Hydrated magnesium silicate	17
Huang bai 黄柏	*Phellodendron chinense* Schneid.	17
Shi wei 石韦	*Pyrrosia* spp.	17
Zhi zi 栀子	*Gardenia jasminoides* Ellis	14
Mu tong 木通	*Akebia* spp.	13
Da huang 大黄	*Rheum* spp.	12
Duration of symptoms: seven meta-analyses, 14 studies		
Gan cao 甘草	*Glycyrrhiza* spp.	7
Jin qian cao 金钱草	*Lysimachia christinae* Hance	7
Che qian zi 车前子	*Plantago* spp.	6

(Continued)

Table 5.22. **(*Continued*)**

Herbs	Scientific Name	Frequency of Use
Qu mai 瞿麦	*Dianthus* spp.	6
Shi wei 石韦	*Pyrrosia* spp.	6
Bian xu 萹蓄	*Polygonum aviculare* L.	5
Mu tong 木通	*Akebia* spp.	5
Che qian cao 车前草	*Plantago* spp.	4
Hua shi 滑石	Hydrated magnesium silicate	4
Zhi zi 栀子	*Gardenia jasminoides* Ellis	4
Biological tests: one meta-analysis, three studies		
Bian xu 萹蓄	*Polygonum aviculare* L.	2
Fu ling 茯苓	*Poria cocos* (Schw.) Wolf	2
Gan cao 甘草	*Glycyrrhiza* spp.	2
Huang bai 黄柏	*Phellodendron chinense* Schneid.	2
Qu mai 瞿麦	*Dianthus* spp.	2
Shi wei 石韦	*Pyrrosia* spp.	2

Composite cure: Refer to Tables 5.4, 5.5, 5.6 and 5.7, and the section 'Oral Chinese Herbal Medicine plus Pharmacotherapy versus Pharmacotherapy Alone' (pp. 103–105).
Duration of symptoms: Tables 5.8, 5.9, 5.10, 5.11, 5.12, 5.13 and 5.14.
Biological tests: Refer to the section 'Pyuria' (pp. 114–115).

All of the studies of oral CHM reported cure, and most studies were included in meta-analyses. Five of the meta-analyses, that included 52 of the 60 RCTs, showed positive benefits for oral CHM used alone or as integrative medicine. The herbs that may have contributed to the positive effects demonstrated are similar to those seen in the overall pool (Table 5.2), which was not surprising. Key herbs included *che qian zi* 车前子, *bian xu* 萹蓄 and *qu mai* 瞿麦.

Seven meta-analyses, including 14 RCTs, showed benefit for oral CHM in reducing the duration of symptoms. The herbs *gan cao* 甘草 and *jin qian cao* 金钱草 were reported in half of the studies that contributed to these results (Table 5.22). One meta-analysis of three studies found oral CHM plus antibiotics to be beneficial in reducing pyuria.

Six herbs were common to two studies: *bian xu* 萹蓄, *fu ling* 茯苓, *gan cao* 甘草, *huang bai* 黄柏, *qu mai* 瞿麦 and *shi wei* 石韦. These herbs may be considered when prescribing or modifying CHM treatments.

Safety of Oral Chinese Herbal Medicine in Randomised Controlled Trials for Acute Urinary Tract Infection

Thirty-two RCTs reported on safety, with ten RCTs (H1, H2, H8, H19, H22, H35, H37, H47, H48, H52) reporting that no adverse events occurred during the trial. Twenty-two RCTs (H9, H14, H15, H18, H21, H24, H26, H30, H31, H36, H42, H43, H46, H49–H51, H53, H55, H57–H60) reported the nature and number of adverse events that occurred.

Six adverse events were reported in groups that received oral CHM alone: two cases of constipation that resolved with treatment, two cases of vomiting and nausea, one case of gastric discomfort and one case of elevated bilirubin. When oral CHM was combined with antibiotics, 59 adverse events were reported. Adverse events included 18 cases of gastrointestinal discomfort, 10 cases of mild diarrhoea, five cases of nausea and stomach upset, four cases of nausea, four cases of rash, four cases of nausea and loss of appetite, three cases of vomiting, three cases of loss of appetite, two mild headaches, two cases of mild nausea and diarrhoea, two cases of nausea and vomiting, and one case each of dizziness, and increased thirst and hunger.

The number of adverse events reported in people who received antibiotics alone was higher, with 93 adverse events reported. Adverse events included 23 cases of gastrointestinal discomfort, 17 cases of nausea, 11 cases of vomiting, 11 cases of diarrhoea, seven cases of nausea and stomach upset, four cases of rash, four cases of loss of appetite, four cases of stomach discomfort and nausea, three cases of worsening backache and mild proteinuria, two cases of mild dizziness, two cases of dizziness and headache, two cases of headache, two cases of nausea and vomiting, and one case of stomachache and diarrhoea.

Controlled Clinical Trials of Oral Chinese Herbal Medicine for Acute Urinary Tract Infection

Three controlled trials (H61–H63) evaluated oral CHM in people with acute UTI. Studies were conducted in China and involved 261 participants with a UTI in the upper or lower urinary tract. In the study that reported duration of infection, this ranged from one to 31 days (H63). None of the studies reported using CM syndrome differentiation as an inclusion criterion or to guide treatment.

The duration of treatment was five days (H63) or two weeks (H61, H62). All studies used manufactured products as integrative medicine with antibiotics: Two studies used *San jin pian* 三金片 (H61, H63), and one used *Ning mi tai jiao nang* 宁泌泰胶囊 (H62). Antibiotics used in the control groups included oral levofloxacin and gatifloxacin and injection of pazufloxacin mesylate. Follow-up assessment was conducted six months after the end of treatment in two studies (H61, H63). One study reported loss to follow-up (H63).

Outcomes

Composite cure was reported by all three studies and all studies reported on adverse events. One study (H62) also reported duration of all urinary symptoms.

Composite Cure

All studies reported short-term composite cure and were pooled for meta-analysis. Oral CHM as integrative medicine was not more effective than antibiotics alone in increasing the chances of a cure of symptoms and infection (261 participants, RR 1.11, [0.86, 1.43], $I^2 = 50\%$).

Duration of All Urinary Symptoms

The duration of all urinary symptoms was assessed in one study (H62). The combination of oral CHM with antibiotics was more effective than antibiotics alone in reducing the duration of all urinary symptoms (112 participants, MD –1.93 days [–2.37, –1.49]).

Safety of Oral Chinese Herbal Medicine in Controlled Clinical Trials for Acute Urinary Tract Infection

All three studies reported on safety of oral CHM for people with acute UTI. No adverse events occurred in one study (H62). Adverse events in people who received oral CHM as integrative medicine included five cases of mild nausea and gastric discomfort and two cases of mild diarrhoea. Adverse events in the antibiotic group included six cases of mild nausea and gastric discomfort, and three cases of loss of appetite.

Non-controlled Studies of Oral Chinese Herbal Medicine for Acute Urinary Tract Infection

Four case series from China evaluated oral CHM (H64–H67). Participants included 338 people with acute UTI. Treatment duration varied from three days (H64) to 84 days (H67), and one study conducted follow-up assessment three months after the end of treatment (H64).

The CM syndrome damp-heat was used as an inclusion criterion in one study (H65). Four of the five studies tested oral CHM alone, while one study (H66) used oral CHM as integrative medicine with guideline-recommended treatments. A different formula was used in all studies, so no overlap in formulas was seen among the studies. Similarly, there was no overlap in herbs among the five studies; each herb was used only once. Herbs included *bai mao gen* 白茅根, *bian xu* 萹蓄, *chai hu* 柴胡, *che qian zi* 车前子, *da huang* 大黄, *da zao* 大枣, *gan cao shao* 甘草梢, *hai jin sha* 海金沙, *hua sheng yi* 花生衣, *hua shi* 滑石, *huang qin* 黄芩, *jin gang chi* 金刚刺, *jin ying gen* 主要由, *qu mai* 瞿麦, *zhi zi* 山栀 and *shi wei* 石韦.

Safety of Oral Chinese Herbal Medicine in Non-controlled Studies for Acute Urinary Tract Infection

One study (H64) reported nine cases of diarrhoea or indigestion.

Persistent Urinary Tract Infection

Fifty-three studies (H68–H120) evaluated the effectiveness of CHM in people with persistent UTI. The majority of studies tested oral CHM

(52 studies) and one study (H120) tested the combination of oral plus topical CHM.

Randomised Controlled Trials of Oral Chinese Herbal Medicine for Persistent Urinary Tract Infection

Thirty-nine RCTs (H68–H106), involving 3,297 participants with persistent UTI, evaluated the effect of oral CHM on clinical outcomes. The majority of studies included participants with an acute infection at the time of randomisation. Two studies included three arms; one study (H105) compared oral CHM alone and oral CHM combined with antibiotics with antibiotics alone, and the second (H106) included two intervention arms with different formulas. All studies were conducted in China. In studies that specified the setting, participants were recruited from hospital inpatient and/or outpatient departments.

Participants had lived with persistent UTI for at least six months in most studies. The longest duration was 31 years (H73). Thirteen studies (H69, H74, H81, H82, H85, H90, H93, H94, H100, H102–H105) focused on women with persistent UTI. The remaining studies either included both females and males or did not provide this information. The site of infection was the upper urinary tract in 19 studies (H68, H69, H72, H74, H75, H79, H80, H83, H88–H91, H93, H94, H97–H99, H104, H105), both the upper and lower urinary tract in three studies (H73, H78, H87), and was not reported in 17 studies (H70, H71, H76, H77, H81, H82, H84–H86, H92, H95, H96, H100–H103, H106).

Treatment duration was as few as ten days (H106) to as long as six months (H94, H97); the median duration of treatment was six weeks. Follow-up assessment was conducted in 28 studies (H68–H70, H72, H76–H78, H80, H81, H84–H86, H88–H90, H92–H94, H96–H98, H100–H106). Assessment was conducted between two weeks (H100) and two years (H102, H103) after the end of treatment, with most studies conducting follow-up assessments at six months.

Chinese medicine syndromes were used as inclusion criteria in 14 studies (H68, H72–H74, H83, H87, H88, H95, H96, H99, H102,

H104–H106) and were used to guide treatment in 16 studies (H70, H72, H74, H76–H78, H81, H90, H98–H105). Syndromes included Spleen and Kidney deficiency syndrome (five RCTs), Kidney deficiency and damp-heat (four RCTs), Liver and Kidney *yin* deficiency (two RCTs), damp-heat in the Lower Energiser (two RCTs), Spleen and Kidney dual deficiency of *qi* and Blood (two RCTs), *yin* deficiency and damp-heat (two RCTs), and retention of damp-heat (two RCTs).

Nineteen studies compared oral CHM with antibiotics alone (H69, H71–H74, H79, H84, H85, H87, H89, H90, H96, H99, H101, H104–H106) or combined with other treatments, such as potassium permanganate topical wash (H98) and sodium bicarbonate tablets (H68). Twenty-one studies (H70, H75–H78, H80–H83, H86, H88, H91–H95, H97, H100, H102, H103, H105) evaluated the combination of oral CHM with antibiotics. Six studies tested formulas developed by the trial investigator, and these were excluded from frequency analysis of formulas. Thirty different oral CHM formulas were described in the 39 RCTs, although only four formulas were evaluated in two or more studies (Table 5.23).

Table 5.23. Frequently Reported Oral Formulas in Randomised Controlled Trials for Persistent Urinary Tract Infection

Most Common Formulas	No. of Studies	Ingredients
Ba zheng san 八正散	3	*Che qian zi* 车前子, *qu mai* 瞿麦, *bian xu* 萹蓄, *hua shi* 滑石, *zhi zi* 栀子, *gan cao* 甘草, *mu tong* 木通 and *da huang* 大黄.
Yi shen xie zhuo hua yu tang 益肾泄浊化瘀汤	3	Variant 1: *Yi yi ren* 薏苡仁, *bai jiang cao* 败酱草, *dan shen* 丹参, *shan yao* 山药, *sheng di huang* 生地黄, *shu di huang* 熟地黄, *xian ling pi* 仙灵脾, *fen bi xie* 粉萆薢, *nv zhen zi* 女贞子, *shan yu rou* 山萸肉 and *hu zhang* 虎杖 (H70, H78).
		Variant 2: *Bai jiang cao* 败酱草, *yi yi ren* 生薏苡仁, *dan shen* 丹参, *shan yao* 怀山药, *xian ling pi* 仙灵脾,

(Continued)

133

5.23. **(Continued)**

Most Common Formulas	No. of Studies	Ingredients
		sheng di huang 生地黄, *shu di huang* 熟地黄 and *bi xie* 萆薢 (H76).
Zhi bai di huang tang 知柏地黄汤	2	*Shu di huang* 熟地黄, *shan zhu yu* 山茱萸, *huai shan yao* 淮山药, *fu ling* 茯苓, *mu dan pi* 牡丹皮, *ze xie* 泽泻, *huang bai* 黄柏, *zhi mu* 知母, *bian xu* 萹蓄, *qu mai* 瞿麦, *che qian zi* 车前子, *hua shi* 滑石 and *sheng gan cao* 生甘草 (H72, H105).
Zi shen qing gan tong lin tang 滋肾清肝通淋汤	2	*Shan zhi zi* 山栀子, *bai mao gen* 白茅根, *sheng gan cao* 生甘草, *chai hu* 柴胡, *che qian zi* 车前子, *sheng di huang* 生地黄, *deng xin cao* 灯心草, *huang qin* 黄芩, *tu fu ling* 土茯苓 and *bai shao* 白芍 (H84, H86).

Ingredients are referenced to the original studies where possible. If herb ingredients varied across studies, the herb ingredients were sourced from *Zhong Yi Fang Ji Da Ci Dian* 中医方剂大辞典.

The use of some herbs may be restricted in some countries. Readers are advised to comply with relevant regulations.

The most frequently used formulas were *Ba zheng san* 八正散 and *Yi shen xie zhuo hua yu tang* 益肾泄浊化瘀汤, used in three studies each. Many different herbs were used in the 39 RCTs; in total 108 different herbs were described. The most frequently reported herbs were *gan cao* 甘草, *sheng di huang* 生地黄, *fu ling* 茯苓 and *shan yao* 山药 (Table 5.24).

Risk of Bias

All RCTs involving adults with persistent UTI were described as using random allocation, but more than half of the studies (27 RCTs, 69.2%; H68, H72–H78, H81–H86, H89–H98, H100, H104, H105) did not provide a description of the method used (Table 5.25). One study (H83) described using sealed envelopes to conceal group allocation and was judged to pose 'low' risk of bias. All but one (H74) of

Table 5.24. Frequently Reported Orally Used Herbs in Randomised Controlled Trials for Persistent Urinary Tract Infection

Most Common Herbs	Scientific Name	Frequency of Use
Gan cao 甘草	*Glycyrrhiza* spp.	18
Sheng di huang 生地黄	*Rehmannia glutinosa* Libosch.	18
Fu ling 茯苓	*Poria cocos* (Schw.) Wolf	17
Shan yao 山药	*Dioscorea opposita* Thunb.	16
Che qian zi 车前子	*Plantago* spp.	11
Huang bai 黄柏	*Phellodendron chinense* Schneid.	11
Huang qi 黄芪	*Astragalus membranaceus* (Fisch.) Bge.	11
Shan zhu yu 山茱萸	*Cornus officinalis* Sieb. et Zucc.	11
Bai mao gen 白茅根	*Imperata cylindrica* Beauv. var. major (Nees) C. E. Hubb.	10
Dan shen 丹参	*Salvia miltiorrhiza* Bge.	9
Pu gong ying 蒲公英	*Taraxacum* spp.	9
Hua shi 滑石	Hydrated magnesium silicate	8
Qu mai 瞿麦	*Dianthus* spp.	8
Shu di huang 熟地黄	*Rehmannia glutinosa* Libosch.	8
Tu fu ling 土茯苓	*Smilax glabra* Roxb.	8
Ze xie 泽泻	*Alisma orientalis* (Sam.) Juzep.	8
Mu dan pi 牡丹皮	*Paeonia suffruticosa* Andr.	7

The use of some herbs may be restricted in some countries. Readers are advised to comply with relevant regulations.

Table 5.25. Risk of Bias of Randomised Controlled Trials for Persistent Urinary Tract Infection: Oral Chinese Herbal Medicine

Risk of Bias Domain	Low Risk n (%)	Unclear Risk n (%)	High Risk n (%)
Sequence generation	12 (30.8)	27 (69.2)	0 (0)
Allocation concealment	1 (2.6)	38 (97.4)	0 (0)
Blinding of participants	0 (0)	1 (2.6)	38 (97.4)
Blinding of personnel	0 (0)	1 (2.6)	38 (97.4)
Blinding of outcome assessors	0 (0)	39 (100)	0 (0)
Incomplete outcome data	36 (92.3)	2 (5.1)	1 (2.6)
Selective outcome reporting	0 (0)	39 (100)	0 (0)

the RCTs lacked blinding of participants and personnel and were judged 'high' risk for these domains. None of the studies provided information about blinding of outcome assessors. Thirty-six (H68–H73, H75–H100, H102–H105) of the 39 studies analysed data for all included participants, posing 'low' risk of bias. Two studies (H74, H101) reported loss to follow-up but did not state the group allocation of withdrawals; these studies were judged as 'unclear' risk of bias. The number of withdrawals in one study (H106) was greater than 15%; this study was judged as 'high' risk for the domain incomplete outcome data. All studies were judged 'unclear' risk for selective outcome reporting as no trial protocols or trial registrations were identified.

Outcomes

The most frequently reported outcome was composite cure, which was reported in 34 studies. Nineteen studies assessed UTI recurrence; two measured duration of urinary symptoms; one measured the number of people with microbiologically positive urine culture; two reported levels of serum creatinine; eight measured levels of urinary β2-MG; ten RCTs reported on safety. Some studies reported results incompletely, thus the results are presented for data that were able to be analysed.

Composite Cure

All 34 studies that assessed cure used a composite measure of resolution of symptoms and biological tests. Fifteen studies (H68, H69, H71–H73, H79, H84, H87, H89, H90, H96, H98, H99, H101, H105) that reported composite cure compared oral CHM with pharmacotherapy, and 20 studies (H70, H75–H78, H80, H82, H83, H86, H88, H91–H95, H97, H100, H102, H103, H105) tested the combination of oral CHM with pharmacotherapy compared to pharmacotherapy alone. All studies used antibiotics as the comparator, with three studies using antibiotics in combination with sodium bicarbonate (H68, H94), potassium permanganate solution (H98) or dietary advice (H94).

Oral Chinese herbal medicine versus antibiotics

Fifteen studies reported composite cure, with eight RCTs (H71–H73, H79, H96, H99, H101, H105) measuring short-term cure (six weeks or less) and seven RCTs (H68, H69, H84, H87, H89, H90, H98) measuring long-term cure (six months or more). The chance of achieving a composite cure was greater with oral CHM than with antibiotics (667 participants, RR 1.68 [1.39, 2.03], I^2 = 11%; Table 5.26). Subgroup analysis showed that people with an upper UTI also received benefit with oral CHM over antibiotics (243 participants, RR 1.54 [1.16, 2.03], I^2 = 0%), while one study that included people with upper or lower UTI showed no such benefit. One study included only women with persistent UTI, and women who received oral CHM were no more or less likely to achieve a cure than women who received antibiotics (35 women, RR 1.32 [0.43, 4.12]). In two studies that tested the combination of *Zhi bai di huang wan* 知柏地黄汤 plus *Ba zheng san* 八正散, there was no difference between CHM and antibiotics (95 participants, RR 1.65 [0.66, 4.13], I^2 = 0%; Table 5.26).

Table 5.26. Oral Chinese Herbal Medicine versus Antibiotics for Persistent Urinary Tract Infection: Short-term Cure

Assessment	No. of Studies (Participants)	Effect Size (RR [95% CI], I^2)	Included Studies
All studies	8 (667)	1.68 [1.39, 2.03]*, 11%	H71–H73, H79, H96, H99, H101, H105
Subgroup analyses			
Upper UTI	4 (243)	1.54 [1.16, 2.03]*, 0%	H72, H79, H99, H105
Both upper and lower UTI	1 (60)	1.44 [0.73, 2.86], NA	H73
Infection site NS	3 (364)	1.79 [1.18, 2.72]*, 65%	H71, H96, H101
Females	1 (35)	1.32 [0.43, 4.12], NA	H105

(Continued)

Table 5.26. (*Continued*)

Assessment	No. of Studies (Participants)	Effect Size (RR [95% CI], I²)	Included Studies
Both females and males	7 (632)	1.69 [1.37, 2.08]*, 22%	H71–H73, H79, H96, H99, H101
Zhi bai di huang tang 知柏地黄汤 plus *Ba zheng san* 八正散	2 (95)	1.65 [0.66, 4.13], 0%	H72, H105

*Statistically significant, see Chapter 4.
Abbreviations: CI, confidence interval; NA, not applicable; NS, not specified; RR, risk ratio; UTI, urinary tract infection.

Table 5.27.   Oral Chinese Herbal Medicine versus Pharmacotherapy for Persistent Urinary Tract Infection: Long-term Cure

Assessment	No. of Studies (Participants)	Effect Size (RR [95% CI], I²)	Included Studies
All studies	7 (592)	1.87 [1.50, 2.32]*, 0%	H68, H69, H84, H87, H89, H90, H98
Subgroup analyses			
Upper UTI	5 (439)	2.37 [1.71, 3.29]*, 0%	H68, H69, H89, H90, H98
Both upper and lower UTI	1 (73)	1.64 [1.04, 2.59]*, NA	H87
Infection site NS	1 (80)	1.47 [1.00, 2.16]#, NA	H84
Females	2 (146)	1.97 [1.20, 3.26]*, 0%	H69, H90
Both females and males	5 (446)	1.91 [1.41, 2.58]*, 26%	H68, H84, H87, H89, H98

*Statistically significant, see Chapter 4. #p = 0.05.
Abbreviations: CI, confidence interval; NA, not applicable; NS, not specified; RR, risk ratio; UTI, urinary tract infection.

Seven studies (H68, H69, H84, H87, H89, H90, H98) that assessed long-term cure used antibiotics alone or combined with other treatments. Oral CHM was more effective than antibiotics in achieving long-term cure, assessed six or more months after the end of treatment (592 participants, RR 1.87 [1.50, 2.32], I² = 0%; Table 5.27). Benefit with oral CHM was seen in studies where infection was in the upper urinary tract (439 participants, RR 2.37 [1.71, 3.29], I^2 = 0%), or in either the upper or lower urinary tract (73 participants, RR 1.64 [1.04, 2.59]). Women who received oral CHM were more likely to achieve a composite cure than women who received pharmacotherapy (146 participants, RR 1.97 [1.20, 3.26], I^2 = 0%).

Oral Chinese herbal medicine plus pharmacotherapy versus pharmacotherapy alone

Twenty RCTs that tested the combination of oral CHM with pharmacotherapy reported composite cure. Eleven studies (H75, H77, H82, H91–H93, H95, H100, H102, H103, H105) assessed short-term cure, three studies (H80, H83, H88) assessed medium-term cure (between six weeks and six months) and six studies (H70, H76, H78, H86, H94, H97) assessed long-term cure. The combination of oral CHM with antibiotics improved chances of achieving a short-term cure compared with antibiotics alone (735 participants, RR 1.30 [1.11, 1.52], I^2 = 0%; Table 5.28). Similar benefits were seen in subgroup analyses of studies where the infection was in the upper urinary tract (205 participants, RR 1.47 [1.04, 2.09], I^2 = 0%) and in studies that did not specify the site of infection (350 participants, RR 1.26 [1.06, 1.50], I^2 = 0%). There was a trend towards significance in studies that included women with persistent UTI (346 women, RR 1.23 [1.00, 1.51], p = 0.05, I^2 = 0%). The result favoured the combination of oral CHM and pharmacotherapy in studies that included both males and females (341 participants, RR 1.52 [1.09, 2.10], I^2 = 28%).

Three RCTs (H80, H83, H88) assessed composite cure between six weeks and six months. All studies included participants with upper UTI. Meta-analysis of these studies showed that the combination of oral CHM with antibiotics increased the chance of achieving a composite cure more than antibiotics alone (368 participants, RR 1.45 [1.05, 2.00], I^2 = 0%).

In six studies that assessed cure after six months or more, the chance of achieving a cure was greater in participants who received oral CHM plus pharmacotherapy, than in participants who received

Table 5.28. **Oral Chinese Herbal Medicine plus Antibiotics versus Antibiotics Alone for Persistent Urinary Tract Infection: Short-term Cure**

Assessment	No. of Studies (Participants)	Effect Size (RR [95% CI], I²)	Included Studies
All studies	11 (735)	1.30 [1.11, 1.52]*, 0%	H75, H77, H82, H91, H92, H93, H95, H100, H102, H103, H105
Subgroup analyses			
Upper UTI	4 (205)	1.47 [1.04, 2.09]*, 0%	H75, H91, H93, H105
Infection site NS	7 (530)	1.26 [1.06, 1.50]*, 0%	H77, H82, H92, H95, H100, H102, H103
Females	5 (346)	1.23 [1.00, 1.51]ⁱ, 0%	H82, H93, H100, H102, H103
Both females and males	5 (341)	1.52 [1.09, 2.10]*, 28%	H75, H91, H92, H95, H105
Gender NS	1 (48)	1.08 [0.63, 1.87], NA	H77

*Statistically significant, ⁱp = 0.05, see Chapter 4.
Abbreviations: CI, confidence interval; NA, not applicable; NS, not specified; RR, risk ratio; UTI, urinary tract infection.

pharmacotherapy alone (470 participants, RR 1.49 [1.24, 1.79], I^2 = 0%; Table 5.29). In subgroup meta-analyses, studies that included people with an upper UTI (148 participants, RR 1.87 [1.19, 2.92], I^2 = 0%) and studies that did not specify the site of infection (252 participants, RR 1.40 [1.11, 1.78], I^2 = 0%) also favoured the combination of oral CHM with pharmacotherapy. In one study, women who received oral CHM plus pharmacotherapy fared no better or worse than those who received pharmacotherapy alone (90 women, RR 1.63 [0.75, 3.54]). Three studies that tested *Yi shen xie zhuo hua yu tang* 益肾泄浊化瘀汤 plus antibiotics found the combination to be superior to antibiotics alone (262 participants, RR 1.41 [1.12, 1.77], I^2 = 0%).

Recurrence

Nineteen studies (H69, H70, H72, H76–H78, H80, H81, H85, H88, H93, H96, H100–H106) assessed UTI recurrence. Fifteen of these studies assessed recurrence in all participants, including

Table 5.29. Oral Chinese Herbal Medicine plus Pharmacotherapy versus Pharmacotherapy Alone for Persistent Urinary Tract Infection: Long-term Cure

Assessment	No. of Studies (Participants)	Effect Size (RR [95% CI], I²)	Included Studies
All studies	6 (470)	1.49 [1.24, 1.79]*, 0%	H70, H76, H78, H86, H94, H97
Subgroup analyses			
Upper UTI	2 (148)	1.87 [1.19, 2.92]*, 0%	H94, H97
Both upper and lower UTI	1 (72)	1.47 [0.98, 2.21], NA	H78
Infection site NS	3 (252)	1.40 [1.11, 1.78]*, 0%	H70, H76, H86
Females	1 (90)	1.63 [0.75, 3.54], NA	H94
Both females and males	5 (380)	1.48 [1.22, 1.79]*, 0%	H70, H76, H78, H86, H97
Yi shen xie zhuo hua yu tang 益肾泄浊化瘀汤	3 (262)	1.41 [1.12, 1.77]*, 0%	H70, H76, H78

*Statistically significant, see Chapter 4.
Abbreviations: CI, confidence interval; NA, not applicable; NS, not specified; RR, risk ratio; UTI, urinary tract infection.

those who did not achieve a cure, or in a subset of participants who achieved some improvement in symptoms. Data from these studies were not analysed. Two studies included participants with persistent UTI who were in remission at the time of randomisation. Data for recurrence in all participants was assessed, and these data were included in analyses. Findings from studies that reported recurrence in patients who achieved a cure at the end of treatment are also described.

Oral Chinese herbal medicine versus antibiotics

Three studies that compared oral CHM with antibiotics assessed recurrence at six months in women who were in remission at the time of randomisation (H85, H104), or in women who achieved a composite cure at the end of treatment (H69). Meta-analysis of recurrence in 261 women in remission at trial onset favoured oral CHM over antibiotics (RR 0.55 [0.43, 0.71], I^2 = 1%). One study that assessed recurrence in people who achieved a cure after treatment found no such benefit (20 women, RR 0.29 [0.06, 1.30]).

Oral Chinese herbal medicine plus antibiotics versus antibiotics alone

Three studies (H80, H100, H102) that tested the combination of oral CHM plus antibiotics assessed recurrence in participants who achieved a cure at the end of treatment. Recurrence was assessed at different time points which prevented meta-analysis. Results from individual studies showed oral CHM as integrative medicine with antibiotics reduced the risk of recurrence at 12 weeks (40 participants, RR 0.40 [9.18, 0.93]; H80) and at two years (29 women, RR 0.61 [0.40, 0.91]; H102). No such benefit was seen in one study when recurrence was assessed at six months (38 women, RR 0.24 [9.06, 1.05]; H100).

Duration of Symptoms

One study involving 198 people with persistent UTI assessed the duration of all urinary symptoms (H96). People who received the oral formula *Jian pi yi shen tong lin tang* 健脾益肾通淋汤 reported resolution of urinary symptoms 2.1 days earlier than those who received norfloxacin ([−2.65, −1.55]).

Microbiologically Positive Urine Culture

The number of people with a positive urine culture at the end of treatment was lower among people who received *Jian pi yi shen tong lin tang* 健脾益肾通淋汤 than in those who received norfloxacin (RR 0.17 [0.09, 0.32]; H96).

Serum Creatinine

Serum creatinine was assessed in two studies (H80, H88) that evaluated oral CHM as integrative medicine with antibiotics plus other treatments. Meta-analysis of results from 308 participants showed serum creatinine to be lower among people who received oral CHM as integrative medicine with antibiotics plus other treatments (MD −29.45 [−58.50, −0.40], I^2 = 95%). While both studies showed benefit individually, the magnitude of the treatment effect varied and there was no overlap in the confidence intervals, which is reflected in the considerable levels of statistical heterogeneity.

Urinary Beta-2 Microglobulin

Seven RCTs reported results for urinary β2-MG that were able to be analysed. Four of the seven studies (H69, H74, H79, H90) compared oral CHM with antibiotics and three (H80, H88, H94) evaluated oral CHM as integrative medicine.

Oral Chinese herbal medicine versus antibiotics

Three of the four studies (H69, H74, H90) reported results in mg/L and one study (H79) reported results in international units (IU). Results were analysed separately. Meta-analysis showed urinary β2-MG was 0.07 mg/L lower in people who received oral CHM compared to antibiotics (204 women, [−0.09, −0.05], I^2 = 0%). Findings from one RCT showed that urinary β2-MG was also lower when measured in IU (MD −0.10 [−0.13, −0.07]).

Oral Chinese herbal medicine plus antibiotics versus antibiotics alone

Three studies (H80, H88, H94) measured urinary β2-MG in people with persistent UTI. All studies included participants with upper UTI. The mean β2-MG at the end of treatment was 0.12 mg/L lower in people who received oral CHM as integrative medicine with antibiotics (398 participants,

[–0.19, –0.04], I^2 = 97%). Subgroup analyses showed results favouring oral CHM as integrative medicine in 90 women (MD –0.22 [–0.26, –0.18]; H94) and in studies that included both men and women (308 participants, MD –0.06 [–0.09, –0.04], I^2 = 71%; H80, H88).

Assessment Using Grading of Recommendations, Assessment, Development and Evaluation: Persistent Urinary Tract Infection

The approach for selecting comparisons for GRADE assessment has been outlined in the section 'Acute Urinary Tract Infection'. The GRADE assessment was conducted for studies that compared oral CHM with antibiotics, and studies that compared oral CHM plus antibiotics with antibiotics alone. The GRADE tables were planned for the formulas *Ba zheng san* 八正散 (alone or as integrative medicine) and *San jin pian* 三金片 (alone or as integrative medicine); however, no studies of these comparisons reported on the outcomes selected by expert consensus.

Oral Chinese Herbal Medicine versus Antibiotics for Persistent Urinary Tract Infection

Thirteen studies (H69, H71–H73, H79, H84, H87, H89, H90, H96, H99, H101, H105), that compared oral CHM with antibiotics, reported on the outcomes: composite cure, recurrence, duration of urinary symptoms and adverse events. Based on 'moderate' certainty evidence, oral CHM was probably more effective than antibiotics in increasing the number of people who achieved short-term cure (Table 5.30). Evidence for long-term cure was 'low' certainty and showed oral CHM may be superior to antibiotics. Based on 'low' certainty evidence from one study, oral CHM may lead to little, or no, change in the chance of recurrence of UTI compared to antibiotics. Oral CHM may reduce the duration of urinary symptoms by 2.1 days ('low' certainty evidence from one study). Safety was reported in five RCTs, with three RCTs (H71, H72, H99) reporting that no adverse events occurred during the trial. Seven adverse events were reported

Table 5.30. GRADE: Oral Chinese Herbal Medicine versus Antibiotics for Persistent Urinary Tract Infection

Outcome	Absolute Effect		Relative effect (95% CI) No. of Participants (Studies)	Certainty of the Evidence (GRADE)
	With Oral CHM	With Antibiotics		
Short-term cure, treatment duration: 2 w to 42 d	**55 per 100** Difference: 22 more per 100 patients (95% CI: 13 to 34 more per 100 patients)	**33 per 100**	**RR 1.68*** (1.39 to 2.03) 667 (8 RCTs)	⊕⊕⊕◯ MODERATE[a]
Long-term cure, treatment duration: 2 w to 12 w	**48 per 100** Difference: 19 more per 100 patients (95% CI: 8 to 33 more per 100 patients)	**29 per 100**	**RR 1.66*** (1.29 to 2.13) 359 (5 RCTs)	⊕⊕◯◯ LOW[a,b]
Recurrence at 6 months, treatment duration: 12 w	**14 per 100** Difference: 36 fewer per 100 patients (95% CI: 47 fewer to 15 more per 100 patients)	**50 per 100**	**RR 0.29** (0.06 to 1.30) 20 (1 RCT)	⊕⊕◯◯ LOW[a,b]
Duration of urinary symptoms, treatment duration: 6 w	**10.2 days** Average difference: 2.1 days lower (95% CI: 2.65 to 1.55 days lower)	**12.3 days**	**MD −2.1*** (−2.65 to −1.55) 198 (1 RCT)	⊕⊕◯◯ LOW[a,b]

*Statistically significant result.

Abbreviations: CI, confidence interval; d, days; GRADE, Grading of Recommendations Assessment, Development and Evaluation; MD, mean difference; RCT, randomised controlled trial; RR, risk ratio; w, weeks.

Notes
[a] High risk of bias due to lack of blinding of participants and personnel.
[b] Small sample size.

Study references
Short-term cure: H71–H73, H79, H96, H99, H101, H105.
Long-term cure: H69, H84, H87, H89, H90.
Recurrence at 6 months: H69.
Duration of urinary symptoms: H96.

in the remaining two RCTs (H96, H106). Adverse events with oral CHM were five cases of increased frequency of bowel movements that resolved after three days. Two cases of mild gastrointestinal discomfort were reported among people who received antibiotics.

Oral Chinese Herbal Medicine plus Antibiotics versus Antibiotics Alone for Persistent Urinary Tract Infection

The certainty of evidence for the comparison oral CHM plus antibiotics versus antibiotics was 'low' (Table 5.31). Adding oral CHM to

Table 5.31. GRADE: Oral Chinese Herbal Medicine plus Antibiotics versus Antibiotics Alone for Persistent Urinary Tract Infection

Outcome	Absolute Effect		Relative Effect (95% CI) No. of Participants (Studies)	Certainty of the Evidence (GRADE)
	With Oral CHM IM	With Antibiotics		
Short-term cure, treatment duration: 3 d to 35 d	**51 per 100**	**39 per 100**	**RR 1.30***	⊕⊕◯◯
	Difference: 12 more per 100 patients (95% CI: 4 to 21 more per 100 patients)		(1.11 to 1.52) 735 (11 RCTs)	LOW^a,b
Medium-term cure, treatment duration: 12 w to 6 m	**33 per 100**	**23 per 100**	**RR 1.45***	⊕⊕◯◯
	Difference: 10 more per 100 patients (95% CI: 1 to 23 more per 100 patients)		(1.05 to 2.00) 368 (3 RCTs)	LOW^a,c
Long-term cure, treatment duration: 2 w to 6 m	**64 per 100**	**43 per 100**	**RR 1.48***	⊕⊕◯◯
	Difference: 21 more per 100 patients (95% CI: 9 to 34 more per 100 patients)		(1.22 to 1.79) 380 (5 RCTs)	LOW^a,c
Recurrence at 12 w, treatment duration: 12 w	**23 per 100**	**57 per 100**	**RR 0.40***	⊕⊕◯◯
	Difference: 34 fewer per 100 patients (95% CI: 47 to 4 fewer per 100 patients)		(0.18 to 0.93) 40 (1 RCT)	LOW^a,c

Table 5.31. (*Continued*)

Outcome	Absolute Effect		Relative Effect (95% CI) No. of Participants (Studies)	Certainty of the Evidence (GRADE)
	With Oral CHM IM	With Antibiotics		
Recurrence at 6 m, treatment duration: 2 w	**9 per 100**	**38 per 100**	**RR 0.24**	⊕⊕◯◯
	Difference: 29 fewer per 100 patients (95% CI: 35 fewer to 2 more per 100 patients)		(0.06 to 1.05) 38 (1 RCT)	LOW[a,c]
Recurrence at 2 y, treatment duration: 6 w	**61 per 100**	**100 per 100**	**RR 0.61***	⊕⊕◯◯
	Difference: 39 fewer per 100 patients (95% CI: 60 to 9 fewer per 100 patients)		(0.40 to 0.91) 29 (1 RCT)	LOW[a,c]

*Statistically significant result.

Abbreviations: CHM, Chinese herbal medicine; CI, confidence interval; d, days; GRADE, Grading of Recommendations Assessment, Development and Evaluation; IM, integrative medicine; m, months; RCT, randomised controlled trial; RR, risk ratio; w, weeks; y, years.

Notes
[a]High risk of bias due to lack of blinding of participants and personnel.
[b]Publication bias suspected.
[c]Small sample size.

Study references
Short-term cure: H75, H77, H82, H91–H93, H95, H100, H102, H103, H105.
Medium-term cure: H80, H83, H88.
Long-term cure: H70, H76, H78, H86, H97.
Recurrence at 12 weeks: H80.
Recurrence at 6 months: H100.
Recurrence at 2 years: H102.

antibiotic therapy may increase the chance of a short-, medium- or long-term cure, and may increase the chance of recurrence assessed at 12 weeks and at two years. The combination of oral CHM plus antibiotics may lead to little, or no, difference in recurrence at six months compared with antibiotics alone. Five studies reported safety, with no adverse events occurring in two RCTS (H70, H103). Three RCTs (H86, H92, H97) reported adverse events in both the treatment and control groups. Nine adverse events in people who received both oral CHM and antibiotics included gastrointestinal discomfort (five cases), nausea (two cases) and one case each of vomiting and mild diarrhoea. Sixteen adverse events were reported in people who received antibiotics. These included vomiting (five cases), gastrointestinal discomfort (four cases), nausea (three cases), mild diarrhoea (two cases) and rash (two cases).

Randomised Controlled Trial Evidence for Individual Oral Formulas for Persistent Urinary Tract Infection

Meta-analysis was possible for two formulas that measured clinical outcomes for people with persistent UTI. The combination of *Zhi bai di huang wan* 知柏地黄汤 and *Ba zheng san* 八正散 was not statistically different to antibiotics in increasing the number of people achieving a short-term cure (95 participants, RR 1.65 [0.66, 4.13], I^2 = 0%; H72, H105). When *Yi shen xie zhuo hua yu tang* 益肾泄浊化瘀汤 was used in combination with antibiotics, the combination increased the chance of a long-term cure more than antibiotics alone (262 participants, RR 1.41 [1.12, 1.77], I^2 = 0%; H70, H76, H78).

Frequently Reported Orally Used Herbs in Meta-analyses Showing Favourable Effect for Persistent Urinary Tract Infection

Studies of oral CHM for persistent UTI have shown benefit in increasing the number of people achieving a composite cure, reducing recurrence and duration of urinary symptoms, and improving results of biological tests. Herb ingredients were analysed to identify which herbs may be contributing to the effects seen in positive meta-analyses (Table 5.32). Five meta-analyses, involving 34 studies, showed positive benefits of oral CHM used alone, or with antibiotics, in terms of composite cure. The herbs most frequently described in these analyses are similar to the herbs used in all studies, given that most studies reported composite cure. Herbs such as *gan cao* 甘草, *fu ling* 茯苓, *sheng di huang* 生地黄 and *shan yao* 山药 may contribute to the positive results seen for composite cure.

Table 5.32. Frequently Reported Orally Used Herbs in Meta-Analyses Showing Favourable Effect for Persistent Urinary Tract Infection

Herbs	Scientific Name	Frequency of Use
Composite cure: five meta-analyses, 34 studies		
Gan cao 甘草	*Glycyrrhiza* spp.	18
Fu ling 茯苓	*Poria cocos* (Schw.) Wolf	17
Sheng di huang 生地黄	*Rehmannia glutinosa* Libosch.	17
Shan yao 山药	*Dioscorea opposita* Thunb.	16
Che qian zi 车前子	*Plantago* spp.	11
Shan zhu yu 山茱萸	*Cornus officinalis* Sieb. et Zucc.	11
Bai mao gen 白茅根	*Imperata cylindrica* Beauv. var. major (Nees) C. E. Hubb.	10
Huang qi 黄芪	*Astragalus membranaceus* (Fisch.) Bge.	10
Huang bai 黄柏	*Phellodendron chinense* Schneid.	9
Biological tests: three meta-analyses, six studies		
Dan shen 丹参	*Salvia miltiorrhiza* Bge.	3
Fu ling 茯苓	*Poria cocos* (Schw.) Wolf	3
Huang qi 黄芪	*Astragalus membranaceus* (Fisch.) Bge.	3
Niu xi 牛膝	*Achyranthes bidentata* Bl.	3
Shan yao 山药	*Dioscorea opposita* Thunb.	2
Shan zhu yu 山茱萸	*Cornus officinalis* Sieb. et Zucc.	2
Shu di huang 熟地黄	*Rehmannia glutinosa* Libosch.	2
Tai zi shen 太子参	*Pseudostellaria heterophylla* (Miq.) Pax ex Pax et Hoffm.	2
Yi yi ren 薏苡仁	*Coix lacryma-jobi* L. var. mayuen (Roman.) Stapf	2

Composite cure: refer to Tables 5.26, 5.27, 5.28, 5.29, section 'Oral Chinese Herbal Medicine plus Antibiotics versus Antibiotics Alone' (pp. 139–140).
Biological tests: refer to sections 'Serum Creatinine' (p. 143) and 'Urinary Beta-2 Microglobulin' (pp. 143–144).

One meta-analysis showed benefit of oral CHM over antibiotics for reducing recurrence. Meta-analysis included two RCTs, but each study used different herbs. As such, no suggestions about the herbs which may have contributed to effects can be made. Biological tests for which meta-analysis results favoured oral CHM included serum creatinine and urinary β2-MG. Analysis of the six RCTs included in these meta-analyses showed that *dan shen* 丹参, *fu ling* 茯苓, *huang qi* 黄芪 and *niu xi* 牛膝 were the most frequently used herbs, used in three studies each. These herbs may contribute to improving results of biological tests.

Safety of Oral Chinese Herbal Medicine in Randomised Controlled Trials for Persistent Urinary Tract Infection

Ten RCTs (H70–H72, H86, H92, H96, H97, H99, H103, H106) reported on safety of oral CHM in people with persistent UTI. Five RCTs (H70, H71, H72, H99, H103) reported that no adverse events occurred. Adverse events among participants who received oral CHM alone included five cases of increased frequency of bowel motions in the first three days that resolved spontaneously. Adverse events among participants who received oral CHM and antibiotics included five cases of gastrointestinal discomfort, two cases of nausea, one case of vomiting and one case of mild diarrhoea. Adverse events in the antibiotics group included six cases of gastrointestinal discomfort, five cases of vomiting, three cases of nausea, two cases of mild diarrhoea and two cases of rash.

Controlled Clinical Trials of Oral Chinese Herbal Medicine for Persistent Urinary Tract Infection

Six CCTs (H107–H112), involving 1,104 participants, tested the effectiveness of oral CHM in people with persistent UTI. All were two-arm trials that compared oral CHM alone (H107, H110, H111) or as integrative medicine (H108, H109, H112) with antibiotics. Studies were conducted in mainland China and recruited participants from hospital inpatient and outpatient departments. The duration of persistent UTI ranged from six months in one study (H112) to 31 years in another (H107), although an infection for 31 years seems unlikely. Four studies (H108, H109, H110, H112) included participants with infections of the upper urinary tract, one (H107) included participants with lower UTI and one (H111) included participants with pyelonephritis and cystitis.

Treatment was provided for between two weeks (H112) and two months (H108); the median treatment duration was two weeks. All but one study (H110) conducted follow-up assessment six months after the end of treatment. One study (H109) used CM syndrome differentiation as an inclusion criterion, which included the syndrome Kidney *yin* deficiency. A second study used CM principles (H111) to determine treatment, although details for this were not described. All studies used different oral CHM formulas. The most frequently used herbs were *fu ling* 茯苓, *bai hua she she cao* 白花蛇舌草, *bai zhu* 白术, *che qian cao* 车前草, *shan yao* 山药 and *sheng di huang* 生地黄 (Table 5.33).

Table 5.33. Frequently Reported Orally Used Herbs in Controlled Clinical Trials for Persistent Urinary Tract Infection

Most Common Herbs	Scientific Name	Frequency of Use
Fu ling 茯苓	*Poria cocos* (Schw.) Wolf	4
Bai hua she she cao 白花蛇舌草	*Hedyotis diffusa* Willd.	3
Bai zhu 白术	*Atractylodes macrocephala* Koidz.	3
Che qian cao 车前草	*Plantago* spp.	3
Shan yao 山药	*Dioscorea opposita* Thunb.	3
Sheng di huang 生地黄	*Rehmannia glutinosa* Libosch.	3
Bai mao gen 白茅根	*Imperata cylindrica* Beauv. var. major (Nees) C. E. Hubb.	2
Du zhong 杜仲	*Eucommia ulmoides* Oliv.	2
Gan cao 甘草	*Glycyrrhiza* spp.	2
Huang bai 黄柏	*Phellodendron chinense* Schneid.	2
Huang qi 黄芪	*Astragalus membranaceus* (Fisch.) Bge.	2
Shan zhu yu 山茱萸	*Cornus officinalis* Sieb. et Zucc.	2

The use of some herbs may be restricted in some countries. Readers are advised to comply with relevant regulations.

Outcomes

All studies reported composite cure, either in the short term (less than six weeks) or long term (more than six months). Two studies (H109, H110) also reported on the safety of oral CHM for people with persistent UTI.

Composite Cure

Oral Chinese herbal medicine versus antibiotics

Three studies that evaluated oral CHM compared to antibiotics reported composite cure. Two studies (H110, H107) involving 150 participants assessed short-term cure and meta-analysis was conducted. Oral CHM was not statistically different to antibiotics (RR 1.70 [0.99, 2.91], I^2 = 0%). However, the wide confidence intervals raise uncertainty of the true treatment effect. When composite cure was assessed at six months in 168 participants (H111), there was no statistical difference between groups (RR 1.19 [1.00, 1.43], p < 0.06).

Oral Chinese herbal medicine plus antibiotics versus antibiotics alone

All three studies (H108, H109, H112) that compared oral CHM as integrative medicine assessed long-term composite cure. Among the 786 participants with pyelonephritis/upper UTI, people who received oral CHM as integrative medicine had a greater chance of achieving a cure than those who received antibiotics alone (RR 1.49 [1.30, 1.70], I^2 = 0%).

Safety of Oral Chinese Herbal Medicine in Controlled Clinical Trials for Persistent Urinary Tract Infection

Two studies (H110, H109) reported on safety. In people who received oral CHM alone, adverse events included one case of loss of appetite and one case of nausea and vomiting. In people who received both oral CHM and antibiotics, adverse events included seven cases of gastrointestinal discomfort and two cases of allergic rash. Adverse events in people who received antibiotics included five cases of gastrointestinal discomfort, three cases of rash, three cases of nausea and vomiting, two cases of loss of appetite and one case of headache.

Non-controlled Studies of Oral Chinese Herbal Medicine for Persistent Urinary Tract Infection

Seven case series (H113–H119) involving 364 participants with persistent UTI evaluated oral CHM. Study participants were recruited from inpatient and outpatient departments in China. Treatment was provided for between 14 days and 18 weeks, with one study (H117) conducting follow-up assessment after one year. Chinese medicine syndrome differentiation was reported as an inclusion criterion in three studies (H113, H118, H119). Syndromes included Spleen and Kidney deficiency with retention of damp-heat and Blood stasis, Spleen and Kidney deficiency, and Spleen and Kidney *yang* deficiency. Two studies (H114, H115) used syndrome differentiation to guide treatment. In one study, syndrome differentiation was individualised. In the second study, syndromes included *qi* deficiency, Blood stasis, *yin* deficiency and Spleen deficiency.

One study (H116) tested oral CHM as integrative medicine and the remaining studies tested oral CHM alone. Most studies used an investigator-developed formula and there was no overlap in formulas used across the studies. Fifty-four different herbs were reported in these studies (Table 5.34); the most frequently used herbs were *fu ling* 茯苓, *bai zhu* 白朮 and *huang qi* 黄芪.

Safety of Oral Chinese Herbal Medicine in Non-controlled Studies for Persistent Urinary Tract Infection

Two studies reported the safety of oral CHM in people with persistent UTI. One study (H118) found that no adverse events occurred and the second reported one case of nausea and diarrhoea (H116) that resolved when the CHM dose was reduced.

Table 5.34. **Frequently Reported Orally Used Herbs in Non-controlled Studies for Persistent Urinary Tract Infection**

Most Common Herbs	Scientific Name	Frequency of Use
Fu ling 茯苓	*Poria cocos* (Schw.) Wolf	5
Bai zhu 白术	*Atractylodes macrocephala* Koidz.	4
Huang qi 黄芪	*Astragalus membranaceus* (Fisch.) Bge.	4
Du zhong 杜仲	*Eucommia ulmoides* Oliv.	3
Gan cao 甘草	*Glycyrrhiza* spp.	3
Dang shen 党参	*Codonopsis* spp.	2
Jin qian cao 金钱草	*Lysimachia christinae* Hance	2
Mu dan pi 牡丹皮	*Paeonia suffruticosa* Andr.	2
Niu xi 牛膝	*Achyranthes bidentata* Bl.	2
Shan yao 山药	*Dioscorea opposita* Thunb.	2
Shu di huang 熟地黄	*Rehmannia glutinosa* Libosch.	2

The use of some herbs may be restricted in some countries. Readers are advised to comply with relevant regulations.

Controlled Clinical Trials of Oral plus Topical Chinese Herbal Medicine for Persistent Urinary Tract Infection

One CCT combined oral and topical CHM for 160 people with persistent UTI (H120). The study included participants with upper and lower UTI who were recruited through hospital outpatient departments in China. Participants had lived with persistent UTI for as little as one year and as many as 22 years. The study used CM syndrome differentiation as an inclusion criterion (H120) with the syndrome Spleen and Kidney deficiency with residual pathogen.

The CHM formula *Jian pi li shui tong ling fang* 健脾利水通淋方 included the herbs *huang qi* 黄芪, *bai zhu* 白术, *fu ling* 茯苓, *dan zhu ye* 淡竹叶, *huang bai* 黄柏, *bai mu tong* 白木通, *liu yi san* 六一散, *zi hua di ding* 紫花地丁, *huang hua di ding* 黄花地丁, *che qian zi* 车前子, *qu mai sui* 瞿麦穗, *ya zhi cao* 鸭跖草, *bai hua she she cao* 白花蛇舌草 and *bai shi ying* 白石英. This formula was taken orally and was also used as a topical wash for the genital area for six weeks. Participants were followed up for a further six months after the end of treatment. The combination of oral and topical CHM was compared with norfloxacin. One outcome of this study was relevant to this review. The combination of oral plus topical CHM was more effective than norfloxacin in reducing the number of people with microbiologically positive urine culture at the end of treatment (RR 0.58 [0.42, 0.80]). The study reported no adverse events in the intervention group and two cases of gastrointestinal discomfort in the norfloxacin group.

Recurrent Urinary Tract Infection

Sixty-seven clinical studies (H121–H187) evaluated the actions of CHM in patients with recurrent UTI. Of these, 66 studies (H121–H186) tested oral CHM and two studies (H164, H187) tested the combination of oral plus topical CHM. One RCT (H164) tested both oral CHM and oral plus topical CHM, and this study has been included in both sections.

Randomised Controlled Trials of Oral Chinese Herbal Medicine for Recurrent Urinary Tract Infection

Oral CHM for the treatment or prevention of recurrent UTI was tested in 47 RCTs that included 4,004 participants (H121–H167). Many studies recruited participants during an acute infection and some recruited participants between active infections. Forty-one RCTs (H121–H161) compared two groups, and six (H162–H167) included three arms. The third arm of one study (H162) was not relevant to this review and data for clinical outcomes were not analysed. One study (H163) compared two different CHM formulas with antibiotics; data for the two arms were merged for analysis. One study (H164) included two treatments arms, one of oral CHM as integrative medicine and one of oral plus topical CHM as integrative medicine. The results for oral plus topical CHM versus antibiotics are presented in the section 'Randomised Controlled Trials of Oral plus Topical Chinese Herbal Medicine for Recurrent Urinary Tract Infection' (pp. 187–188). One study (H165) compared oral CHM with a group that received antibiotics and with another group who received antibiotics plus estriol cream. Data for the control groups were merged for analysis. Oral

CHM was used alone and as integrative medicine with antibiotics in one three-arm study (H167). One study (H166) included a treatment group that received oral CHM and a second treatment group that received oral CHM plus moxibustion. Data for the comparison of oral CHM plus moxibustion versus antibiotics are presented in Chapter 8.

Participants were recruited from hospital inpatient and outpatient departments or community clinics in China. Participants had lived with recurrent UTI for as little as six months (H126, H144, H150, H153) and as many as 28 years (H150). Treatment ranged from two weeks to one year; the median duration of treatment was three weeks. Thirty-six studies (H121–H123, H125–H128, H130–H133, H135–H139, H141, H143, H145–H149, H151, H153–H158, H160–H162, H164–H166) conducted follow-up assessment after the end of treatment. There was diversity in the time at which follow-up assessment was conducted, ranging from six weeks (H133) to two years (H138). The most common time for follow-up was six months after the end of treatment (24 studies). Ten studies (H123–H125, H128, H132–H134, H141, H161, H163) reported loss to follow-up, which was generally small and balanced across groups.

The majority of studies included only women (35 studies; H121–H126, H128, H132, H135–H138, H142–H146, H148–H157, H159, H161–H167). Eleven studies (H127, H129, H130, H131, H133, H134, H139–H141, H147, H158) included both females and males and the remaining studies did not report this information. Participant age ranged from 18 years (H127) to 85 years (H126, H127) and 23 studies (H121–H126, H135, H138, H142, H145, H148, H149, H151, H153–H157, H162–H166) focused on recurrent UTI in postmenopausal women. One study (H136) only included women with upper UTI, four studies (H145, H159, H165, H166) included women with lower UTI, two studies (H138, H147) included participants with either upper or lower UTI and the remaining studies did not specify the location of infection.

Chinese medicine syndromes were used as an inclusion criterion or to guide treatment in 31 studies (H122–H128, H132–H136, H138, H141–H146, H149, H150, H153, H155–H160, H164–H166). Syndromes described concepts of dampness, heat and deficiency of *qi*, *yin* or *yang*. The most frequently described syndromes were retained dampness-heat (six studies), and Spleen and Kidney deficiency syndrome (four studies). Other syndromes included Bladder dampness-heat (three studies), Kidney *yin* deficiency (three studies), Kidney deficiency and dampness-heat (three studies), *yin* deficiency and dampness-heat (three studies), cold-heat complex syndrome (two studies), dampness-heat syndrome (two studies), Kidney *yang* deficiency (two studies) and dual deficiency of *qi* and *yin* (two studies); and one study each described syndromes Kidney essence insufficiency, Kidney *qi* deficiency, Spleen and Kidney *yang* deficiency, and *yang* deficiency with dampness.

Twenty-two studies (H124, H126–H128, H132, H137, H138, H143, H145–H147, H149, H152–H154, H157, H159–H161, H163, H165, H167) compared oral CHM alone with antibiotic-based therapy, and oral CHM was used as integrative medicine with antibiotic-based therapy in 26 RCTs (H121–H123, H125, H129–H131, H133–H136, H139–H142, H144, H148, H150, H151, H155, H156, H158, H162, H164, H166, H167). Four RCTs tested an investigator-developed formula, and these studies were excluded from formula frequency analysis. Thirty-four named formulas were described, but only ten formulas were used in two or more studies (Table 5.35). The most

Table 5.35. Frequently Reported Oral Formulas in Randomised Controlled Trials for Recurrent Urinary Tract Infection

Most Common Formulas	No. of Studies	Ingredients
Qing xin lian zi yin 清心莲子饮	5	*Huang qin* 黄芩, *mai dong* 麦冬, *di gu pi* 地骨皮, *che qian zi* 车前子, *zhi gan cao* 炙甘草, *shi lian zi* 石莲肉, *fu ling* 茯苓, *huang qi* 黄芪 and *ren shen* 人参.
Er ding er xian tang 二丁二仙方	3	Variant 1: *Yin yang huo* 淫羊藿, *xian mao* 仙茅, *ba ji tian* 巴戟天, *dang gui* 当归, *huang bai* 黄柏, *zhi mu* 知母, *pu gong ying* 蒲公英 and *di ding cao* 地丁草 (H123). Variant 2: *Zhi mu* 知母, *huang bai* 黄柏, *pu gong ying* 蒲公英, *di ding cao* 地丁草, *xian mao* 仙茅, *xian ling pi* 仙灵脾, *ba ji tian* 巴戟天 and *dang gui* 当归 (H124).

(Continued)

Table 5.35. (Continued)

Most Common Formulas	No. of Studies	Ingredients
		Variant 3: *Xian mao* 仙茅, *yin yang huo* 淫羊藿, *dang gui* 当归, *huang bai* 黄柏, *zhi mu* 知母, *pu gong ying* 蒲公英, *di ding cao* 地丁草 and *hong teng* 红藤 (H132).
Ning mi tai jiao nang 宁泌泰胶囊	3	*Si ji hong* 四季红, *bai mao gen* 白茅根, *da feng teng* 大风藤, *san ke zhen* 三颗针, *xian he cao* 仙鹤草, *fu rong ye* 芙蓉叶 and *lian qiao* 连翘 (H159, H162, H163).
San jin pian 三金片	2	*Jin ying gen* 金樱根, *ba qia* 菝葜, *yang kai kou* 羊开口, *jin sha teng* 金沙藤 and *ji xue cao* 积雪草 (H154, H167).
Er xian tang 加味二仙汤	2	*Zi hua di ding* 紫花地丁, *pu gong ying* 蒲公英, *dang gui* 当归, *zhi mu* 知母, *huang bai* 黄柏, *ba ji tian* 巴戟天, *xian ling pi* 仙灵脾 and *xian mao* 仙茅 (H125, H163).
He fa tong lin tang 和法通淋汤	2	*Huang qin* 黄芩, *jin yin hua* 金银花, *zi hua di ding* 紫花地丁, *qu mai* 瞿麦, *bian xu* 篇蓄, *bai hua she she cao* 白花蛇舌草, *bai mao gen* 白茅根, *dan zhu ye* 淡竹叶, *ye ju hua* 野菊花, *ban zhi liang* 半枝莲, *che qian zi* 车前子, *lian qiao* 连翘, *ze xie* 泽泻, *niu xi* 牛膝, *jin qian cao* 金钱草, *yi mu cao* 益母草 and *gan cao* 甘草 (H126, H127).
Tong lin 1 hao fang 通淋1号方	2	*Zhi mu* 知母, *huang bai* 黄柏, *dang gui* 当归, *sheng di huang* 生地黄, *zhu ling* 猪苓, *fu ling* 茯苓, *ze xie* 泽泻, *dan shen* 丹参, *da huang* 大黄, *che qian zi* 车前子, *tong cao* 通草, *bian xu* 篇蓄 and *hua shi* 滑石 (H143, H146).
Tong lin 2 hao fang 通淋2号方	2	*Shan yao* 山药, *zhu ling* 猪苓, *fu ling* 茯苓, *ze xie* 泽泻, *sheng di huang* 生地黄, *shu di huang* 熟地黄, *shan zhu yu* 山茱萸, *ba ji tian* 巴戟天, *tu si zi* 菟丝子, *du zhong* 杜仲, *chuan niu xi* 川牛膝, *tai zi shen* 太子参, *tong cao* 通草, *bian xu* 蓄篇, *qu mai* 瞿麦, *hua shi* 滑石, *da huang* 大黄 and *che qian zi* 车前子 (H143, H146).

Table 5.35. (*Continued*)

Most Common Formulas	No. of Studies	Ingredients
Zhi bai di huang tang/wan 知柏地黄汤/丸	2	*Shu di huang* 熟地黄, *shan zhu yu* 山茱萸, *shan yao* 山药, *ze xie* 泽泻, *fu ling* 茯苓, *mu dan pi* 牡丹皮, *zhi mu* 知母 and *huang bai* 黄柏.
Zi shen tong guan fang/jiao nang 滋肾通关方/胶囊	2	*Huang bai* 黄柏, *zhi mu* 知母 and *rou gui* 肉桂.

1. Ingredients are referenced to the original studies where possible. If herb ingredients varied across studies, the herb ingredients were sourced from *Zhong Yi Fang Ji Da Ci Dian* 中医方剂大辞典.

2. The use of some herbs may be restricted in some countries. Readers are advised to comply with relevant regulations.

frequently tested formula was *Qing xin lian zi yin* 清心莲子饮, used in five RCTs for recurrent UTI.

There was considerable diversity in the herbs used in the 47 RCTs, with 106 different herbs reported in the studies. Many of the herbs are similar to those used in studies for acute and persistent UTI. The most frequently reported herbs were *fu ling* 茯苓, *sheng di huang* 生地黄, *huang bai* 黄柏, *qu mai* 瞿麦 and *shan yao* 山药 (Table 5.36).

All studies used antibiotics in the comparator group. In five studies antibiotics were combined with other treatments, such as estriol cream (H162, H165), oral oestrogen tablets (H122), oral enalapril maleate tablets (H124) or oral sodium bicarbonate tablets (H150). Three studies (H132, H143, H146) included a placebo CHM tablet in the comparator group, in addition to antibiotics, and one study (H161) used a 'double dummy' design where placebo tablets were used in both the treatment and control groups.

Risk of Bias

Although all studies were described as using random allocation, few described the process in detail (Table 5.37). Nineteen RCTs (H122–H128, H132, H134, H135, H136, H137, H144, H146, H150, H157, H159, H162, H163) used a random number table and one study

Table 5.36. Frequently Reported Orally Used Herbs in Randomised Controlled Trials for Recurrent Urinary Tract Infection

Most Common Herbs	Scientific Name	Frequency of Use
Fu ling 茯苓	*Poria cocos* (Schw.) Wolf	25
Sheng di huang 生地黄	*Rehmannia glutinosa* Libosch.	20
Huang bai 黄柏	*Phellodendron chinense* Schneid.	19
Qu mai 瞿麦	*Dianthus* spp.	18
Shan yao 山药	*Dioscorea opposita* Thunb.	18
Che qian zi 车前子	*Plantago* spp.	17
Gan cao 甘草	*Glycyrrhiza* spp.	17
Shan zhu yu 山茱萸	*Cornus officinalis* Sieb. et Zucc.	16
Huang qi 黄芪	*Astragalus membranaceus* (Fisch.) Bge.	15
Zhi mu 知母	*Anemarrhena asphodeloides* Bge.	14
Bian xu 萹蓄	*Polygonum aviculare* L.	13
Ze xie 泽泻	*Alisma orientalis* (Sam.) Juzep.	12
Dang gui 当归	*Angelica sinensis* (Oliv.) Diels	11
Shu di huang 熟地黄	*Rehmannia glutinosa* Libosch.	11
Bai mao gen 白茅根	*Imperata cylindrica* Beauv. var. major (Nees) C. E. Hubb.	10
Bai zhu 白术	*Atractylodes macrocephala* Koidz.	10
Ba ji tian 巴戟天	*Morinda officinalis* How	9
Niu xi 牛膝	*Achyranthes bidentata* Bl.	9
Pu gong ying 蒲公英	*Taraxacum* spp.	9

The use of some herbs, such as *mu tong* 木通, may be restricted in some countries. Readers are advised to comply with relevant regulations.

Table 5.37. Risk of Bias of Randomised Controlled Trials for Recurrent Urinary Tract Infection: Oral Chinese Herbal Medicine

Risk of Bias Domain	Low Risk *n* (%)	Unclear Risk *n* (%)	High Risk *n* (%)
Sequence generation	20 (42.6)	27 (57.4)	0 (0)
Allocation concealment	1 (2.1)	46 (97.9)	0 (0)
Blinding of participants	3 (6.4)	0 (0)	44 (93.6)
Blinding of personnel	1 (2.1)	2 (4.3)	44 (93.6)
Blinding of outcome assessors	1 (2.1)	46 (97.9)	0 (0)
Incomplete outcome data	43 (91.5)	4 (8.5)	0 (0)
Selective outcome reporting	1 (2.1)	45 (95.7)	1 (2.1)

(H161) used computer-generated block randomisation. These 20 studies were judged as 'low' risk of bias (Table 5.36). One study (H161)
used sealed sequentially numbered envelopes to conceal group allocation and was judged 'low' risk of bias. Three studies (H132, H146,
H161) included a placebo in the control group to blind participants,
with one study (H161) also using a placebo in the treatment arm. Two
of these three studies did not provide sufficient detail to determine
whether personnel were blind to group allocation. The remaining
studies were judged 'high' risk due to a lack of blinding of participants
and personnel. Outcome assessors were blind to group allocation in
one RCT (H161), posing 'low' risk of bias. Most studies (43 RCTs)
either did not report any missing data, or the amount of missing data
was small, considered unlikely to influence results, or was accounted
for using intention-to-treat analysis. For four studies it was not possible to determine the impact of missing data on outcomes; these were
judged as 'unclear' risk of bias. One trial (H161) was registered and
reported all pre-specified outcomes. In one study report the outcomes
described in the methods differed to those reported in the results
(H129). This study was judged as 'high' risk of bias.

Outcomes

The most frequently reported outcome was composite cure, reported
in 38 studies. Recurrence was reported in 34 RCTs, of which seven
RCTs reported recurrence among people who had achieved a cure at
the end of treatment. Data for these seven studies were analysed,
while data for the remaining 27 studies were excluded from analysis.
Five studies reported usable data on the duration of symptoms, which
included duration of all urinary symptoms, urinary urgency, flank
pain, suprapubic pain, haematuria and general symptoms. Four RCTs
reported usable data on the number of people with a positive urine
culture, three RCTs reported pyuria, two reported usable data for
serum creatinine, four reported β2-MG and two reported alpha-1
microglobulin (α1-MG). Health-related quality of life using the
Medical Outcome Study 36-item Short Form Health Survey (SF-36)[9]
was reported in two studies, but data were inconsistent with the

recommended reporting for the scale and were excluded. Fifteen studies reported on safety.

Composite Cure

Among the 38 RCTs that reported on composite cure in people with recurrent UTI, two studies (H143, H146) compared oral CHM with antibiotics plus CHM placebo, one study (H161) compared CHM plus placebo with antibiotics plus CHM placebo, 14 studies (H126–H128, H138, H145, H147, H149, H152, H153, H157, H159, H160, H163, H165) compared oral CHM with antibiotic-based therapy and 21 RCTs (H121–H123, H129–H131, H133–H136, H139–H142, H144, H148, H150, H156, H158, H164, H166) compared oral CHM as integrative medicine to antibiotic-based therapy. Results for these comparisons are presented separately.

Oral Chinese herbal medicine versus antibiotics plus placebo

In the two studies that compared oral CHM with antibiotics plus placebo for recurrent UTI, the short-term cure rate was not statistically different between the two groups (134 participants, RR 1.32 [0.78, 2.25], I^2 = 72%; H143, H146).

Oral Chinese herbal medicine plus placebo versus antibiotics plus placebo

One study (H161) used a 'double dummy' design with placebo used in both groups. Oral CHM plus placebo was not superior to antibiotics plus placebo in improving the chances of a short-term cure (122 participants, RR 1.06 [0.62, 1.81]).

Oral Chinese herbal medicine versus pharmacotherapy

Three (H128, H152, H160) of the 14 studies that compared oral CHM with antibiotic-based therapy reported short-term cure. Oral

Table 5.38. Oral Chinese Herbal Medicine versus Antibiotics for Recurrent Urinary Tract Infection: Short-term Cure

Assessment	No. of Studies (Participants)	Effect Size (RR [95% CI], I^2)	Included Studies
All studies	3 (255)	2.06 [1.36, 3.11]*, 0%	H128, H152, H160
Subgroup analyses			
Females	2 (196)	2.44 [1.36, 4.38]*, 0%	H128, H152
Gender NS	1 (59)	1.74 [0.97, 3.11], NA	H160

*Statistically significant, see Chapter 4.
Abbreviations: CI, confidence interval; NA, not applicable; NS, not specified; RR, risk ratio.

CHM increased the chance of a short-term cure at the end of treatment, compared with antibiotics (255 participants, RR 2.06 [1.36, 3.11], I^2 = 0%; Table 5.38). Subgroup analyses for gender showed the treatment effect to be positive in females, but not in one study where gender was not specified. One study (H128) assessed short-term cure at follow-up. The result favoured oral CHM (126 participants, RR 3.25 [1.12, 9.43]), although the magnitude of the effect and wide confidence intervals lower confidence in this result.

Three RCTs (H145, H163, H165) that assessed medium-term cure (between six weeks and six months) included only women with recurrent UTI. One study (H163) included two treatment arms which were merged for analysis, and one study (H165) included two control groups (antibiotics, and antibiotics plus estriol cream) which were also merged for analysis. Oral CHM was not statistically different to antibiotic-based therapy in meta-analysis of all three studies (290 participants, RR 2.30 [0.77, 6.88], I^2 = 85%). Statistical heterogeneity was considerable and was not reduced in subgroup analyses according to infection site (Table 5.39).

Eight RCTs (H126, H127, H138, H147, H149, H153, H157, H159) tested the effect of oral CHM on long-term cure. Oral CHM was superior to antibiotics in increasing the chance of achieving a long-term cure (881 participants, RR 1.49 [1.33, 1.67], I^2 = 0%; Table 5.40). In one study that included women with lower UTI, there was no

Table 5.39. Oral Chinese Herbal Medicine versus Pharmacotherapy for Recurrent Urinary Tract Infection: Medium-term Cure

Assessment	No. of Studies (Participants)	Effect Size (RR [95% CI], I^2)	Included Studies
All studies	3 (290)	2.30 [0.77, 6.88], 85%	H145, H163, H165
Subgroup analyses			
Lower UTI	2 (201)	2.91 [0.49, 17.30], 92%	H145, H165
Infection site NS	1 (89)	1.45 [0.58, 3.60], NA	H163

Abbreviations: CI, confidence interval; NA, not applicable; NS, not specified; RR, risk ratio; UTI, urinary tract infection.

Table 5.40. Oral Chinese Herbal Medicine versus Antibiotics for Recurrent Urinary Tract Infection: Long-term Cure

Assessment	No. of Studies (Participants)	Effect Size (RR [95% CI], I^2)	Included Studies
All studies	8 (881)	1.49 [1.33, 1.67]*, 0%	H126, H127, H138, H147, H149, H153, H157, H159
Subgroup analyses			
Lower UTI	1 (140)	1.57 [0.83, 2.96], NA	H159
Both upper and lower UTI	2 (195)	1.93 [1.22, 3.07]*, 0%	H138, H147
Infection site NS	5 (546)	1.46 [1.30, 1.65]*, 0%	H126, H127, H149, H153, H157
Females	6 (545)	1.48 [1.25, 1.76]*, 0%	H126, H138, H149, H153, H157, H159
Both females and males	2 (336)	1.64 [1.11, 2.42]*, 57%	H127, H147

*Statistically significant, see Chapter 4.
Abbreviations: CI, confidence interval; NA, not applicable; NS, not specified; RR, risk ratio; UTI, urinary tract infection.

difference between oral CHM and antibiotics in long-term cure (140 participants, RR 1.57 [0.83, 2.96]; H159). Other subgroup analyses for location site and gender showed oral CHM to be superior to antibiotics (Table 5.41).

Table 5.41. Oral Chinese Herbal Medicine plus Pharmacotherapy versus Pharmacotherapy Alone for Recurrent Urinary Tract Infection: Short-term Cure

Assessment	No. of Studies (Participants)	Effect Size (RR [95% CI], I²)	Included Studies
All studies	12 (932)	1.65 [1.36, 2.00]*, 45%	H121, H123, H130, H131, H133, H136, H139, H141, H142, H150, H156, H164
Subgroup analyses			
Upper UTI	1 (243)	1.87 [1.40, 2.51]*, NA	H136
Infection site NS	11 (689)	1.62 [1.31, 2.00]*, 41%	H121, H123, H130, H131, H133, H139, H141, H142, H150, H156, H164
Females	7 (634)	1.57 [1.15, 2.16]*, 60%	H121, H123, H136, H142, H150, H156, H164
Both females and males	5 (298)	1.80 [1.45, 2.24]*, 0%	H130, H131, H133, H139, H141
Qing xin lian zi yin 清心莲子饮 (modified)	2 (99)	1.39 [0.87, 2.24], 0%	H133, H164

*Statistically significant, see Chapter 4.
Abbreviations: CI, confidence interval; NA, not applicable; NS, not specified; RR, risk ratio; UTI, urinary tract infection.

Oral Chinese herbal medicine plus pharmacotherapy versus pharmacotherapy alone

The effect of oral CHM plus antibiotic-based therapy on short-term cure was tested in 12 studies (H121, H123, H130, H131, H133, H136, H139, H141, H142, H150, H156, H164). Benefit was seen with adding oral CHM to antibiotic treatments in increasing the chances of a short-term cure (932 participants, RR 1.65 [1.32, 2.00], I² = 45%; Table 5.41). Similar results were seen in subgroup analyses according to the location of infection, and regardless of gender. Meta-analysis was possible with two studies (H133, H164) that tested the original or modified formula, *Qing xin lian zi yin* 清心莲子饮. In these studies, *Qing xin lian zi yin* 清心莲子饮 as integrative medicine was no more effective than using antibiotics alone (99 participants, RR 1.39 [0.87, 2.24], I² = 0%).

Two studies (H148, H158) examined the effect of oral CHM plus antibiotics on medium-term cure. Meta-analysis showed the benefit of combining oral CHM with antibiotics in increasing the chance of a cure between six weeks and six months (118 participants, RR 1.86 [1.20, 2.88], I^2 = 0%).

Long-term cure was assessed in seven studies (H122, H129, H134, H135, H140, H144, H166) involving 504 participants. Oral CHM combined with antibiotic-based therapy increased the chances of a long-term composite cure, compared to antibiotic-based therapy alone (504 participants, RR 1.97 [1.58, 2.46], I^2 = 0%; Table 5.42). Similar results were seen in subgroup analyses, with the greatest effect seen in one study that included participants with lower UTI (H166). The wide confidence intervals in this study limit certainty about the results.

Recurrence

Urinary tract infection recurrence was assessed in studies that compared oral CHM plus placebo with antibiotics plus placebo (H161),

Table 5.42. Oral Chinese Herbal Medicine plus Pharmacotherapy versus Pharmacotherapy for Recurrent Urinary Tract Infection: Long-term Cure

Assessment	No. of Studies (Participants)	Effect Size (RR [95% CI], I^2)	Included Studies
All studies	7 (504)	1.97 [1.58, 2.46]*, 0%	H122, H129, H134, H135, H140, H144, H166
Subgroup analyses			
Lower UTI	1 (86)	2.52 [1.41, 4.51]*, NA	H166
Infection site NS	6 (418)	1.89 [1.49, 2.40]*, 0%	H122, H129, H134, H135, H140, H144
Females	4 (334)	1.92 [1.40, 2.63]*, 23%	H122, H135, H144, H166
Both females and males	3 (170)	2.15 [1.48, 3.14]*, 0%	H129, H134, H140

*Statistically significant, see Chapter 4.

Abbreviations: CI, confidence interval; NA, not applicable; NS, not specified; RR, risk ratio; UTI, urinary tract infection.

oral CHM with antibiotic-based therapy (H128, H137, H167, H154) and oral CHM as integrative medicine (H121, H130, H131, H141, H151, H155, H156, H166, H167).

Oral Chinese herbal medicine plus placebo versus antibiotics plus placebo

Recurrence was assessed six months after the end of treatment in one RCT (H161). Oral CHM plus placebo did not result in a reduction in recurrence compared to antibiotics plus placebo (37 participants, RR 0.68 [0.26, 1.75]).

Oral Chinese herbal medicine versus pharmacotherapy

Meta-analysis was possible with two studies (H154, H167) that recruited people with recurrent UTI who were in remission at the time of study enrolment. *San jin pian* 三金片 was not statistically different to antibiotics in reducing the chance of recurrence six months after the end of treatment (163 participants, RR 0.63 [0.29, 1.41], I^2 = 57%).

One study (H128) recruited participants with recurrent UTI who had an active infection at the time of study enrolment. The chance of recurrence at six months among participants who obtained a cure at the end of treatment was not statistically different between the two groups (36 participants, RR 0.71 [0.30, 1.68]).

The number of recurrent episodes within 12 months was reported in one study (H137). The mean number of UTI episodes was similar in people who received oral CHM and people who received antibiotics (60 participants, MD 0.30 episodes [–0.05, 0.65]).

Oral Chinese herbal medicine plus pharmacotherapy versus pharmacotherapy alone

Seven studies that tested oral CHM as integrative medicine assessed recurrence, and five of these (H121, H130, H131, H141, H156) included participants with an active infection at the time of

Table 5.43. **Oral Chinese Herbal Medicine plus Antibiotics versus Antibiotics Alone for Recurrent Urinary Tract Infection: Recurrence**

Assessment	No. of Studies (Participants)	Effect Size (RR [95% CI], I^2)	Included Studies
All studies	4 (206)	0.17 [0.06, 0.50]*, 56%	H121, H130, H131, H141
Subgroup analyses			
Females	1 (100)	0.37 [0.20, 0.71]*, NA	H121
Both females and males	3 (106)	0.11 [0.03, 0.35]*, 21%	H130, H131, H141

*Statistically significant, see Chapter 4.
Abbreviations: CI, confidence interval; NA, not applicable; RR, risk ratio.

study enrolment. Meta-analysis was possible for four studies (H121, H130, H131, H141) that assessed recurrence between six and 12 months in people who achieved a cure at the end of treatment. The addition of oral CHM to antibiotics reduced the chance of recurrence between six and 12 months from the end of treatment (206 participants, RR 0.17 [0.06, 0.50], I^2 = 56%; Table 5.43). Statistical heterogeneity was lower in three studies that included both females and males (106 participants, RR 0.11 [0.03, 0.35], I^2 = 21%).

One study (H156) that included women with active infection assessed recurrence six weeks after the end of treatment. Results showed no difference between women who received oral CHM plus antibiotics and women who received antibiotics alone (24 participants, RR 0.50 [0.11, 2.31]). Recurrence between six months and one year was assessed in women who were in the remission stage at the time of study enrolment (H155, H167). Women who received oral CHM plus antibiotics were less likely to have a recurrent episode than women who received antibiotics alone (103 participants, RR 0.33 [0.19, 0.59], I^2 = 0%). The number of episodes of recurrence within 12 months was reported in two RCTs (H151, H166). Oral CHM combined with antibiotics reduced the number of UTI episodes compared to antibiotics alone (154 participants, MD –0.81 episodes [–1.03, –0.60], I^2 = 0%).

Duration of Symptoms

Duration of symptoms was reported in a way that could be analysed in five studies (H151, H158, H159, H165, H166).

Oral Chinese herbal medicine versus pharmacotherapy

In two studies of women with active lower UTI, oral CHM resulted in a reduction in the duration of all urinary symptoms by 2.2 days (237 participants, [–3.39, –0.98], I^2 = 83%; H159, H165). Oral CHM also reduced the duration of haematuria in one study (97 participants, MD –0.83 days [–1.06, –0.60]; H165).

Oral Chinese herbal medicine plus antibiotics versus antibiotics alone

Three studies (H151, H158, H166) that compared oral CHM plus antibiotics with antibiotics alone assessed the duration of symptoms. Adding oral CHM to antibiotics reduced the duration of all urinary symptoms (86 participants, MD –1.30 days [–1.88, –0.72]; H166), urinary urgency (60 participants, MD –0.78 days [–0.95, –0.61]; H158), flank pain (60 participants, MD –0.86 days [–1.09, –0.63]; H158) and suprapubic pain (60 participants, MD –0.45 days [–0.67, –0.23]; H158). Oral CHM plus antibiotics was no different to antibiotics alone in reducing the duration of all general symptoms (68 participants, MD –1.60 days [–3.24, 0.04]).

Microbiologically Positive Urine Culture

Urine culture was assessed in four studies (H128, H143, H144, H161). Pathogens were reported in two studies (H143, H161) and included methicillin-resistant coagulase-negative *Staphylococcus, Escherichia coli, Enterococcus faecalis, Staphylococcus aureus, Staphylococcus epidermidis, Klebsiella pneumoniae, Streptococcus* and *Proteus mirabilis*.

Oral Chinese herbal medicine versus antibiotics plus placebo

The number of people with a positive urine culture at the end of treatment was no different between people who received oral CHM and people who received antibiotics plus placebo (74 participants, RR 0.96 [0.19, 4.88]; H143).

Oral Chinese herbal medicine plus placebo versus antibiotics plus placebo

When combined with placebo, oral CHM was not superior to antibiotics plus placebo in reducing the number of people with a positive urine culture (122 participants, RR 0.83 [0.27, 2.59]; H161).

Oral Chinese herbal medicine versus antibiotics

Results from one study showed oral CHM was not superior to antibiotics in reducing the number of people with a positive urine culture (126 participants, RR 0.75 [0.34, 1.65]; H128).

Oral Chinese herbal medicine plus antibiotics versus antibiotics alone

The addition of oral CHM to antibiotics did not reduce the number of people with a positive urine culture compared to antibiotics alone (60 participants, RR 0.36 [0.13, 1.01]; H144).

Pyuria

The presence of white blood cells in the urine at the end of treatment was assessed in three studies (H143, H144, H167).

Oral Chinese herbal medicine versus antibiotics plus placebo

In one study that compared oral CHM with antibiotics plus placebo, there was no statistical difference in the number of people with pyuria at the end of treatment (74 participants, RR 0.55 [0.23, 1.34]; H143).

Oral Chinese herbal medicine versus antibiotics

Oral CHM was not superior to antibiotics in reducing the number of people with pyuria at the end of treatment in one study (63 women, RR 1.13 [0.63, 2.04]; H167).

Oral Chinese herbal medicine plus antibiotics versus antibiotics alone

Meta-analysis of two RCTs showed that adding oral CHM to antibiotics reduced the number of people with pyuria at the end of treatment, compared to antibiotics alone (123 women, RR 0.49 [0.29, 0.84], $I^2 = 0\%$; H144, H167).

Serum Creatinine

Serum creatinine was assessed in two RCTS (H136, H157).

Oral Chinese herbal medicine versus antibiotics

Results from one study found no difference between oral CHM and antibiotics in serum creatinine level at the end of treatment (82 women, MD −2.69 mg/L [−13.82, 8.44]; H157).

Oral Chinese herbal medicine plus antibiotics versus antibiotics alone

Oral CHM used as integrative medicine with antibiotics resulted in lower serum creatinine at the end of treatment compared to antibiotics alone (243 women, MD −13.14 mg/L, [−13.87, −12.40]; H136).

Urinary Beta-2 Microglobulin

Urinary β2-MG was assessed in two studies (H124, H136, H157, H158) that compared oral CHM with antibiotics. Meta-analysis was possible for studies that compared oral CHM with antibiotics and those that compared oral CHM plus antibiotics to antibiotics alone.

Oral Chinese herbal medicine versus pharmacotherapy

When oral CHM was compared with antibiotic-based therapy, there was no difference between groups in the level of urinary $\beta2$-MG at the end of treatment (143 women, MD -0.03 mg/L [-0.07, 0.01], $I^2 = 86\%$; H124, H157).

Oral Chinese herbal medicine plus antibiotics versus antibiotics alone

In two studies that compared oral CHM as integrative medicine with antibiotics, the level of urinary $\beta2$-MG at the end of treatment was not statistically different between the two groups (303 participants, MD -0.30 mg/L, [-0.81, 0.20], $I^2 = 86\%$; H124, H157).

Urinary Alpha-1 Microglobulin

Urinary $\alpha1$-MG was assessed in two studies (H124, H158). Meta-analysis was not possible due to differences in the comparisons.

Oral Chinese herbal medicine versus pharmacotherapy

Oral CHM resulted in a lower urinary $\alpha1$-MG at the end of treatment than antibiotics combined with enalapril maleate (61 women, MD -0.04 ng/L, [-0.08, -0.001]; H124).

Oral Chinese herbal medicine plus antibiotics versus antibiotics alone

Findings from one study that compared the combination of oral CHM and antibiotics with antibiotics alone showed oral CHM plus antibiotics to be superior in reducing urinary levels of $\alpha1$-MG (60 participants, MD -0.54 mg/L [-0.85, -0.23]; H158).

Assessment Using Grading of Recommendations Assessment, Development and Evaluation

Assessment of the strength and quality (certainty) of evidence in RCTs of recurrent UTI was conducted using the approach outlined in Chapter 4. The GRADE assessment was possible for studies that compared oral CHM with antibiotics and oral CHM plus antibiotics with antibiotics alone. Evidence for the formulas *Ba zheng san* 八正散 and *San jin pian* 三金片 was also assessed.

Oral Chinese Herbal Medicine versus Antibiotics for Recurrent Urinary Tract Infection

Fourteen studies (H126–H128, H138, H145, H147, H149, H152, H153, H157, H159, H160, H163, H165) that compared oral CHM with antibiotics reported on the selected important clinical outcomes. Oral CHM may improve short-term ('low' certainty evidence) and may probably improve long-term cure ('moderate' certainty evidence), and may make little, or no, difference to medium-term cure ('low' certainty evidence; Table 5.44). Oral CHM may make little, or no,

Table 5.44. GRADE: Oral Chinese Herbal Medicine versus Antibiotics for Recurrent Urinary Tract Infection

Outcome	Absolute Effect		Relative Effect (95% CI) No. of Participants (Studies)	Certainty of the Evidence (GRADE)
	With Oral CHM	With Antibiotics		
Short-term cure, treatment duration: 3 w to 12 w	37 per 100	18 per 100	RR 2.06*	⊕⊕○○
	Difference: 19 more per 100 patients (95% CI: 7 to 38 more per 100 patients)		(1.36 to 3.11) 255 (3 RCTs)	LOW[a,b]
Medium-term cure, treatment duration: 4 w to 12 w	51 per 100	22 per 100	RR 2.30	⊕⊕○○
	Difference: 29 more per 100 patients (95% CI: 5 fewer to 100 more per 100 patients)		(0.77 to 6.88) 290 (3 RCTs)	LOW[a,b]

(Continued)

Table 5.44. (*Continued*)

| Outcome | Absolute Effect | | Relative Effect (95% CI) No. of Participants (Studies) | Certainty of the Evidence (GRADE) |
	With Oral CHM	With Antibiotics		
Long-term cure, treatment duration: 4 w to 16 w	**58 per 100** Difference: 19 more per 100 patients (95% CI: 13 to 26 more per 100 patients)	**39 per 100**	**RR 1.49*** (1.33 to 1.67) 881 (8 RCTs)	⊕⊕⊕◯ MODERATE[a]
Recurrence at 6 m, treatment duration: 3 w	**36 per 100** Difference: 14 fewer per 100 patients (95% CI: 35 fewer to 34 more per 100 patients)	**50 per 100**	**RR 0.71** (0.30 to 1.68) 36 (1 RCT)	⊕⊕◯◯ LOW[a,b]
Duration of symptoms, treatment duration: 4 w to 2 m	**4.74 days** Average difference: 2.18 days lower (95% CI: 3.39 to 0.98 days lower)	**6.92 days**	**MD −2.18*** (−3.39 to −0.98) 237 (2 RCTs)	⊕⊕◯◯ LOW[a,b]

*Statistically significant result.

Abbreviations: CHM, Chinese herbal medicine; CI, confidence interval; d, days; GRADE, Grading of Recommendations Assessment, Development and Evaluation; m, months; MD, mean difference; RCT, randomised controlled trial; RR, risk ratio; w, weeks.

Notes
[a]High risk of bias due to lack of blinding of participants and personnel.
[b]Small sample size.

Study references
Short-term cure: H128, H152, H160.
Medium-term cure: H145, H163, H165.
Long-term cure: H126, H127, H138, H147, H149, H153, H157, H159.
Recurrence at 6 months: H128.
Duration of symptoms: H159, H165.

difference to the rate of recurrence ('low' certainty evidence). Oral CHM may reduce the duration of all urinary symptoms by two days ('low' certainty evidence). Four studies (H137, H145, H163, H167) reported on safety, with adverse events reported in one RCT (H167). No adverse events occurred with oral CHM, and three cases of elevated alanine aminotransferase and aspartate aminotransferase were reported with antibiotics; these events resolved with treatment.

Oral Chinese Herbal Medicine plus Antibiotics versus Antibiotics for Recurrent Urinary Tract Infection

The evidence for oral CHM plus antibiotics, compared to antibiotics, came from 19 RCTS (H121, H123, H129–H131, H133–H136, H139–H142, H144, H148, H156, H158, H164, H166). 'Moderate' certainty evidence showed the oral CHM as integrative medicine to be superior to antibiotics alone in improving short-term and long-term cure, while 'low' certainty evidence showed oral CHM as integrative medicine may be effective in improving the chances of a medium-term cure (Table 5.45). Oral CHM as integrative medicine may make little, or no, difference to

Table 5.45. GRADE: Oral Chinese Herbal Medicine plus Antibiotics versus Antibiotics for Recurrent Urinary Tract Infection

Outcome	Absolute Effect		Relative Effect (95% CI) No. of Participants (Studies)	Certainty of the Evidence (GRADE)
	With Oral CHM IM	With Antibiotics		
Short-term cure, treatment duration: 2 w to 12 w	**66 per 100**	**40 per 100**	**RR 1.65***	⊕⊕⊕◯
	Difference: 26 more per 100 patients (95% CI: 14 to 40 more per 100 patients)		(1.35 to 2.02) 866 (11 RCTs)	MODERATEa
Medium-term cure, treatment duration: 12 w to 3 m	**58 per 100**	**31 per 100**	**RR 1.86***	⊕⊕◯◯
	Difference: 27 more per 100 patients (95% CI: 6 to 58 more per 100 patients)		(1.20 to 2.88) 118 (2 RCTs)	LOWa,b
Long-term cure, treatment duration: 15 d to 14 w	**59 per 100**	**30 per 100**	**RR 1.95***	⊕⊕⊕◯
	Difference: 29 more per 100 patients (95% CI: 16 to 44 more per 100 patients)		(1.53 to 2.49) 406 (6 RCTs)	MODERATEa

(Continued)

Table 5.45. (*Continued*)

Outcome	Absolute Effect		Relative Effect (95% CI) No. of Participants (Studies)	Certainty of the Evidence (GRADE)
	With Oral CHM IM	With Antibiotics		
Recurrence rate at 6 w, treatment duration: 6 w	17 per 100	33 per 100	RR 0.50	⊕⊕◯◯
	Difference: 16 fewer per 100 patients (95% CI: 30 fewer to 44 more per 100 patients)		(0.11 to 2.31) 24 (1 RCT)	LOW[a,b]
Recurrence rate at 6 to 12 m, treatment duration: 2 w	9 per 100	54 per 100	RR 0.17*	⊕⊕◯◯
	Difference: 45 fewer per 100 patients (95% CI: 51 to 27 fewer per 100 patients)		(0.06 to 0.50) 206 (4 RCTs)	LOW[a,b]
Duration of symptoms, treatment duration: 4 w to 2 m	4.00 days	5.3 days	MD –1.30*	⊕⊕◯◯
	Average difference: 1.3 days lower (95% CI: 1.88 to 0.72 days lower)		(–1.88 to –0.72) 86 (1 RCT)	LOW[a,b]

*Statistically significant result.
Abbreviations: CHM, Chinese herbal medicine; CI, confidence interval; d, days; GRADE, Grading of Recommendations Assessment, Development and Evaluation; IM, integrative medicine; m, months; MD, mean difference; RCT, randomised controlled trial; RR, risk ratio; w, weeks.

Notes
[a]High risk of bias due to lack of blinding of participants and personnel.
[b]Small sample size.

Study references
Short-term cure: H121, H123, H130, H131, H133, H136, H139, H141, H142, H156, H164.
Medium-term cure: H148, H158.
Long-term cure: H129, H134, H135, H140, H144, H166.
Recurrence at 6 weeks: H156.
Recurrence at 6–12 months: H121, H130, H131, H141.
Duration of symptoms: H166.

short-term recurrence (six weeks after the end of treatment; 'low' certainty evidence) but may increase the chance of recurrence between six and 12 months ('low' certainty evidence). The combination of oral CHM and antibiotics may slightly reduce the duration of all urinary symptoms by 1.3 days ('low' certainty evidence). Nine RCTs reported on safety, with five (H123, H133, H134, H144, H158) reporting no adverse events. The number of adverse events was greater among people who received antibiotics in the remaining four RCTs (H141, H142, H166, H167). One adverse event occurred in people who received oral CHM and antibiotics, although the details of this were not specified. In the antibiotics group, adverse events were three cases of elevated alanine aminotransferase and aspartate aminotransferase which resolved with treatment, one case of nausea and unspecified events in four participants.

Ba Zheng San 八正散 plus Antibiotics versus Antibiotics Alone for Recurrent Urinary Tract Infection

One study (H130) addressed the comparison of *Ba zheng san* 八正散 as integrative medicine versus antibiotics and reported on the selected outcomes. *Ba zheng san* 八正散 plus antibiotics may increase the chances of a short-term cure and may reduce the chance of recurrence (both 'low' certainty evidence; Table 5.46). The study did not report on safety.

San Jin Pian 三金片 versus Antibiotics for Recurrent Urinary Tract Infection

The manufactured product *San jin pian* 三金片 was tested against antibiotics in two studies (H154, H167) that reported on relevant outcomes. Both studies included participants who did not have an active infection at the time of study enrolment. The effect of *San jin pian* 三金片 on reducing recurrence six months after the end of treatment is unclear, as the certainty of the evidence is 'very low' (Table 5.47). One study reported on safety (H167) with no adverse events in the treatment group. Adverse events among people who received antibiotics alone were three cases of elevated elevated alanine aminotransferase and aspartate aminotransferase which returned to normal levels after treatment.

San Jin Pian 三金片 plus Antibiotics versus Antibiotics Alone for Recurrent Urinary Tract Infection

One study that tested *San jin pian* 三金片 plus antibiotics included participants in remission at the time of study enrolment (H167). 'Low'

Table 5.46. GRADE: *Ba Zheng San* 八正散 plus Antibioics versus Antibiotics Alone for Recurrent Urinary Tract Infection

Outcome	Absolute Effect		Relative Effect (95% CI) No. of Participants (Studies)	Certainty of the Evidence (GRADE)
	With *Ba Zheng San* 八正散 IM	With Antibiotics		
Short-term cure, treatment duration: 4 w	**79 per 100** Difference: 41 more per 100 patients (95% CI: 10 to 93 more per 100 patients)	**38 per 100**	**RR 2.09*** (1.27 to 3.45) 58 (1 RCT)	⊕⊕◯◯ LOW[a,b]
Recurrence at 6 to 12 m, treatment duration: 4 w	**4 per 100** Difference: 78 fewer per 100 patients (95% CI: 81 to 52 fewer per 100 patients)	**82 per 100**	**RR 0.05*** (0.01 to 0.37) 34 (1 RCT)	⊕⊕◯◯ LOW[a,b]

*Statistically significant result.

Abbreviations: CI, confidence interval; GRADE, Grading of Recommendations Assessment, Development and Evaluation; IM, integrative medicine; m, months; RCT, randomised controlled trial; RR, risk ratio; w, weeks.

Notes
[a]High risk of bias due to lack of blinding of participants and personnel.
[b]Small sample size.

Study references
Short-term cure: H130.
Recurrence at 6–12 months: H130.

certainty evidence showed the combination of *San jin pian* 三金片 and antibiotics may reduce the chance of recurrence at six months (Table 5.48).

Randomised Controlled Trial Evidence for Individual Oral Formulas

Compared to studies of oral CHM for acute UTI, there were few meta-analyses possible with multiple studies testing the same formula for recurrence of UTI. Two formulas were tested in meta-analyses: *Qing xin lian zi yin* 清心莲子饮 (as the original or modified formula) and *San jin pian* 三金片. The combination of *Qing xin lian zi yin* 清

Table 5.47. **GRADE:** *San Jin Pian* 三金片 **versus Antibiotics for Recurrent Urinary Tract Infection**

Outcome	Absolute Effect		Relative Effect (95% CI) No. of Participants (Studies)	Certainty of the Evidence (GRADE)
	With *San Jin Pian* 三金片	With Antibiotics		
Recurrence at 6 m, treatment duration: 8 w to 6 m	**22 per 100** Difference: 13 fewer per 100 patients (95% CI: 25 fewer to 14 more per 100 patients)	**35 per 100**	**RR 0.63** (0.29 to 1.41) 163 (2 RCTs)	⊕◯◯◯ VERY LOW[a,b,c]

Abbreviations: CI, confidence interval; GRADE, Grading of Recommendations Assessment, Development and Evaluation; m, months; RCT, randomised controlled trial; RR, risk ratio; w, weeks.

Notes
[a]High risk of bias due to lack of blinding of participants and personnel.
[b]Small sample size.
[c]Wide variance in effect estimates.

Study references
Recurrence at 6 months: H154, H167.

Table 5.48. **GRADE:** *San Jin Pian* 三金片 **plus Antibioics versus Antibiotics Alone for Recurrent Urinary Tract Infection**

Outcome	Absolute Effect		Relative Effect (95% CI) No. of Participants (Studies)	Certainty of the Evidence (GRADE)
	With *San Jin Pian* 三金片 IM	With Antibiotics		
Recurrence at 6 m, treatment duration: 6 m	**13 per 100** Difference: 29 fewer per 100 patients (95% CI: 37 to 8 fewer per 100 patients)	**42 per 100**	**RR 0.30*** (0.11 to 0.82) 63 (1 RCT)	⊕⊕◯◯ LOW[a,b]

*Statistically significant result.
Abbreviations: CI, confidence interval; GRADE, Grading of Recommendations Assessment, Development and Evaluation; IM, integrative medicine; m, months; RCT, randomised controlled trial; RR, risk ratio.

Notes
[a]High risk of bias due to lack of blinding of participants and personnel.
[b]Small sample size.

Study references
Recurrence at 6 months: H167.

心莲子饮 with antibiotics was not statistically different to antibiotics alone in improving the chances of achieving a short-term cure in two RCTs (99 participants, RR 1.39 [0.87, 2.24], I^2 = 0%; H133, H164).

Two studies that tested *San jin pian* 三金片 assessed recurrence six months after the end of treatment (H154, H167). *San jin pian* 三金片 was not statistically different to antibiotics in reducing the chance of recurrence six months after the end of treatment (163 participants, RR 0.63 [0.29, 1.41], I^2 = 57%).

Frequently Reported Orally Used Herbs in Meta-analyses Showing Favourable Effect

Studies of oral CHM for people with recurrent UTI have shown benefits in increasing the chance of a composite cure, reducing recurrence and duration of symptoms, and improving outcomes of biological tests. The herb ingredients of studies included in meta-analyses showing favourable results for oral CHM were analysed to identify the herbs that may be contributing to the positive effects.

Five meta-analyses, involving 34 RCTs, showed a benefit of oral CHM used alone, or as integrative medicine with antibiotic-based therapy. The herb most frequently used in these studies was *fu ling* 茯苓, described in 22 studies (Table 5.49). Other frequently used herbs

Table 5.49. Frequently Reported Orally Used Herbs in Meta-Analyses Showing Favourable Effect for Recurrent Urinary Tract Infection

Herbs	Scientific Name	Frequency of Use
Composite cure: five meta-analyses, 34 studies		
Fu ling 茯苓	*Poria cocos* (Schw.) Wolf	22
Sheng di huang 生地黄	*Rehmannia glutinosa* Libosch.	18
Gan cao 甘草	*Glycyrrhiza* spp.	17
Qu mai 瞿麦	*Dianthus* spp.	17
Che qian zi 车前子	*Plantago* spp.	15
Shan yao 山药	*Dioscorea opposita* Thunb.	15
Huang bai 黄柏	*Phellodendron chinense* Schneid.	14

Table 5.49. (*Continued*)

Herbs	Scientific Name	Frequency of Use
Bian xu 萹蓄	*Polygonum aviculare* L.	13
Huang qi 黄芪	*Astragalus membranaceus* (Fisch.) Bge.	13
Shan zhu yu 山茱萸	*Cornus officinalis* Sieb. et Zucc.	13
Recurrence: three meta-analyses, eight studies		
Fu ling 茯苓	*Poria cocos* (Schw.) Wolf	5
Shan yao 山药	*Dioscorea opposita* Thunb.	5
Shan zhu yu 山茱萸	*Cornus officinalis* Sieb. et Zucc.	5
Huang qi 黄芪	*Astragalus membranaceus* (Fisch.) Bge.	4
Shu di huang 熟地黄	*Rehmannia glutinosa* Libosch.	4
Bai zhu 白术	*Atractylodes macrocephala* Koidz.	3
Che qian zi 车前子	*Plantago* spp.	3
Huang bai 黄柏	*Phellodendron chinense* Schneid.	3
Mu dan pi 牡丹皮	*Paeonia suffruticosa* Andr.	3
Sheng di huang 生地黄	*Rehmannia glutinosa* Libosch.	3
Ze xie 泽泻	*Alisma orientalis* (Sam.) Juzep.	3
Duration of symptoms: one meta-analysis, two studies		
Che qian zi 车前子	*Plantago* spp.	2
Biological tests: one meta-analysis, two studies, no overlap in herb ingredients		

Composite cure: Refer to Tables 5.38, 5.40, 5.41, 5.42, section 'Oral Chinese Herbal Medicine plus Pharmacotherapy versus Pharmacotherapy Alone' (pp. 165–166). Duration of symptoms: Refer to section 'Duration of Symptoms' (p. 169). Biological tests: Refer to section 'Pyuria' (pp. 170–171).

were *sheng di huang* 生地黄, *gan cao* 甘草 and *qu mai* 瞿麦. Among the three meta-analyses with eight studies that showed a benefit of oral CHM in preventing recurrence, the most frequent herbs were *fu ling* 茯苓, *shan yao* 山药 and *shan zhu yu* 山茱萸. These three herbs were used in five of the eight studies and were also found in the list of most frequently used herbs in meta-analyses for composite cure.

Only one meta-analysis of two studies was conducted for duration of symptoms, and this showed a positive result for oral CHM. There was very little overlap in herb ingredients; *che qian zi* 车前子 was the only herb common to both studies (Table 5.49). There were no herbs common to both studies included in a meta-analysis favouring oral CHM for pyuria.

Analysis of the herb ingredients in meta-analyses that favoured oral CHM may explain how the treatments exert their effects. Practitioners may wish to consider formulas that include herbs, such as *fu ling* 茯苓, *sheng di huang* 生地黄, *gan cao* 甘草, *qu mai* 瞿麦, *shan yao* 山药 or *shan zhu yu* 山茱萸, or modify existing formulas to include these herbs.

Safety of Oral Chinese Herbal Medicine in Randomised Controlled Trials for Recurrent Urinary Tract Infection

Fifteen studies (H122–H124, H133, H134, H137, H141, H142, H144, H145, H158, H161, H163, H166, H167) reported on the safety of oral CHM in people with recurrent UTI. Nine studies (H123, H124, H133, H134, H137, H144, H145, H158, H163) reported that no adverse events occurred. In the two studies where oral CHM was used alone, one study (H167) reported no adverse events with oral CHM and the other (H161) reported that no significant side effects were observed, although no details were provided about mild adverse events. Seven adverse events were reported in people who received oral CHM plus antibiotics, which included three cases of gastrointestinal discomfort, two cases of headache, one case of dizziness and one unspecified adverse event. More adverse events were reported in people who received antibiotics. Twelve adverse events included three cases of elevated alanine aminotransferase and aspartate aminotransferase which resolved after treatment, two cases of gastrointestinal discomfort, two cases of headache, one case of nausea and four unspecified adverse events.

Controlled Clinical Trials of Oral Chinese Herbal Medicine for Recurrent Urinary Tract Infection

Nine CCTs (H168–H176) evaluated the effectiveness of oral CHM for prophylaxis in 1,447 people with recurrent UTI. All studies were conducted in China. One study (H174) included people with upper UTI, two studies (H171, H175) included people with lower UTI and all other studies included people with an infection anywhere in the urinary tract. The duration of recurrent UTI ranged from three weeks (H174) to 23 years (H168) in studies that reported this information.

Chinese medicine syndrome differentiation was reported in two studies (H168, H173). Syndromes included Kidney deficiency and *yin* deficiency with damp-heat. Several studies reported using CM syndromes to guide treatment. One study (H175) described tailoring treatment for people with syndromes of damp-heat pouring downward, Liver and Gallbladder damp-heat, and Liver and Kidney *yin* deficiency. Details were not described for other studies that modified treatment according to the participant's clinical presentation (H168–H172).

Three studies (H168, H170, H176) tested oral CHM alone and six (H169, H171–H175) used oral CHM as integrative medicine with antibiotics. All studies compared oral CHM with antibiotic treatment. Oral CHM was administered for between seven days (H170, H175) and three months (12 weeks) (H173, H176). Formulas varied among the included CCTs and only one formula was described in multiple studies: *Zhi bai di huang tang/wan* 知柏地黄汤/丸. One study (H171) used this formula as integrative medicine and the second (H175) used it with a second formula, *Er zhi wan* 二至丸, as integrative medicine. The herbs used in CCTs were similar to those used in RCTs (Table 5.36). The most common herbs were *huang bai* 黄柏, *qu mai* 瞿麦, *bian xu* 萹蓄 and *gan cao* 甘草 (Table 5.50).

Outcomes

The outcome composite cure was reported by all studies; one study (H170) reported recurrence and one study (H171) reported duration of all urinary symptoms. None of the studies reported on safety.

Composite Cure

Oral Chinese herbal medicine versus antibiotics

Three studies (H168, H170, H176,) measured the number of people who achieved a short- or long-term composite cure. Long-term

Table 5.50. Frequently Reported Orally Used Herbs in Controlled Clinical Trials for Recurrent Urinary Tract Infection

Most Common Herbs	Scientific Name	Frequency of Use
Huang bai 黄柏	*Phellodendron chinense* Schneid.	5
Qu mai 瞿麦	*Dianthus* spp.	5
Bian xu 萹蓄	*Polygonum aviculare* L.	5
Gan cao 甘草	*Glycyrrhiza* spp.	5
Hua shi 滑石	Hydrated magnesium silicate	4
Bai mao gen 白茅根	*Imperata cylindrica* Beauv. var. major (Nees) C. E. Hubb.	4
Che qian zi 车前子	*Plantago* spp.	4
Zhi zi 栀子	*Gardenia jasminoides* Ellis	4
Chai hu 柴胡	*Bupleurum* spp.	3
Huang qin 黄芩	*Scutellaria baicalensis* Georgi	3
Jin yin hua 金银花	*Lonicera japonica* Thunb.	3
Pu gong ying 蒲公英	*Taraxacum* spp.	3
Sheng di huang 生地黄	*Rehmannia glutinosa* Libosch.	3
Tu fu ling 土茯苓	*Smilax glabra* Roxb.	3

The use of some herbs may be restricted in some countries. Readers are advised to comply with relevant regulations.

cure with oral CHM was greater than that seen with antibiotics (648 participants, RR 2.24 [1.41, 3.55], $I^2 = 47\%$; H168, H176). In the one study that reported short-term cure, oral CHM was more effective than antibiotics (300 participants, RR 1.62 [1.31, 2.01]; H170).

Oral Chinese herbal medicine plus antibiotics versus antibiotics alone

Six studies (H169, H171–H175) that used oral CHM as integrative medicine with antibiotics measured composite cure. Five studies (H169, H171, H173–H175) measured short-term cure and meta-analysis was possible. The combination of oral CHM plus antibiotics increased the chance of achieving a clinical and microbiological cure (427 participants, RR 1.62 [1.32, 1.99], I^2 = 0%; H169, H171, H173–H175). Results from one CCT showed that the chance of achieving a long-term cure was greater when oral CHM was combined with antibiotics, compared to antibiotics alone (72 participants, RR 2.17 [1.21, 3.88]; H172).

Recurrence

The number of cases of recurrence was lower six months after the end of treatment in people who received oral CHM alone but was not statistically different to those who received antibiotics (300 participants, RR 0.84 [0.50, 1.41]; H170).

Duration of All Urinary Symptoms

One study of 96 women with lower UTI compared the combination of oral CHM and antibiotics with antibiotics alone (H171). Women who received the combination reported a shorter duration of all urinary symptoms by 1.6 days ([–1.96, –1.24]).

Safety of Oral Chinese Herbal Medicine in Controlled Clinical Trials for Recurrent Urinary Tract Infection

None of the CCTs that evaluated oral CHM in people with recurrent UTI reported on safety.

Non-controlled Studies of Oral Chinese Herbal Medicine for Recurrent Urinary Tract Infection

Ten case series studies (H177–H186) evaluated oral CHM in people with recurrent UTI. Four hundred and forty-one people were recruited from hospital inpatient and outpatient departments in China. Chinese medicine syndrome differentiation was described in two studies (H183, H184) and included damp-heat in the Bladder combined with both deficiency and excess, dual deficiency of *qi* and *yin*, and damp-heat in the Bladder.

Duration of treatment ranged from two weeks to six months, and all but one study (H183) conducted follow-up assessments at either six months or one year. Seven studies (H177, H178, H180, H181, H183, H184, H186) used oral CHM alone and three (H179, H182, H185) used oral CHM as integrative medicine with guideline-recommended treatments. Two studies (H179, H181) tested the manufactured product *San jin pian* 三金片, otherwise there was no overlap in formulas. Fifty different herbs were used, and 18 were used in two or more studies (Table 5.51). The three most frequently reported herbs were *gan cao* 甘草, *fu ling* 茯苓 and *huang qi* 黄芪.

Table 5.51. Frequently Reported Herbs in Non-controlled Studies for Recurrent Urinary Tract Infection

Most Common Herbs	Scientific Name	Frequency of Use
Gan cao 甘草	*Glycyrrhiza* spp.	5
Fu ling 茯苓	*Poria cocos* (Schw.) Wolf	4
Huang qi 黄芪	*Astragalus membranaceus* (Fisch.) Bge.	4
Bian xu 萹蓄	*Polygonum aviculare* L.	3
Hua shi 滑石	Hydrated magnesium silicate	3
Huang bai 黄柏	*Phellodendron chinense* Schneid.	3
Pu gong ying 蒲公英	*Taraxacum* spp.	3
Qu mai 瞿麦	*Dianthus* spp.	3
Bai hua she she cao 白花蛇舌草	*Hedyotis diffusa* Willd.	2
Bai zhu 白术	*Atractylodes macrocephala* Koidz.	2
Chai hu 柴胡	*Bupleurum* spp.	2
Che qian zi 车前子	*Plantago* spp.	2
Dan shen 丹参	*Salvia miltiorrhiza* Bge.	2
Dan zhu ye 淡竹叶	*Lophatherum gracile* Brongn.	2
Dang gui 当归	*Angelica sinensis* (Oliv.) Diels	2
Shi wei 石韦	*Pyrrosia* spp.	2
Shan yu rou 山萸肉	*Cornus officinalis* Sieb. et Zucc.	2
Zhi mu 知母	*Anemarrhena asphodeloides* Bge.	2

The use of some herbs may be restricted in some countries. Readers are advised to comply with relevant regulations.

Safety of Oral Chinese Herbal Medicine in Non-controlled Studies for Recurrent Urinary Tract Infection

One study (H186) reported on safety of oral CHM for recurrent UTI, with no adverse events occurring.

Randomised Controlled Trials of Oral plus Topical Chinese Herbal Medicine for Recurrent Urinary Tract Infection

One three-arm study (H164) compared a group who received oral CHM and a group who received oral plus topical CHM with a third group who received antibiotics. This section summarises the findings for the comparison of oral plus topical CHM and antibiotics. The study was conducted in China and included 60 women aged between 43 and 60 years. The location of UTI was not reported, and data were available for all women at the end of treatment. The treatment group received oral *Qing xin lian zi yin* 清心莲子饮 and topical wash *Ku shen huang bai xi ye* 苦参柏洗液 as integrative medicine with levofloxacin. Treatment was provided for one month and participants were followed up six months after the end of treatment.

The study was not free from risk of bias. Although it was described as randomised, no details were provided about the method used to randomise participants or to conceal the group allocation. The study was judged as 'unclear' risk for sequence generation and allocation concealment. Blinding of participants and personnel were unlikely due to the nature of the intervention and comparator ('high' risk of bias). No information was provided as to whether the outcome assessor was blinded, resulting in a judgment of 'unclear' risk. The study was 'low' risk for incomplete outcome data as all data were available and 'unclear' risk for selective outcome reporting as no trial protocol or registration was identified.

Outcome data were reported for short-term cure and recurrence. *Qing xin lian zi yin* 清心莲子饮 and *Ku shen huang bai xi ye* 苦参柏洗液 used as integrative medicine was not statistically different to antibiotics alone in increasing the number of women achieving a short-term cure (RR 1.83 [0.84, 3.99]) or reducing the chance of recurrence at six months (RR 0.20 [0.30, 1.56]). The study did not report on adverse events.

Controlled Clinical Trials of Oral plus Topical Chinese Herbal Medicine for Recurrent Urinary Tract Infection

The combination of oral plus topical CHM for recurrent UTI was tested in one CCT (H187). Fifty-six women with pyelonephritis or cystitis were recruited from inpatient and outpatient departments in China. Women had been living with recurrent UTI for one to 16 years but were likely menopausal or postmenopausal when recruited (age range 50 to 73 years).

The formula *Qing re bu shen tang* 清热补肾汤 was used orally and prepared as a wash for the vulva. Herbs used in the formula were *jin qian cao* 金钱草, *pu gong ying* 蒲公英, *zhi mu* 知母, *huang bai* 黄柏, *hua shi* 滑石, *gan cao* 甘草, *shi wei* 石苇, *wang bu liu xing* 王不留行, *che qian zi* 车前子, *chi shao* 赤芍, *tao ren* 桃仁, *xian mao* 仙茅, *xian ling pi* 仙灵脾, *ba ji tian* 巴戟天 and *shan zhi zi* 山栀子. Treatment was administered for four weeks, with a follow-up assessment conducted after six months. This treatment was compared with the antibiotic levofloxacin.

Oral and topical *Qing re bu shen tang* 清热补肾汤 was not statistically different to levofloxacin in improving the number of people achieving a short-term composite cure (RR 1.41 [0.69, 2.86]). The duration of urinary symptoms was lower among those who received the combination of oral plus topical CHM. People who received CHM had a shorter duration of all urinary symptoms by 1.84 days ([–2.42, –1.26]), shorter duration of suprapubic pain by 2.0 days ([–3.16, –0.84]), and shorter duration of haematuria by 0.90 days ([–1.55, –0.25]). The study did not report on safety of oral plus topical CHM.

Clinical Evidence for Commonly Used Chinese Herbal Medicine Treatments

Clinical textbooks and guidelines that provided the content for Chapter 2 recommend the traditional formulas *Ba zheng san* 八正散,

Chen xiang san 沉香散, *Wu bi shan yao wan* 无比山药丸 and *Zhi bai di huang tang* 知柏地黄汤 based on syndrome differentiation. Manufactured products can also be used for specific syndromes, and include *Ba zheng he ji* 八正合剂, *Jin gui shen qi wan* 金匮肾气丸, *Niao gan ning ke li* 尿感宁颗粒, *Re lin qing ke li* 热淋清颗粒, *San jin pian* 三金片, *Shen shu ke li* 肾舒颗粒and *Zhi bai di huang wan* 知柏地黄丸. With the exception of *Ba zheng he ji* 八正合剂 and *Jin gui shen qi wan* 金匮肾气丸, all other formulas were tested in at least one clinical study included in this review. Results for each formula are presented below.

Ba Zheng He Ji 八正合剂

One study (H35) tested the manufactured product *Ba zheng he ji* 八正合剂 as integrative medicine with cefuroxime. In people with acute UTI, the chance of achieving a medium-term cure was greater with *Ba zheng he ji* 八正合剂 plus antibiotics, than with antibiotics alone (92 participants, RR 1.55 [1.05, 2.28]). People who received *Ba zheng he ji* 八正合剂 plus antibiotics also reported shorter duration of suprapubic pain (MD –2.07 days [–3.19, –0.95]), haematuria (MD –0.92 days [–1.57, –0.27]) and all urinary symptoms (MD –1.55 days [–2.05, –1.05]) compared to people who received antibiotics alone. The study reported that no adverse events occurred during the trial.

Ba Zheng San 八正散

Ba zheng san 八正散 was tested in 13 RCTs (H5, H14, H22, H31, H34, H47, H52, H54, H72, H100, H105, H130, H161), one CCT (H175), and one non-controlled study (H183). Several studies (H14, H31, H100) used *Ba zheng san* 八正散 as one of several formulas to treat individual syndromes, or with other formulas that are not recommended in guideline and textbooks (H175); evidence from these studies will not be described here.

Two studies (H72, H105) combined *Ba zheng san* 八正散 with *Zhi bai di huang tang* 知柏地黄汤 for people with persistent UTI. Meta-analysis was possible for the outcome short-term cure when *Ba zheng san* 八正散 plus *Zhi bai di huang tang* 知柏地黄汤 was compared with ciprofloxacin. The two formulas combined were not superior to ciprofloxacin in increasing the chance of a short-term cure (95 participants, RR 1.65 [0.66, 4.13], I^2 = 0%). One study tested the two formulas used as integrative medicine, finding the combination was not superior to ciprofloxacin alone in improving chances of a short-term cure (37 participants, RR 1.89 [0.69, 5.21]; H105). One study (H72) described that no adverse events were reported during the trial.

Evidence was available from three studies (H5, H34, H161) that compared *Ba zheng san* 八正散 with antibiotics. In people with acute UTI, *Ba zheng san* 八正散 was more effective than levofloxacin in increasing chance of a short-term cure (70 participants, RR 2.20 [1.23, 3.94]; H34), but was not different to levofloxacin in achieving long-term cure (100 participants, RR 1.50 [0.86, 2.60]; H5). In people with recurrent UTI (H161), *Ba zheng san* 八正散 did not increase the chance of a short-term cure (122 participants, RR 1.06 [0.62, 1.81], nor did it reduce the chance of recurrence (37 participants, RR 0.68 [0.26, 1.75]) or positive urine culture (122 participants, RR 0.83 [0.27, 2.59]).

Five studies tested *Ba zheng san* 八正散 as integrative medicine with antibiotics, four of which included participants with acute UTI (H22, H47, H52, H54) and one (H130) which tested *Ba zheng san* 八正散 in people with recurrent UTI. In people with acute UTI, the chance of achieving a short-term cure was greater with *Ba zheng san* 八正散 plus antibiotics than with antibiotics alone (268 participants, RR 1.32 [1.12, 1.55], I^2 = 0%). The risk of recurrence one month after the end of treatment was not statistically different to ceftriaxone sodium injection in people who achieved a cure at the end of treatment (108 participants, RR 0.47 [0.21, 1.05]; H52). Three studies (H22, H47, H52) reported that no adverse events occurred in people with acute UTI.

One study (H130) tested *Ba zheng san* 八正散 as integrative medicine in people with recurrent UTI. The number of people achieving a short-term cure was higher in the treatment group than the antibiotics group (58 participants, RR 2.09 [1.27, 3.45]), and rate of recurrence was lower (34 participants, RR 0.05 [0.01, 0.37]). Safety was not reported in this study, nor was it reported in the non-controlled study (H183).

Chen Xiang San 沉香散

One RCT (H31) used *Chen xiang san* 沉香散 as one of five formulas according to syndrome differentiation in people with acute UTI. As the outcome data were reported in aggregate, it was not possible to determine the evidence for *Chen xiang san* 沉香散.

Niao Gan Ning Ke Li 尿感宁颗粒

One RCT (H36) tested *Niao gan ning ke li* 尿感宁颗粒 as integrative medicine with levofloxacin and sodium chloride injection in 69 people with acute UTI. The combination increased the chance of achieving a short-term cure more than levofloxacin and sodium chloride injection alone (RR 1.67 [1.15, 2.42]). The combination also provided a reduction in urinary frequency (MD –1.92 days, [–2.48, –1.36]), urinary urgency (MD –1.91 days, [–2.47, –1.35]), dysuria (MD –1.74 days [–2.20, –1.28]) and fever (MD –2.24 days [–2.81, –1.67]) compared with levofloxacin and sodium chloride injection alone. Adverse events were reported in both groups. One case of vomiting and one case of rash were reported in the CHM as integrative medicine group, and two cases of vomiting and one case of mild dizziness were reported in the control group.

Re Lin Qing Ke Li 热淋清颗粒

Re lin qing ke li 热淋清颗粒 was tested as integrative medicine in three RCTs (H9, H18, H27) for acute UTI. The results for *Re lin qing ke li* 热淋清颗粒 as integrative medicine were superior to those of antibiotics alone (222 participants, RR 1.42 [1.14, 1.78], $I^2 = 17\%$). One study, with 112 participants, reported duration of symptoms (H27) with *Re lin qing ke li* 热淋清颗粒 as integrative medicine reducing the duration of urinary frequency (MD –1.90 days [–2.38, –1.42]), urinary urgency (MD –1.90 days [–2.41, –1.39]), dysuria

(MD –1.80 days [–2.16, –1.44]) and fever (MD –2.20 days [–2.72, –1.68]). Meta-analysis with two of the three studies (H9, H18) showed a reduction in the number of people with a positive urine culture at the end of treatment, compared to antibiotics alone (110 participants, RR 0.31 [0.12, 0.80], I^2 = 0%). Adverse events in people who received *Re lin qing ke li* 热淋清颗粒 included four cases of gastric discomfort, while adverse events among people who received antibiotics included five cases of vomiting and four cases of nausea (H9, H18).

San Jin Pian 三金片

Thirteen studies tested *San jin pian* 三金片. Of these, eight (H12, H41, H56, H58, H59, H106, H154, H167) were RCTs, three (H61, H63, H108) were CCTs and two (H179, H181) were case series. One study (H58) compared *San jin pian* 三金片 plus a placebo antibiotic tablet with levofloxacin plus a placebo CHM tablet. There was no difference between groups in the number of people with a short-term cure after treatment (141 participants, RR 0.94 [0.71, 1.25]), nor was there a difference in the number of people with a positive urine culture (141 participants, RR 0.65 [0.27, 1.57]).

Short-term cure in participants with acute UTI was not statistically different between people who received *San jin pian* 三金片 and those who received antibiotics (250 participants, RR 0.99 [0.81, 1.22], I^2 = 0%; H41, H56, H59). One study found no difference between *San jin pian* 三金片 and antibiotics in recurrence at an unspecified time point (58 participants, RR 0.54 [0.21, 1.37]; H41).

Two studies (H154, H167) tested *San jin pian* 三金片 in people with recurrent UTI. Meta-analysis showed *San jin pian* 三金片 was no more effective than antibiotics in reducing recurrence six months after the end of treatment (163 participants, RR 0.63 [0.29, 1.41], I^2 = 57%; H154, H167). *San jin pian* 三金片 was not different to antibiotics in the number of people with pyuria at the end of treatment (63 participants, RR 1.13 [0.63, 2.04]; H167).

Five RCTs (H12, H41, H58, H59, H167) tested the combination of *San jin pian* 三金片 and antibiotics. In participants with acute

UTI, *San jin pian* 三金片 plus antibiotics was more effective than antibiotics alone in improving the chance of short-term cure (244 participants, RR 1.24 [1.06, 1.44], I^2 = 0%; H12, H41, H59) and reduced the chance of recurrence at an unspecified time point (124 participants, RR 0.20 [0.05, 0.88]; H41), compared with antibiotics alone. When *San jin pian* 三金片 plus antibiotics was compared with antibiotics plus CHM placebo, there was no difference between groups in short-term cure (143 participants, RR 1.15 [0.90, 1.48]; H58) or the number of people with a positive urine culture at the end of treatment (RR 0.45 [0.16, 1.22], 143 participants; H58). One RCT (H167) tested *San jin pian* 三金片 plus antibiotics in people with recurrent UTI. The combination reduced the chance of recurrence between six and 12 months (RR 0.33 [0.19, 0.59], 63 participants; H167) but did not reduce the chance of a positive urine culture at the end of treatment (RR 0.57 [0.26, 1.25], 63 participants; H167).

Two of the three CCTs (H61, H63) that tested *San jin pian* 三金片 as integrative medicine reported short-term cure in people with acute UTI. There was no statistical difference in the number of people achieving a short-term cure between the two groups (49 participants, RR 1.01 [0.87, 1.18], I^2 = 0%). The third study (H108) included people with persistent UTI. Among the 600 participants, people who received *San jin pian* 三金片 as integrative medicine had a higher chance of achieving a short-term cure than people who received lomefloxacin plus cefaclor (RR 1.51 [1.31, 1.74]).

Adverse events were reported in three RCTs (H58, H59, H167) and one case series (H181). Adverse events among people who received *San jin pian* 三金片 alone were one case of elevated total bilirubin and one case of gastric discomfort. In people who received *San jin pian* 三金片 as integrative medicine, adverse events included three cases of gastric discomfort, one case of rash and one case of increased thirst and appetite. Adverse events in people who received antibiotics alone, or with placebo, included three cases of elevated alanine aminotransferase and aspartate aminotransferase, two cases of gastric discomfort, one case of headache and one case of stomachache.

Shen Shu Ke Li 肾舒颗粒

Shen shu ke li 肾舒颗粒 was tested in three studies: two RCTs (H57, H140) and one case series (H185). When *Shen shu ke li* 肾舒颗粒 was compared with norfloxacin in people with acute UTI, there was no statistical difference between groups (128 participants, RR 1.86 [0.91, 3.80]; H57). However, when *Shen shu ke li* 肾舒颗粒 was combined with norfloxacin, the chance of achieving a short-term cure was greater than that with norfloxacin alone (124 participants, RR 2.29 [1.15, 4.57]; H57). In people with recurrent UTI with an active infection at the time of study enrolment, the combination of *Shen shu ke li* 肾舒颗粒 and levofloxacin plus cefixime increased the chance of achieving a short-term cure, compared with levofloxacin plus cefixime alone (66 participants, RR 2.44 [1.33, 4.49]; H140). One three-arm study (H57) reported on safety. Two cases of vomiting and nausea were reported in people who received *Shen shu ke li* 肾舒颗粒 alone, and three cases of gastric discomfort were reported in people who received the combination of *Shen shu ke li* 肾舒颗粒 and norfloxacin. Adverse events with norfloxacin included four cases of gastrointestinal discomfort.

Wu Bi Shan Yao Wan 无比山药丸

One RCT (H31) used *Wu bi shan yao wan* 无比山药丸 with another formula, *Bu zhong yi qi tang* 补中益气汤, as integrative medicine with cefuroxime axetil. As participants in the treatment group received both formulas, the evidence for *Wu bi shan yao wan* 无比山药丸 remains uncertain.

Zhi Bai Di Huang Tang 知柏地黄汤

The traditional formula *Zhi bai di huang tang* 知柏地黄汤 was used in three RCTs (H72, H100, H105). In one study (H100), *Zhi bai di huang tang* 知柏地黄汤 was one of several formulas used according to individual syndrome diagnosis in the remission stage for people with persistent UTI. Data for this study were presented in aggregate, so the evidence for *Zhi bai di huang tang* 知柏地黃汤 from this study is not able to be determined. In the other two RCTs (H72, H105), *Zhi bai di huang tang* 知柏地黃汤 was combined with *Ba zheng san* 八正散, another formula recommended in clinical textbooks and guidelines. The findings for this study have been described in the section for *Ba zheng san* 八正散 (pp. 189–191).

Zhi Bai Di Huang Wan 知柏地黄丸

Zhi bai di huang wan 知柏地黄丸 is a commercially available product based on *Zhi bai di huang tang* 知柏地黄汤 and was tested in four RCTs (H14, H31, H72, H105) and one CCT (H175). *Zhi bai di huang wan* 知柏地黄丸 was combined with *Ba zheng san* 八正散 in two RCTs (H72, H105) and findings for these studies are described in the section for *Ba zheng san* 八正散 (pp. 189–191). One RCT (H31) used *Zhi bai di huang wan* 知柏地黄丸 with *Xiao ji yin zi* 小蓟饮子 as integrative medicine. As *Xiao ji yin zi* 小蓟饮子 was not included in guidelines and textbooks that informed Chapter 2, results for this combination of formulas are not reviewed in this section. One RCT (H14) used *Zhi bai di huang wan* 知柏地黄丸 as one of many treatments selected based on syndrome differentiation. As results were presented in aggregate, it was not possible to assess the potential benefit of *Zhi bai di huang wan* 知柏地黄丸 in this study. Finally, one CCT (H175) combined *Zhi bai di huang wan* 知柏地黄丸 with *Er zhi wan* 二至丸. Again, the data were presented in aggregate and the benefit of *Zhi bai di huang wan* 知柏地黄丸 alone was not able to be determined.

Summary of Chinese Herbal Medicine Clinical Evidence

Urinary tract infections pose a significant health burden for patients and health care services. Antibiotic resistance poses a challenge for the management of UTI, and non-pharmacological approaches may offer a solution. Chinese herbal medicine has been evaluated in many clinical studies from 'low-' to 'high-' level evidence. A selection of studies that met the inclusion criteria outlined in Chapter 4 have shown some promising results for people with acute, persistent and recurrent UTI. Most research has focused on oral administration of CHM, which is the main method used in clinical practice. Oral CHM was combined with a topical CHM wash in three studies, although there is insufficient information to support the routine use of such a combination.

Syndrome differentiation is an important feature of CM, allowing treatment to be tailored according to the presentation of each individual patient. Many of the clinical studies described used syndrome differentiation as an inclusion criterion for the study, or to guide treatment. Concepts such as damp(ness)-heat and *yin* deficiency were common. Syndromes in clinical studies of acute UTI tended to be excess patterns. The most frequently described syndromes included damp-heat generally, or damp-heat in the Lower Energiser or Bladder more specifically, damp-heat and *yin* deficiency, and CM disease diagnoses such as heat strangury (*re lin* 热淋) and fatigue strangury (*lao lin* 劳淋).

Syndromes in studies of persistent and recurrent UTI also reported excess patterns, but also emphasised the importance of organ dysfunction. Some of the key syndromes in studies of persistent UTI included Spleen, Kidney (*yin*) and Liver deficiency combined with damp-heat, and *qi* deficiency. Syndromes for recurrent UTI were similar to those seen for persistent UTI, and included others such as Kidney *yang* deficiency, Kidney essence (*jing* 精) deficiency, Bladder damp-heat, and Liver and Gallbladder damp-heat. Syndromes for all three categories of UTI were broadly consistent with those described in contemporary clinical textbooks and guidelines included in Chapter 2.

Chinese herbal medicine treatments were analysed to identify the most common formulas and herbs tested in the included studies. Analysis of formulas was based on the formula name, not herb ingredients, due to the complexity of distinguishing formulas once modifications are made. Several studies tested formulas that were developed by study investigators. These may have been modifications of traditional formulas; however, it is impossible to be certain about the origins of the formula. Hence, such formulas were excluded from frequency analyses.

Few formulas were used in multiple studies, reflecting diversity in formula names. There were some similarities in formulas used in clinical studies of acute, persistent and recurrent UTI. *Ba zheng san* 八正散 was the most frequently used formula in RCTs of acute and persistent UTI and was used in 15 studies overall. *Zhi bai di huang tang* 知柏地黄汤 and the commercial preparation, *Zhi bai di huang wan* 知柏地黄丸, were used in multiple studies for persistent and recurrent UTI and were used in eight studies overall. Both formulas were recommended in clinical guidelines and textbooks described in Chapter 2, and are used for syndromes damp-heat and *yin* deficiency.[10]

Where few formulas were evaluated in multiple studies, analysis of herb ingredients may provide greater insight into the key actions of CHM. There was overlap in some of the most common herbs in RCTs, which constituted the majority of the clinical evidence, across the three UTI types. The herbs *che qian zi* 车前子, *qu mai* 瞿麦, *gan cao* 甘草, *huang bai* 黄柏, *fu ling* 茯苓, *huang qi* 黄芪 and *sheng di huang* 生地黄 were among the most frequently used herbs for all categories of UTI. *Che qian zi* 车前子, *fu ling* 茯苓 and *qu mai* 瞿麦 have actions to drain dampness while *huang bai* 黄柏 clears heat. *Huang qi* 黄芪 tonifies *qi* and promotes Spleen function, which assists in resolving damp. *Sheng di huang* 生地黄 nourishes *yin* and clears heat and *gan cao* 甘草 is widely known to harmonise the actions of all herbs in a formula. The actions of these frequently used herbs address the syndromes described in trials and reflect the treatment principles described in Chapter 2.

Clinical outcomes were reported in included studies, with the majority focusing on cure and recurrence. Diversity existed in definitions for these outcomes. Moves are underway to develop a core outcome set for uncomplicated UTI in adults.[11] In the absence of a core outcome set, several decisions were made to categorise data for analysis. For the outcome composite cure, results were analysed according to the time when cure was assessed: short-term (six weeks or less), medium-term (between six weeks and six months) and long-term (six months or more). It is possible that the findings would change if different criteria were used.

Similarly, assumptions were made in relation to UTI recurrence. Studies reported recurrence in all participants, in those who achieved some improvement in symptoms and in those that achieved a composite cure. It is possible that for participants who received some improvement in symptoms, a cure was not achieved, thus any 'recurrence' may have been residual infection rather than true recurrence. For this reason, we only analysed data for studies that reported recurrence in people who achieved a composite cure. In addition, the time point at which recurrence was assessed was diverse and studies were grouped according to when recurrence was assessed: less than six months, between six and 12 months, and 12 months or beyond. Different groupings may alter the findings.

Randomised controlled trials provide evidence that is least likely to be affected by selection bias and upon which clinical decisions are often made. Findings from meta-analyses of acute UTI RCTs showed oral CHM used alone to be superior to antibiotic-based treatment in achieving short- and long-term cure. When oral CHM was combined with antibiotics, improvements were seen in short-, medium- and long-term cure. Furthermore, the duration of all urinary symptoms was reduced, as was duration of urinary frequency, urinary urgency, dysuria, fever, suprapubic pain and haematuria. The number of people with pyuria at the end of treatment was lower in people who received oral CHM plus antibiotics, compared to those who received antibiotics alone.

Findings from meta-analyses of persistent UTI RCTs found that oral CHM provided a greater chance of short- and long-term cure than antibiotics, and reduced the chance of recurrence. Oral CHM also reduced the levels of β2-MG compared to antibiotics. Oral CHM combined with antibiotic-based treatment showed benefits superior to antibiotic-based treatment alone in short-, medium- and long-term cure. Benefits were also seen for serum creatinine and β2-MG.

Findings from meta-analyses of recurrent UTI RCTs suggested oral CHM used alone increased the chance of short- and long-term cure. As integrative medicine to antibiotic-based treatment, oral

CHM improved the chance of a short-, medium- and long-term cure. The combination of oral CHM and antibiotics reduced recurrence between six and 12 months and reduced the mean number of UTI episodes within 12 months.

Meta-analysis of formulas used in multiple RCTs showed promising results for *Jin qian cao ke li* 金钱草颗粒 used alone, and for *Ba zheng san* 八正散, *Ning mi tai jiao nang* 宁泌泰胶囊, *Re lin qing ke li/pian* 热淋清颗粒/片, *San jian pian* 三金片 and *Yin hua mi yan ling pian* 银花泌炎灵片 used as integrative medicine in improving short-term cure for people with acute UTI. *Yi shen xie zhuo hua yu tang* 益肾泄浊化瘀汤 used as integrative medicine may provide improvements in long-term cure for people with persistent UTI. Several of these formulas were recommended in clinical guidelines and textbooks described in Chapter 2, and practitioners may consider these as treatment options where relevant to the individual patient's CM syndrome.

Safety was reported in one-third of all clinical studies (69 studies; 36.7%) with no serious adverse effects reported. Most adverse events were mild and several studies reported that side effects resolved with treatment. Gastrointestinal adverse events were frequently reported and patients should be informed about the possibility of such events occurring.

While some positive results have been found, the evidence is not free from bias. The results of many analyses were of 'low' or 'very low' certainty. Few studies used appropriate methods of randomisation or adequately described how group allocation was concealed. A 'double dummy' design, where placebos were used in both the treatment and control groups, in addition to oral CHM or antibiotics, was used in several studies. These studies were judged as 'low' risk of bias for blinding of participants and personnel. Most studies compared oral CHM with antibiotic therapy and participants and personnel were unlikely to be blind. The lack of blinding may influence results. Finally, the vast majority of studies were conducted in China and were published in Chinese language journals. This suggests that publication bias may exist.

References

1. 康林之. (2007) 中西医结合治疗尿路感染的系统评价: 成都中医药大学.

2. 石珺, 范可. (2010) 三金片治疗尿路感染的疗效及安全性评价. *中国药房* **21**(11): 1034–1036.

3. 张韬, 陶红. (2010) 中药与抗菌药物随机对照治疗尿路感染的系统评价. *中国药房* **21**(27): 2569–2572.

4. 蒲翔, 张丽艳, 张俊华. (2016) 三金片治疗单纯性尿路感染随机对照试验的系统评价. *时针国医国药* **27**(4): 1012–1014.

5. 蒲翔, 张丽艳, 杨丰文, *et al.* (2016) 热淋清制剂治疗单纯性尿路感染随机对照试验的系统评价. *天津医药* **44**(8): 1048–1052.

6. Flower A, Wang LQ, Lewith G, *et al.* (2015) Chinese herbal medicine for treating recurrent urinary tract infections in women. *Cochrane Database Syst Rev* **(6):** Cd010446.

7. 王琳, 阎姝, 张津平. (2013) 血必净注射液联合左氧氟沙星治疗泌尿系统感染的临床观察. *中国药房* **24**(44): 4187–4189.

8. 郭银雪, 詹继红, 毕莲, *et al.* (2012) 活血化瘀法治疗绝经后妇女慢性尿路感染. *内蒙古中医药* **31**(17): 8–9.

9. Ware JJ, Sherbourne C. (1992) The MOS 36-item short-form health survey (SF-36). I. Conceptual framework and item selection. *Med Care* **30:** 473–483.

10. 中华中医药学会. (2017) 中医药单用/联合抗生素治疗常见感染性疾病临床实践指南-单纯性下尿路感染 (中华中医药学会团体标准). 中国中医药出版社; 北京.

11. Duane S, Vellinga A, Murphy AW, *et al.* (2019) COSUTI: A protocol for the development of a core outcome set (COS) for interventions for the treatment of uncomplicated urinary tract infection (UTI) in adults. *Trials* **20**(1): 106.

References for Included Chinese Herbal Medicine Clinical Studies

Study No.	References
H1	安玲, 胡文博. (2016) 泻热散瘀通淋汤治疗膀胱湿热型急性肾盂肾炎的疗效观察. 中药材 **39**(1): 203–205.
H2	陈博, 万敬员. (2016) 中西医结合治疗老年女性泌尿系感染的疗效观察. 中华全科医学 **14**(3): 420–422.

(Continued)

Study No.	References
H3	陈飞 (2015) 滋阴益肾清利湿热法治疗阴虚湿热型围绝经期尿路感染的临床观察. 学位论文.
H4	陈刚毅, 林莹莹. (2009) 滋肾清淋汤治疗老年尿路感染的临床观察. 按摩与导引 **25**(8): 58–59.
H5	陈晖, 赵星海, 高履冰. (2012) 八正散治疗女性尿路感染临床观察. 辽宁中医药大学学报 **14**(8): 215–216.
H6	陈辉. (2006) 泌宁方治疗老年尿路感染 46 例临床观察. 临床肾脏病杂志 **6**(3): 128.
H7	邓巍. (2016) 中西医结合治疗急性肾盂肾炎 30 例观察. 实用中医药杂志 **32**(4): 354.
H8	董安民. (2014) 补肾清热利湿汤治疗尿路感染随机平行对照研究. 实用中医内科杂志 **28**(6): 81–82.
H9	房辉, 钱辉军. (2014) 热淋清联合左氧氟沙星治疗泌尿系感染的疗效临床研究. 时珍国医国药 **25**(4): 899–900.
H10	宫伟. (2014) 清心莲子饮加减治疗老年女性下尿路泌尿系感染的疗效分析. 内蒙古医学杂志 **46**(1): 89–92.
H11	巩楠, 段丽萍, 郑朝霞, *et al.* (2010) 癃清片治疗老年女性下尿路感染的疗效观察. 实用心脑肺血管病杂志 **18**(10): 1486–1487.
H12	何红花. (2014) 左氧氟沙星联合三金片治疗更年期妇女尿路感染疗效观察. 北方药学 **11**(11): 29–30.
H13	李琛, 于得水, 吴岩, *et al.* (2014) 左氧氟沙星与银花泌炎灵联用治疗女性下尿路感染的疗效分析. 抗感染药学 **11**(5): 468–470.
H14	李翠云. (2003) 中医辨证治疗尿路感染 72 例疗效观察. 湖南中医药导报 **9**(3): 24.
H15	李红羽. (2006) 中西医结合治疗老年女性下尿路感染疗效观察. 中国老年学杂志 **26**(11): 1573–1574.
H16	李怀斌, 袁素民. (2017) 扶正祛湿方加玉米须治疗老年泌尿系感染 59 例疗效观察. 湖南中医杂志 **33**(5): 16–17.
H17	梁淼, 熊玮. (2010) 三金片治疗更年期妇女尿路感染阴虚湿热证 50 例疗效观察. 中国医院用药评价与分析 **10**(7): 616–619.
H18	梁秀芳. (2010) 热淋清颗粒治疗泌尿系感染 30 例临床观察. 医学信息: 中旬刊 **5**(9): 2505–2506.
H19	刘红芸. (2008) 自拟祛淋汤治疗湿热型急性下尿路感染 60 例. 中国药业 **17**(11): 58–59.

(Continued)

(Continued)

Study No.	References
H20	刘洪林. (2005) 中西医结合治疗急性肾盂肾炎疗效观察. 牡丹江医学院学报 **26**(3): 26–27.
H21	卢晓丰. (2015) 宁泌泰胶囊联合左氧氟沙星片治疗泌尿系感染下焦湿热证临床研究. 河南中医 **35**(11): 2713–2715.
H22	罗璟. (2017) 八正散加减联合左氧氟沙星治疗淋证的疗效观察. 贵阳中医学院学报 **39**(5): 59–61.
H23	孟冬冬, 黄群, 吴军, *et al.* (2016) 结石通胶囊联合左氧氟沙星治疗泌尿系感染的疗效探讨. 中外医疗 **35**(13): 163–165.
H24	渠武帅. (2017) 金钱草颗粒联合加替沙星治疗尿路感染的疗效观察. 现代药物与临床 **32**(6): 1097–1100.
H25	商惠萍, 张蓓茹, 刘大军, *et al.* (2009) 头孢妥仑匹脂片联用清淋颗粒治疗非复杂性尿路感染疗效. 实用药物与临床 **12**(3): 182–184.
H26	申俊岭. (2009) 中西医结合治疗尿路感染 38 例. 河南中医 **29**(4): 389–390.
H27	沈银奎. (2014) 热淋清颗粒联合左氧氟沙星治疗泌尿系感染 56 例. 中国药业 **23**(8): 66–67.
H28	宋万雄. (2014) 金钱草颗粒治疗急性下尿路感染的临床疗效. 中国卫生产业 **11**(29): 13–14.
H29	唐桂军, 郭泉滢, 杨玉廷. (2003) 银花泌炎灵片治疗急性泌尿系感染 26 例. 中医研究 **16**(3): 33–34.
H30	王梦旻, 江厚敏, 陶智. (2017) 宁泌泰胶囊联合头孢哌酮舒巴坦钠治疗急性肾盂肾炎的临床研究. 现代药物与临床 **32**(6): 1074–1077.
H31	王慎鸿, 高云球, 谭洪鳌, *et al.* (2013) 中西医结合治疗下尿路感染临床治疗方案的规范化研究及疗效分析. 浙江中医药大学学报 **37**(10): 1197–1200.
H32	王祥生, 曹爱国, 刘志华. (2010) 清利健肾汤治疗尿路感染 40 例. 现代中医药 **30**(2): 21–22.
H33	魏道祥. (2011) 开泄复方治疗尿路感染热淋证 55 例. 辽宁中医杂志 **38**(3): 497–499.
H34	温广学. (2014) 八正散加减治疗泌尿系感染 35 例观察. 实用中医药杂志 **30**(11): 1020.
H35	徐卫刚, 浦裕美, 裴彬, *et al.* (2009) 中西医结合治疗老年人下尿路感染 46 例疗效观察. 世界感染杂志 **9**(4): 258–260.
H36	杨海帆. (2015) 尿感宁颗粒联合左氧氟沙星治疗尿路感染的疗效观察. 现代药物与临床 **30**(11): 1370–1373.

(Continued)

Study No.	References
H37	杨蕾. (2016) 健脾益肾清热利湿方辅助治疗急性肾盂肾炎的疗效观察. 湖南中医药大学学报 **36**(12): 52–54.
H38	杨梅. (2015) 复方石韦片治疗湿热下注型尿路感染. 吉林中医药 **35**(6): 587–589.
H39	杨宁宁, 管敏昌, 彭苍骄, *et al.* (2011) 金钱草颗粒治疗急性下尿路感染疗效观察. 现代中西医结合杂志 **20**(21): 2629–2630.
H40	杨卫平, 黄敏, 夏滨祥, *et al.* (2012) 四妙散加味治疗下焦湿热型尿路感染 65 例临床观察. 山西中医学院学报 **13**(3): 85–86.
H41	杨银桂, 郑宝寿. (2011) 左氧氟沙星联合三金片治疗女性尿路感染的疗效观察. 临床合理用药杂志 **4**(21): 76–77.
H42	杨迎. (2015) 萆薢分清丸联合乳酸左氧氟沙星治疗急性下尿路感染的疗效观察. 现代药物与临床 **30**(4): 436–440.
H43	姚丹萍, 孟鑫鑫. (2015) 中西医结合治疗急性尿路感染临床观察. 中国中医急症 **24**(1): 149–150.
H44	叶蕾, 郑慧文. (2003) 益气清热养阴法治疗绝经期妇女尿路感染. 浙江中医学院学报 **27**(3): 52.
H45	袁素民, 李怀斌. (2016) 扶正祛湿方联合阿莫西林胶囊治疗老年性泌尿系感染 45 例. 中医临床研究 **8**(6): 103–104.
H46	张晖辉, 费奎琳, 曹友汉, *et al.* (2017) 舒泌通胶囊联合左氧氟沙星片治疗泌尿系感染 35 例. 中国民族民间医药杂志 **26**(9): 88–90.
H47	张文青, 左琪. (2006) 加味八正散治疗湿热下注型急性下尿路感染的临床观察. 中国医药导报 **3**(23): 142–143.
H48	张亚琦. (2008) 清热利湿方治疗尿路感染湿热证的中医临床研究. 学位论文.
H49	张作营. (2013) 龙胆泻肝片治疗急性膀胱炎的疗效分析. 现代诊断与治疗 **24**(5): 1008–1009.
H50	赵婧. (2017) 左氧氟沙星与银花泌炎灵对女性下尿路感染临床观察. 深圳中西医结合杂志 **27**(1): 33–34.
H51	郑诗凯, 黄笑芝. (2017) 芩翘四妙汤联合呋喃妥因肠溶片治疗尿路感染效果观察. 新中医 **49**(11): 53–55.
H52	钟财根, 李小琴, 陈炜. (2012) 八正散联合头孢曲松钠治疗急性肾盂肾炎疗效观察. 中西医结合研究 **4**(4): 182–183.
H53	周燕萍, 白海燕. (2013) 热淋清片联合诺氟沙星片治疗单纯性尿路感染的疗效观察. 中国药师 **16**(4): 580–581.

(Continued)

(*Continued*)

Study No.	References
H54	朱伟珍, 钟贤. (2014) 中西医结合治疗尿路感染临床研究. 河南中医 **34**(3): 506–507.
H55	朱雯雯, 余洋, 彭芝萍. (2017) 银花泌炎灵联合左氧氟沙星治疗急性单纯下尿路感染疗效观察. 现代中西医结合杂志 **26**(31): 3517–3519.
H56	邹萍. (2007) 三金片合百合固金口服液治疗中老年女性尿路感染 30 例. 现代中西医结合杂志 **16**(35): 5287–5288.
H57	康永胜, 唐云峰, 李华强, *et al.* (2016) 肾舒颗粒联合诺氟沙星治疗尿路感染疗效分析. 深圳中西医结合杂志 **26**(19): 26–27.
H58	刘皓, 谢建兴, 徐钊斯. (2017) 中西医结合治疗急性单纯性细菌性下尿路感染临床研究. 中医学报 **32**(12): 2489–2492.
H59	梅雪峰, 张传涛. (2008) 三金片治疗急性单纯性下尿路感染的临床观察. 现代中西医结合杂志 **17**(26): 4085–4086.
H60	米杰, 焦安钦. (2008) 癃清片治疗尿路感染 126 例临床观察. 山东中医药大学学报 **32**(2): 132–133.
H61	李树堂. (2008) 三金片联合抗生素治疗尿路感染在巩固疗效和减少复发率方面的作用. 实用心脑肺血管病杂志 **16**(12): 20–21.
H62	王正军. (2016) 宁泌泰胶囊联合帕珠沙星治疗泌尿系统感染的疗效观察. 现代药物与临床 **31**(4): 488–491.
H63	郑翰英, 胡建国. (2013) 三金片联合加替沙星治疗单纯急性下尿路感染疗效观察. 浙江中西医结合杂志 **23**(9): 724–726.
H64	欧阳勇, 徐彦刚, 梁敏, *et al.* (2016) 金砂通淋合剂治疗急性膀胱炎疗效和安全性观察. 现代医院 **16**(3): 378–380.
H65	叶陶. (2002) 十味通淋散疗尿路感染100例疗效观察. 中国中医急症 **11**(4): 268.
H66	张全文. (2008) 中西医结合治疗泌尿系感染 23 例报告. 中国民康医学 **20**(22): 2665.
H67	钟先阳, 胡学军, 潘华新. (1997) 三金片治疗尿路感染临床总结及免疫学实验研究. 中草药 **28**(12): 731–734.
H68	曹汉金. (2000) 益肾宁治疗慢性肾盂肾炎 46 例临床观察. 湖南中医杂志 **16**(3): 14–15.
H69	曹和欣, 何立群, 侯卫国, *et al.* (2010) 补肾活血法治疗慢性肾盂肾炎的临床研究. 上海中医药大学学报 **24**(3): 37–39.
H70	褚鸳, 坑蓉, 赵延. (2015) 抗生素联合益肾泄浊化瘀汤治疗慢性尿路感染临床研究. 中国微生态学杂志 **27**(7): 813–815.

Study No.	References
H71	邓剑波, 沈莉, 童心, *et al.* (2015) 利尿通淋调血汤治疗慢性尿路感染随机平行对照研究. 实用中医内科杂志 **29**(10): 45–46.
H72	邓茜, 李顺民. (2013) 知柏地黄汤合八正散治疗慢性肾盂肾炎疗效观察. 广州中医药大学学报 **30**(3): 309–311.
H73	冯继伟, 高继宁. (2007) 滋阴疏肝通淋方对慢性尿路感染患者TNF-a、MCP-1的影响. 北京中医 **26**(9): 591–593.
H74	龚学忠, 郑平东, 杨践, *et al.* (2007) 益气滋肾清利法对慢性肾盂肾炎患者肾小管功能的影响. 江苏中医药 **39**(8): 19–21.
H75	胡献荣. (2015) 补肾健脾清淋汤治疗慢性肾盂肾炎疗效观察. 亚太传统医药 **11**(11): 124–125.
H76	黄松华. (2016) 益肾泄浊化瘀汤联合抗生素治疗慢性尿路感染临床疗效观察. 基层医学论坛 **20**(29): 4132–4133.
H77	金钲铎. (2016) 益肾清利法治疗老年慢性尿路感染疗效观察. 内蒙古中医药 **35**(11): 11–12.
H78	李靖. (2012) 益肾泄浊化瘀汤联合抗生素治疗慢性尿路感染随机对照临床研究. 实用中医内科杂志 **26**(10): 52–53.
H79	李玉芳. (2015) 益气养阴通淋活血法治疗慢性肾盂肾炎的临床研究. 中华中医药学刊 **33**(2): 492–494.
H80	练英, 王意兰, 李雅君, *et al.* (2014) 通淋补肾方联合西药治疗慢性肾盂肾炎 90 例. 上海中医药杂志 **48**(7): 41–43.
H81	梁传军, 郭秋萍, 李建香. (2016) 中药加味二仙汤配合抗菌药物治疗女性患者慢性尿路感染的临床疗效评价. 抗感染药学 **13**(6): 1433–1435.
H82	廖锦芳. (2005) 中西医结合治疗慢性尿路感染 40 例. 福建中医药 **36**(2): 29–30.
H83	刘晓丽. (2016) 中药复方清淋煎治疗慢性肾盂肾炎的临床观察. 中国现代药物应用 **10**(23): 11–12.
H84	钱妍, 吴整军. (2011) 滋肾清肝通淋汤治疗老年慢性泌尿系统感染疗效观察. 人民军医 **54**(2): 128–129.
H85	任飞, 周家俊. (2011) 开郁补肾方治疗老年女性慢性尿路感染伴发抑郁倾向的临床研究. 辽宁中医杂志 **38**(11): 2229–2231.
H86	石彬. (2015) 滋肾清肝通淋汤对慢性泌尿系统感染高龄患者的临床治疗效果分析. 北方药学 **12**(9): 157.
H87	孙利丽. (2012) 加味寒淋汤辨证治疗慢性泌尿系感染临床疗效观察. 中华中医药学刊 **30**(5): 1178–1179.

(*Continued*)

Study No.	References
H88	汤归春, 鲁桂春, 夏良洪. (2014) 杞菊地黄丸辅助治疗慢性肾盂肾炎的疗效及对复发的影响. 新中医 **46**(1): 77–80.
H89	唐志医, 王琼艳. (2008) 滋肾通淋汤治疗慢性肾盂肾炎 30 例临床观察. 中医药导报 **14**(4): 28–29.
H90	田晓翔. (2013) 中医治疗慢性肾盂肾炎的临床疗效探讨. 中国保健营养 (上旬刊) (6): 3360.
H91	王冬燕, 靳宪芳. (2009) 清化益肾颗粒治疗慢性肾盂肾炎临床研究. 山东中医杂志 **28**(6): 381–382.
H92	王建国. (2015) 清热通淋片联合左氧氟沙星治疗泌尿系感染的有效性和安全性探析. 陕西中医 **36**(2): 164–166.
H93	王身菊, 陈岱, 张福产. (2009) 益肾清利活血法治疗中老年女性慢性肾盂肾炎 35 例临床观察. 四川中医 **27**(1): 71–72.
H94	王伟荣, 罗静, 王韶军. (2014) 中西医结合治疗慢性肾盂肾炎45 例临床研究. 江苏中医药 **46**(7): 25–26.
H95	王文海, 靳锋. (2016) 中西医结合治疗慢性泌尿系感染疗效观察. 实用中医药杂志 **32**(11): 1080–1081.
H96	文先惠. (2002) 健脾益肾通淋汤治疗慢性尿路感染 115 例总结. 湖南中医杂志 **18**(1): 22–23.
H97	徐野, 伞春雨. (2009) 中西医结合治疗慢性肾盂肾炎 28 例临床观察. 吉林医学 **30**(13): 1366.
H98	俞娜珍, 王光德. (2002) 益肾排毒疗法治疗慢性肾盂肾炎 104 例. 实用中医药杂志 **18**(3): 16.
H99	张爱国. (2014) 辨证分型联合西药治疗慢性肾盂肾炎随机平行对照研究. 实用中医内科杂志 **28**(10): 133–134, 153.
H100	张莉, 金伟民. (2007) 益气补肾中药治疗老年尿路感染疗效观察. 现代中西医结合杂志 **16**(13): 1794–1795.
H101	张炜晗. (2015) 加味猪苓汤治疗老年慢性泌尿系统感染临床研究. 亚太传统医药 **11**(18): 120–121.
H102	赵洁萍, 李莉, 王晓丽. (2012) 补肾疏肝通淋法治疗更年期的慢性尿路感染. 中医临床研究 **4**(24): 48–49.
H103	赵洁萍, 王晓丽, 李莉. (2013) 温肾通淋法治疗老年女性慢性尿路感染. 光明中医 **28**(6): 1266–1268.
H104	周家俊, 郭华伟, 王昌明, *et al.* (2009) 益气滋肾清利方降低慢性肾盂肾炎复发率的多中心随机对照研究. 上海中医药杂志 **43**(1): 46–48.

(Continued)

Study No.	References
H105	周荣峰. (2014) 中西医结合治疗慢性肾盂肾炎疗效观察. 中国保健营养 (中旬刊) (3): 1219–1220.
H106	周贤慧, 孙怡婕, 高建东, *et al.* (2010) 尿感方治疗慢性尿路感染 (下焦湿热证) 的临床疗效观察. 时珍国医国药 **21**(3): 688–689.
H107	冯继伟. (2007) 补肾清热利湿法治疗慢性尿路感染的临床研究. 辽宁中医药大学学报 **9**(6): 134–135.
H108	武桂霞. (2003) 中西医结合治疗慢性肾盂肾炎 320 例. 中医杂志 **44**(3): 174–174.
H109	叶乙. (2012) 滋阴通淋汤治疗慢性尿路感染的临床疗效. 中国医学工程 **20**(12): 52–52.
H110	余鹏. (2016) 补肾健脾清淋汤治疗慢性肾盂肾炎的临床疗效观察. 文摘版: 医药卫生 **17**: 183.
H111	张素梅, 黄凌. (1997) 补肾活瘀清利法治疗老年慢性肾盂肾炎116 例临床观察. 中国中医药科技 **4**(3): 184–185.
H112	张亚敏, 陈雷, 王无忌. (2006) 中西医结合治疗慢性肾盂肾炎40 例疗效观察. 中华临床医学研究杂志 **12**(21): 2935–2936.
H113	高景环, 杨玉兰, 侯长青, *et al.* (2007) 止淋Ⅰ号胶囊治疗慢性肾盂肾炎急性发作期临床观察. 河北中医 **29**(3): 211–212.
H114	何小萍. (2002) 清疏法治疗慢性肾盂肾炎 40 例. 山东中医杂志 **21**(7): 408–409.
H115	黄春水, 樊文朝, 余安胜. (2016) 益气活血, 清热通淋法治疗慢性尿路感染 40 例的临床观察. 内蒙古中医药 **35**(7): 17.
H116	李晓霞. (2010) 中成药联合左氧氟沙星治疗老年女性尿路感染 28 例. 中国中医药现代远程教育 **8**(9): 148–149.
H117	宋东眷, 程卫东. (1997) 肾康丸治疗慢性肾盂肾炎 36 例疗效观察. 甘肃中医 **10**(6): 28–29.
H118	王婕. (2012) "假后天以济先天" 治疗脾肾两虚型慢性肾盂肾炎临床观察. 学位论文.
H119	王震. (2011) 温补脾肾法对慢性肾盂肾炎的临床观察及对尿N 乙酰 B-D 氨基葡萄糖苷酶的影响. 学位论文.
H120	卢巧珍. (2004) 健脾利水通淋方治疗慢性尿路感染疗效观察. 辽宁中医杂志 **31**(6): 493–494.
H121	曹宠华. (2013) 知柏地黄丸为主治疗老年女性复发性尿路感染 68 例. 浙江中医杂志 **48**(11): 815.

(Continued)

(Continued)

Study No.	References
H122	陈静鸳, 傅文君. (2016) 黄葵胶囊联合结合雌激素治疗绝经后女性复发性尿路感染疗效观察. 医学理论与实践 **29**(10): 1346–1348.
H123	陈敏, 刘蕊. (2016) 从补肾清热论二丁二仙方防治再发性尿路感染的临床疗效. 辽宁中医杂志 **43**(6): 1217–1220.
H124	陈敏, 王怡, 顾向晨. (2008) 加味二仙汤结合抗生素治疗中老年女性慢性尿路感染的疗效观察. 上海中医药杂志 **42**(1): 48–49.
H125	陈敏, 王怡, 徐震宇, *et al.* (2012) 二丁二仙汤治疗中老年妇女反复尿路感染肾小管间质损伤的临床研究. 浙江中医杂志 **47**(11): 784–786.
H126	董园莉, 李玫, 王少杰, *et al.* (2014) 和法通淋汤治疗绝经期女性寒热错杂型复发性泌尿系感染中医证候疗效观察. 北京中医药 **33**(9): 680–682.
H127	董园莉, 王少杰, 段振静, *et al.* (2014) 和法通淋汤治疗寒热错杂型复发性泌尿系感染 108 例. 环球中医药 **7**(2): 130–132.
H128	段苇, 黄秀贞, 董彬. (2017) 猪苓汤加减治疗女性反复尿路感染疗效观察. 云南中医学院学报 **40**(2): 58–61.
H129	方宏. (2012) 中西医结合治疗复发性尿路感染的疗效观察. 现代中西医结合杂志 **21**(9): 956–957.
H130	方文娟, 郭伟, 马居里. (2010) 八正散化裁治疗复发性尿路感染疗效观察. 山东中医杂志 **29**(7): 448–449.
H131	高立超, 李平, 李燕, *et al.* (2011) 益肾化湿通淋法治疗老年复发性尿路感染的临床观察. 中国医药指南 **9**(24): 310–311.
H132	顾向晨, 仇美思, 王怡. (2017) 二丁二仙汤及滋肾清利方中医辨证治疗慢性尿路感染的疗效评价. 中国中西医结合肾病杂志 **18**(7): 582–585.
H133	郝飞. (2016) 加味清心莲子饮治疗中老年再发性尿路感染的临床疗效观察. 学位论文.
H134	蒋春波, 宋永亮, 任燕, *et al.* (2015) 加味滋肾通关方治疗肾虚湿热型淋证临床疗效观察. 中国中西医结合肾病杂志 **16**(8): 712–714.
H135	孔敏, 程皖, 金华, *et al.* (2016) 益肾清热通淋法治疗中老年女性尿路感染的疗效分析. 安徽中医药大学学报 **35**(6): 33–36.
H136	李晨. (2010) 中西医结合治疗慢性肾盂肾炎的临床研究. 学位论文.
H137	李华伟. (2014) 滋肾通关胶囊对尿路感染的预防作用. 河南中医 **34**(5): 971–972.
H138	李建平, 马艳华, 马余鸿. (2009) 二归补肾通淋方加减治疗中老年女性慢性尿路感染疗效观察. 中国中医药信息杂志 **16**(9): 63–64.

(Continued)

Study No.	References
H139	李士旭, 杨静. (2015) 肾气丸加减治疗反复发作性尿路感染临床疗效观察. 医学信息 (西安) **28**(44): 409–410.
H140	李文豪, 谢文博. (2015) 肾舒颗粒治疗慢性尿路感染的临床疗效研究. 中西医结合研究 **7**(5): 246, 249.
H141	李星. (2017) 益肾健脾、清热利湿法治疗再发性尿路感染的临床观察. 学位论文.
H142	刘建月. (2013) 中西药联合治疗老年复发性尿路感染 22 例. 中国中医药现代远程教育 **11**(2): 32–33.
H143	刘世巍, 罗燕楠, 张宁, *et al.* (2012) 扶正清热利湿法防治再发性尿路感染随机对照研究. 北京中医药 **31**(9): 651–654.
H144	罗曼. (2011) 补肾通淋方治疗女性慢性尿路感染的临床研究. 学位论文.
H145	沈以理, 要全保. (2007) 白头翁汤合二仙汤治疗绝经后妇女下尿路感染 52 例. 上海中医药杂志 **41**(12): 37–38.
H146	王鑫. (2011) 中医药辩证论治防治再发性尿路感染的临床研究. 学位论文.
H147	邢跃文. (2005) 中西药合用治疗反复性尿路感染临床研究. 中国临床保健杂志 **8**(2): 161.
H148	许田俊. (2013) 清心莲子饮治疗老年女性复发性尿路感染 30 例观察. 实用中医药杂志 **29**(1): 9–10.
H149	杨耀忠. (2007) 二仙通关汤治疗更年期后女性复发性尿路感染. 中医文献杂志 **25**(2): 42–43.
H150	杨智玮. (2012) 滋阴通淋法治疗 36 例女性复发性尿路感染的临床观察. 中外医疗 **31**(13): 48, 50.
H151	翟晓丽. (2006) 六味地黄丸对绝经期后反复尿路感染防治作用的临床研究. 世界科学技术•中医药现代化 **8**(2): 99–101.
H152	张春艳, 吉勤. (2011) 滋肾通淋汤加减治疗中老年女性反复尿路感染疗效观察. 医学信息•中旬刊 **24**(2): 466–467.
H153	张春艳, 王坤, 王建明, *et al.* (2015) 用黄芪六味生脉汤加减治疗复发性尿路感染的效果观察. 当代医药论丛 **13**(24): 32–34.
H154	张凤, 赵翼洪, 汤学军. (2016) 三金片治疗中老年女性再发性泌尿道感染的临床疗效分析. 中国医药指南 **14**(28): 203–204.
H155	张莉, 王宏燕. (2008) 中西医结合治疗老年女性尿路感染 58 例. 光明中医 **23**(10): 1556–1557.
H156	张晓蕾. (2012) 补肾中药联合抗生素治疗女性绝经后复发性泌尿系感染的疗效观察. 现代中西医结合杂志 **21**(17): 1861–1862.

(Continued)

(Continued)

Study No.	References
H157	赵凯声, 刘宝利, 魏巍, *et al.* (2011) 清肝利湿、健脾益肾法用于中老年女性慢性尿路感染的临床研究. 国际中医中药杂志 **33**(11): 976–978.
H158	赵莉. (2015) 益气滋肾清利方治疗反复发作性尿路感染临床观察. 学位论文.
H159	钟明. (2014) 中药治疗反复发作膀胱炎 80 例观察. 实用中医药杂志 **30**(5): 399–400.
H160	周育锋. (2010) 清心莲子饮加减治疗复发性尿路感染 30 例. 吉林中医药 **30**(12): 1061–1062.
H161	Liu SW, Guo J, Wu WK, *et al.* (2017) Treatment of uncomplicated recurrent urinary tract infection with Chinese medicine formula: A randomized controlled trial. *Chin J Integr Med* **25**(1): 16–22.
H162	唐开发, 石家齐, 乔筠, *et al.* (2014) 雌三醇软膏联合宁泌泰胶囊治疗女性复发性尿路感染临床疗效观察. 现代泌尿外科杂志 **19**(3): 167–169.
H163	徐震宇, 陈敏. (2013) 二丁二仙汤治疗慢性尿路感染临床疗效评价及免疫调节作用研究. 上海中医药大学学报 **27**(1): 30–33.
H164	姚丽娟, 杨浩, 王勇伟, *et al.* (2014) 清心莲子饮加减联合参柏洗液坐浴治疗复发性尿路感染 20 例. 浙江中医杂志 **49**(9): 648–649.
H165	周健淞, 杜浩昌. (2017) 补肾益气通淋方治疗绝经后妇女尿路感染的疗效及其对雌激素水平的影响. 中医药导报 **23**(5): 66–67, 70.
H166	刘麒, 全宇, 文光, *et al.* (2015) 中西医结合联合外治对中老年女性复发性尿路感染的疗效影响研究. 辽宁中医杂志 **42**(2): 358–361.
H167	吕勇, 赵莉, 王东. (2008) 三金片在女性慢性尿路感染抑菌治疗阶段作用观察. 中国中药杂志 **33**(21): 2554–2555.
H168	高继宁, 于尔康, 李宜放, *et al.* (1996) 滋阴通淋方治疗复发性尿路感染 50 例临床观察. 中国中西医结合杂志 **16**(12): 752–753.
H169	黄金明. (2016) 复发性尿路感染的中西医结合治疗的临床效果研究. 中国现代药物应用 **10**(18): 8–10.
H170	黄慕姬. (2007) 三苓解毒汤治疗女性复发性下尿路感染的临床观察. 湖北中医杂志 **29**(6): 38.
H171	李杰伟. (2015) 中西医结合治疗女性复发性下尿路感染 48 例临床研究. 现代医药卫生 **31**(18): 2810–2812.
H172	李永泰, 董凤琴. (1997) 中西医结合治疗反复性泌尿系感染 49 例. 长春中医学院学报 **13**(2): 30.
H173	刘晓晶. (2013) 滋肾清利方治疗再发性尿路感染肾虚湿热证的疗效观察, 学位论文.

Study No.	References
H174	岳志琦, 邹祥发. (2007) 中西医结合治疗复发性肾盂肾炎 36 例. 河南中医 **27**(5): 68.
H175	张隶. (2014) 中西医结合治疗女性复发性下尿路感染临床研究. 中外医学研究 **12**(36): 145–146.
H176	张淑梅, 黄凌. (2001) 抗感染冲剂治疗尿路反复感染 416 例临床观察. 中国中医药科技 **8**(5): 327–328.
H177	康豪鹏, 侯玉晋, 吕昆, *et al.* (2009) 运用滋肾通关丸加减治疗中老年女性尿路感染临床观察 68 例. 辽宁中医杂志 **36**(7): 1163–1164.
H178	刘丽. (2011) 补中益气汤加减治疗老年女性患者反复发作性尿路感染 35 例疗效观察. 中国社区医师·医学专业 **13**(19): 191.
H179	曲黎, 尚敏. (2011) 三金片治疗再发性尿路感染 50 例. 实用心脑肺血管病杂志 **19**(2): 297–298.
H180	孙建实, 魏星珠. (1990) 反复发作性尿路感染的临床与免疫学研究. 中华肾脏病杂志 **6**(3): 157–158.
H181	王君武, 王晓君. (2009) 三金片治疗女性复发尿路感染疗效观察. 临床合理用药杂志 **2**(18): 51.
H182	王娜. (1996) 中西医结合防治尿路感染复发 41 例疗效观察. 成都医药 **22**(4): 214.
H183	杨俊, 张胜容. (2011) 中医药辨证治疗慢性尿路感染临床疗效分析. 北京中医药 **30**(4): 265–267.
H184	张越州, 郝迎秋, 迟继铭. (2013) 清心莲子饮加减治疗气阴两虚型再发性尿路感染 40 例. 黑龙江中医药 **1**: 15.
H185	赵亚清. (2008) 肾舒冲剂治疗复发性尿路感染 18 例临床观察. 牡丹江医学院学报 **29**(6): 65.
H186	Zhang N, Huang L, Liu S, *et al.* (2013) Traditional Chinese medicine: An alternative treatment option for refractory recurrent urinary tract infections. *Clin Infect Dis* **56**(9): 1355.
H187	禹宏. (2009) 清热补肾汤内服外洗治疗绝经后妇女复发性尿路感染临床观察. 中医药临床杂志 **21**(4): 306–308.

6

Pharmacological Actions of Frequently Used Herbs

OVERVIEW

The therapeutic effects of Chinese herbal formulas and herbs in the prevention and treatment of human urinary tract infection have been attracting attention due to increasing antibiotic resistance. Therapeutic effects of these treatments can be attributed to their active compounds. This chapter reviews the available experimental evidence to explore the possible biological activities and mechanisms of the ten most frequently used Chinese herbs from the randomised clinical trials in Chapter 5.

Introduction

As mentioned in Chapter 2, Chinese herbal therapies have been used for a thousand years in eastern Asia for alleviating symptoms of urinary tract infection (UTI). A number of publications have reviewed the potential effects of Chinese herbal medicine (CHM) for UTI[1,2] with some promising results found. The evidence from clinical studies included in Chapter 5 have also shown some benefits of CHM in increasing the chance of a cure and reducing the risk of recurrence, albeit with some limitations in study quality. If such treatments are to play a role in clinical management of UTI, it is important to examine how CHM exerts its clinical effects. This chapter reviews experimental evidence from *in vitro* and *in vivo* models for some of the most frequently used herbs in clinical trials.

The pathological processes and mechanisms of UTI have been described in Chapter 1. Microorganisms that typically inhabit the gut invade the periurethral area and establish (colonise) in the urinary tract. Uropathogenic *Escherichia coli* (UPEC) is the leading cause of UTIs, followed by *Klebsiella pneumoniae (K. pneumoniae)*, *Staphylococcus saprophyticus (S. saprophyticus)*, *Enterococcus faecalis (E. faecalis)*, group B *Streptococcus, Proteus mirabilis (P. mirabilis), Pseudomonas aeruginosa (P. aeruginosa), Staphylococcus aureus (S. aureus)* and *Candida* species. Among its multifactorial pathogenesis, UPEC possesses both structural (such as fimbriae, pili, curli and flagella) and secreted (such as toxins and iron-acquisition systems) mechanisms to adhere to host epithelial cells. These represent an essential step in the progression of a UTI.

Methods

This chapter provides a general overview of a selection of experimental studies relating to the pharmacology of herbs and their constituent compounds for UTI. The most frequently cited herbs in randomised controlled trials were reviewed by the research team and expert urologists. Key herbs used for acute, persistent and recurrent UTI were selected based on their clinical importance. The key herbs were *di huang* 地黄, *fu ling* 茯苓, *gan cao* 甘草, *shan yao* 山药, *bian xu* 萹蓄, *che qian zi* 车前子, *hua shi* 滑石, *huang bai* 黄柏, *huang qi* 黄芪 and *qu mai* 瞿麦.

The extracts and/or isolated compounds from each herb have shown their vast pharmacological effects. To identify experimental studies on their pharmacological actions of relevance to UTI, the activities of each herb and/or main compounds were examined to identify their therapeutic effects on inflammation, microbial activity, bacterial adherence and colonisation, and the innate immune response.

The constituent compounds were identified by searching herbal monographs, high-quality reviews of CHM, *materia medica* and PubMed. To identify pre-clinical studies, a literature search in PubMed, Google Scholar and PubMed Central was undertaken.

Search terms included the names of the plant in Chinese *pinyin* and scientific names, as well as the names of the main compounds contained in the plant/mineral. These were combined with terms for UTI, inflammation, antimicrobial, antiadhesive and immunity.

Experimental Studies on *Di Huang* 地黄

Di huang 地黄, the rhizome of *Rehmannia glutinosa* Libosch, has been used for treatment of a variety of disorders to maintain haemostasis, promote blood circulation and improve kidney function in Chinese medicine (CM). Currently about 140 compounds have been identified from *R. glutinosa,* including monoterpenoids, polysaccharides, triterpenes, flavonoid glycosides, phenethyl alcohol glycosides, phenolic acid glycosides and lignans. Iridoid glycosides, such as catalpol, aucubin and acetoside, are considered to be one of abundant monoterpenoids. The level of catalpol in the extract is an indicator of the quality of *R. glutinosa*. In addition to iridoid glycosides, polysaccharides are also one of the main active constituents of *R. glutinosa.*[3,4]

Biological actions of *di huang* have been examined in many experimental studies. It has been demonstrated that *R. glutinosa* exhibits beneficial activities on the blood system, immune system, endocrine system, cardiovascular system and nervous system.[3,4] Despite *di huang* being one of the most commonly used herbs in clinical studies included in Chapter 5, there is little experimental evidence of *di huang* relevant to UTI. Actions that may be relevant to the pathogenesis of UTI, including anti-inflammatory, antimicrobial and immunomodulatory actions, have been summarised below.

Anti-inflammatory Actions

There are a great number of *in vitro* and/or *in vivo* studies that have demonstrated that various crude extracts and/or compounds of *R. glutinosa* possess strong anti-inflammatory activities in various inflammatory diseases. Such actions are mostly through downregulating the production of pro-inflammatory cytokines and mediators.[5]

Iridoids, secondary metabolites from *R. glutinosa,* exhibited promising anti-inflammatory activity *in vitro* and/or *in vivo*.[6] More recently, catalpol, a major iridoid glycoside, was reported to attenuate inflammatory responses induced by lipopolysaccharide (LPS) in BV2 microglia via suppression of the Toll-like receptor (TLR) 4-mediated nuclear factor kappa-light-chain-enhancer of activated B cells (NF-κB) pathway[7] and via peroxisome proliferator-activated receptors (PPAR)-γ activation in human intestinal Caco-2 cells.[8]

Antimicrobial Actions

Iridoid glycosides are common to many plant species. One study suggested that iridoid glycosides from *Eremostachys laciniata* (L) Bunge had antimicrobial actions against *Bacillus cereus (B. cereus),* penicillin-resistant *E. coli, P. mirabilis,* and *S. aureus* with a minimum inhibitory concentration (MIC) at a value of 0.05 mg/mL assessed by the resazurin microtitre assay.[9]

Immunomodulatory Actions

It has been demonstrated that *R. glutinosa* and its bioactive compounds exhibited both immune-enhancing and immune-suppressing responses. Different solvent extracts of *R. glutinosa* acted on different aspects of the immune system.[4] The aqueous extract of *R. glutinosa* could accelerate the number of periphery leucocytes and concanavalin A (Con A)-activated lymphocytes in the mouse spleen, potentiate the functions of T and B lymphocytes of the spleen, as well as overall non-specific immunity in *yin* deficiency-like mice. In addition, aqueous extract of prepared *Rehmannia* root was also reported to suppress the immune response by inhibiting secretion of interleukin (IL)-1 and tumour necrosis factor (TNF)-α.[10]

In addition to the crude extract of *R. glutinosa,* a series of phenethyl alcohol glycoside-like compounds, such as acetoside, rehmannan SA and SB from *R. glutinosa,* demonstrated immune-enhancing effects.[4] In addition, polysaccharides from *R. glutinosa* also show an immunity excitatory effect. It could activate cellular and humoral immune activity in mice through increasing B and T lymphocyte proliferation and upregulating IL-2 and interferon (IFN)-γ in T cells, and induce maturation of dendritic cells (DCs) to enhance immunity.[11–13]

Experimental Studies on *Fu Ling* 茯苓

Fu ling 茯苓 (*Poria cocos*) is a well-known medicinal fungus that has been used in CM for its diuretic, sedative and tonic effects. The major phytochemical compounds present in *P. cocos* are triterpenoids (lanostane and 3,4-secolanostane skeletons) and polysaccharides (beta-pachyman). Other minor compounds are hyperin, ergosterol, amino acids, choline, histidine and potassium salt.[14,15] These compounds and their derivatives have various pharmacological effects, including anti-inflammatory, antioxidative, antiapoptotic and antiviral activities. Triterpenoids have been shown to exhibit various beneficial biological effects on rheumatoid arthritis, septic shock, psoriasis, auto-immune uveitis and bronchial asthma; and polysaccharides have actions that inhibit tumour activity and potentiate the immune response. Both classes of compounds possess anti-inflammatory, anti-oxidant, antiviral and antibacterial activities.[14,15] Other pharmacological effects in relation to UTI are discussed.

Anti-inflammatory Actions

The crude extract of *P. cocos* has been demonstrated to promote inducible nitric oxide synthase (iNOS) transcription to produce nitric oxide (NO) through activation of NF-κB/Rel in the mouse macrophage line RAW 264.7.[16] Anti-inflammatory activity of *P. cocos* was also reported in a repeated sodium lauryl sulphate-induced irritation model.[17]

Many active compounds isolated from *P. cocos* have been reported to have anti-inflammatory potency in various acute and chronic inflammation models. The hydroalcoholic extract of *P. cocos* inhibits acute ear oedema induced by 12-O-tetradecanoylphorbol 13- acetate (TPA) and arachidonic acid, paw oedema induced by carrageenan, dermatitis induced by TPA and delayed-type hypersensitivity induced by oxazolone. Two triterpenoids, pachymic acid and dehydrotumulosic acid, inhibit TPA-induced acute ear oedema and acute phospholipase A2 (PLA2) and serotonin-induced paw oedema.[18] The possible mechanism of action of the major triterpenoids was confirmed to be associated with phospholipase A2 inhibitors (PLA2) which play a pathogenic role by causing direct/ indirect damage to the cellular membrane.[19] In parallel, a larger group of triterpenes showed similar effects on TPA/arachidonic acid-induced ear oedema via inhibitory activity against PLA2.[20,21] A polysaccharide from *P. cocos*, PC-II, was also involved in inflammatory-related diseases by regulating human interferon-inducible protein 10 (IP-10 or CXCL10) translation.[22] It is notable that CXCL10 is a member of the CXC chemokine family with pro-inflammatory properties.

Immunomodulatory Actions

P. cocos is often referred to as an immunomodulator; the crude extracts of *P. cocos* and its compounds have beneficial activities in enhancing immunity. The various extracts of *P. cocos* have been demonstrated to modulate the immune response by enhancing the production of immune stimulators (IL-1β, IL-6 and TNF-α) secreted by activated neutrophils and macrophages in serum. They also inhibit the production of an immune suppressor (TGF-β) which reduces the inflammatory response by suppressing macrophage activation and the secretion of other cytokines.[23,24]

A new immunomodulatory protein (PCP) from the dried sclerotium of *P. cocos*, glycoprotein, has been found to induce the expression of TNF-α and IL-1β via regulation of NF-κB expression in RAW 264.7 macrophages and the TLR4-mediated myeloid differentiation factor 88 (MyD88) pathway in peritoneal macrophages.[25]

Similarly, a β-(1→3)-D-glucan, PCS3-II showed immunopotentiation activity by increasing the carbon clearance index of macrophages and the spleen and thymus weight index, enhancing haemolytic activity and the production of antibodies, and the delaying-type hypersensitivity responses in mice.[26]

Diuretic Actions

In addition to general anti-inflammatory and immunomodulatory actions of *P. cocos,* its diuretic activity may contribute to UTI treatment. Flushing of uropathogens from the urethra during urination is one of the protective factors to prevent bacteria from colonising in the urinary tract.[27]

The diuretic activity of the epidermis of *P. cocos* has been extensively studied. In inner medullary collecting duct cell lines (IMCD-3), pre-treatment with the sclerotia of *P. cocos* could attenuate the hypertonicity-induced increased expression of aquaporin-2 (AQP2) in a concentration-dependent manner.[28] Aquaporin-2 contributes to regulating water balance in the kidney and assists in concentrating urine. Saline-loaded rats were given oral doses of ethanol and aqueous extracts from the epidermis of *P. cocos.* The urinary extraction rate, with a notable excretion of sodium (Na^+) but not potassium (K^+), was significantly increased by the ethanol extracts, while no such change was seen with the aqueous extracts.[29] After oral administration of the ethyl acetate and n-butanol fractions of the epidermis of *P. cocos*, these fractions demonstrated a diuretic effect, showing a remarkable increase in the urinary excretion rate, Na^+ and chloride (Cl^-) excretion and enhanced Na^+/K^+ value.[30]

Experimental Studies on *Gan Cao* 甘草

The three plant sources of *gan cao* 甘草 (licorice) are *Glycyrrhiza uralensis* Fisch., *Glycyrrhiza inflata* Bat. and *Glycyrrhiza glabra* L. Among at least 400 isolated compounds, the main bioactive constituents of licorice include more than 20 triterpene saponins and more than 300 flavonoids.[31-33] These compounds exhibit extensive pharmacological properties such as anti-inflammatory, antiallergic, antioxidative, antiviral, anticarcinogenic, antithrombotic, antiulceric, immunoregulatory, hepatoprotective and cardioprotective effects.[31-34] Other pharmacological effects in relation to UTI are reviewed below.

Anti-inflammatory Actions

The anti-inflammatory activity of licorice has been well documented due to its use in treatment of inflammatory-related diseases throughout CM history. The extract of licorice and its compounds, such as triterpenes and flavonoids, showed anti-inflammatory properties by decreasing pro-inflammatory cytokines and inflammatory mediators.[35] Glycyhrritinic acid has also exhibited anti-inflammatory properties in different animal models. Inhibition of glucocorticoid metabolism was seen, which enhanced their effects on inflammation. Other derivatives, such as glycyrrhizin, glyderinine, lichochalocone A and isoliquiritigenin, have been also reported to exert anti-inflammation actions through different pathways.[31]

Antimicrobial Actions

Numerous studies have demonstrated that both crude extracts of licorice and its bioactive constituents possess an antimicrobial effect. The ether–water extracts of *G. glabra* have been reported to have effective antibacterial activity against five bacteria: *E. coli, Bacillus subtilis (B. subtilis), Enterobacter aerogenes (E. aerogenes), K. pneumoniae* and *S. aureus.*[36]

A group of flavonoids containing C5 side chains isolated from *G. uralensis,* including licochalcone A, gancaonin G, isoangustone, glyasperins C and D, glabridin, licoricidin, glycycoumarin and licocoumarone have been shown to inhibit clinical isolated methicillin-resistant *S. aureus* (MRSA) strains with minimal inhibitory concentrations (MICs) of 16 µg/ml. The antibacterial effect might be via the lipophilic C5 residues, which could interfere with the cell membrane of the MRSA.[37] In addition, this group of flavonoids could also restore the effects of oxacillin and β-lactam antibiotic against MRSA.[38] The findings from the above compounds against MRSA have been confirmed by several similar studies.[39–43]

Antiadhesive Actions

P fimbriae, type 1 fimbriae (such as FimH) and Dr adhesins have been considered to be the most frequent colonisation factors among UPEC.[44] Carbenoxolone, a drug derived from licorice, has been shown to be effective in clearing experimentally induced UTI in oophorectomised rabbits by blocking the attachment of the bacteria to the bladder cells.[45] This action was mediated by producing the mucopolysaccharide (GAG) layer, a barrier thought to prevent the adherence of bacteria to the transitional cells lining the bladder. More recently, it has been demonstrated that the ethanol-water extract of *G. glabra* exerted maximum antibacterial activity to be effective against seven isolated bacterial strains, including two Gram-positive (*S. aureus* and *Bacillus cereus*), five Gram-negative (*E. coli*, *K. pneumonia*, *E. aerogenes*, *P. aeruginosa* and *Proteus vulgaris*) and commercial *E. coli* (UTI89/UPEC) strains, through inhibiting adhesin FimH, a two-domain proteinaceous filament at the tip of type 1 pili of UPEC. The silico antiadhesive molecular docking studies further confirmed that two identified compounds, quercetin-3-glucoside and ethyl caffeate, could be UPEC FimH antagonists to form H-bonds with the FimH protein ligand.[46]

Immunomodulatory Actions

The immunomodulatory activities of licorice have been attributed to its bioactive ingredients, such as glycyrrhizin, glycyrrhetinic acid, lichochalchone A, isoliquiritigenin (ISL) and polysaccharide. Both glycyrrhizin and glycyrrhetinic acid could induce interferon activity and enhance natural killer cell activity; lichochalocone A inhibited proliferation of T cells and production of cytokines; ISL could decrease the production of NF-κB and interferon regulatory factor 3 activation, cyclooxygenase (COX)-2 and iNOS via toll-interleukin-1 receptor domain-containing adapter inducing interferon-beta (TRIF) -dependent signalling pathways of TLRs.[31,34]

Experimental Studies on *Shan Yao* 山药

Shan yao 山药, the rhizome of *Dioscorea opposita* Thunb. (also called Chinese yam), is one of the well-known edible and pharmaceutical foods in China used for treatment of haemorrhoids, sore throat and struma, lung disease and pancreatic disease, as well as enhancing immunity and lowering blood sugar, among others. Key chemical components and nutrients include polysaccharides, flavonoids, dopamine, allantoin, batatasin and other active ingredients.[47,48]

Anti-inflammatory Actions

There are a great number of *in vitro* and/or *in vivo* studies that have demonstrated that the crude extracts and/or compounds of *D. opposita* have strong anti-inflammatory activity to prevent various inflammatory diseases. This occurs mostly through downregulation of the production of pro-inflammatory cytokines and mediators.[47–49] In particular, the potential anti-inflammatory action has been proven in many constituents from the ethanol extract of *Dioscorea* rhizome in RAW 264.7 macrophage cells, with significant inhibitory activities on LPS-induced NO production.[48,49]

Antimicrobial Actions

A polysaccharide containing 1,3-linked-glucose, 1-linked-galactose and 1,6- linked-galactose glycosidic bonds isolated from *D. opposita* exerted antibacterial activity.[50] The purified polysaccharide showed a certain inhibitory activity against *E. coli* and this inhibitory activity was further improved in the higher concentration with an MIC of 2.5 mg/mL.

Immunomodulatory Actions

YP-1, a homogeneous polysaccharide containing glucose, mannose and galactose (molar ratio of 1:0.37:0.11) purified from the root powder of *D. opposita*, could enhance Con A-induced T lymphocyte proliferation in spleen cells of mice by the ^{3}H-TdR-incorporation method, indicating a strong immune-stimulatory effect of *D. opposita*.[51] More interestingly, D-mannose has been reported to inhibit FimH adhesion to the urothelium by competitively binding to the invariant lectin pocket of FimH.[44]

Experimental Studies on *Bian Xu* 萹蓄

Bian xu 萹蓄 (*Polygonum aviculare* L.), a member of the *Polygonaceae* family, has been traditionally used for improving urinary problems, removing kidney stones, and treating kidney, bladder and UTIs. The active components of *P. aviculare* consist of large quantities of phenolic and flavonoid constituents, including flavonoids (avicularin, kaempferol, quercetin and myricetin), tannins, saponins, alkaloids, quercitrin hydrate, mucilage, caffeic acid, chlorogenic acid, gallic acid, oxalic acid, coumaric acid and rutin, with various biological activities including anti-inflammation, antioxidant, anticancer and antibiotic properties.[52,53]

Anti-inflammatory Actions

The anti-inflammatory potential of *P. aviculare* was studied in combination with extracts of *M. officinalis* in human gingival fibroblast (HGF)-1 and human U-937 monocytes. Results showed that secretion of inflammatory cytokines from LPS-induced HGF-1 and U-937 cells was inhibited and accompanied by reduced IL-6 and IL-8 secretion from HGF-1 cells, and matrix metalloproteinase 2 (MMP-2) and MMP-9 secretion from U-937 cells.[54] By using one dimensional (1D) and two dimensional (2D) nuclear magnetic resonance (NMR) spectra and high-resolution mass spectrometry, the active compounds of flavonol glucuronides were demonstrated to be responsible for anti-inflammation.[55] In addition to flavonol glucuronides, compounds quercitrin hydrate, caffeic acid and rutin from *P. aviculare* have been reported to exert anti-inflammatory actions as well.[56]

Antimicrobial Actions

It was shown that organic (such as acetone, chloroform and ethanolic) and aqueous solvent extracts and fractions of *P. aviculare* demonstrated bacterial inhibitory effects on several microorganisms including *E. coli, P. mirabilis, P. aeruginosa, Salmonella typhi, Salmonella paratyphi* and *Shigella flexneri* for Gram-negative bacteria and *S. aureus, B. subtili* and *Streptococcus pyogenes (S. pyogenes)* for Gram-positive bacteria. It was observed that the chloroform extract had the strongest antimicrobial activity against all tested bacteria with a zone of inhibition diameter between 14 and 28 mm. The aqueous extract had the second highest antimicrobial activity, followed by the ethanol, and finally the acetone extracts. The phytochemical analysis indicated that tannins, saponins, flavonoids, alkaloids and sesquiterpenes could be the responsible constituents against both Gram-negative and Gram-positive bacteria. Furthermore, a new compound, panicudine (6-hydroxy-11-deoxy-13 dehydrohetisane), was identified as one of the active substances in the chlorotorm extract which showed the lowest MIC and minimum bactericidal concentration (MBC) against *S. paratyphi, B. subtilis* and *S. typhi,* and the highest MIC and MBC against *S. aureus.*[57]

Experimental Studies on *Che Qian Zi* 车前子

The sources of *che qian zi* 车前子 consist of *Plantago major* L. (PML), *Plantago asiatica* L. (PAL) and *Plantago depressa* Willd. (PDW). Among them, PDW exhibits wound healing, anti-inflammatory, antioxidant, antibiotic, antiulcerative, antidiabetic, antidiarrhoeal, antinociceptive, and antiviral activities. *Plantago asiatica* L. and PDW are used to treat acute glomerulonephritis, hypertension and liver injury. A total of 108 compounds have been identified from PAL, PDW and PML, including phenylethanoid glycosides (PhGs), flavonoids, triterpenes, caffeic acid derivatives, guanidine derivatives, iridoid glycosides, terpenoids, polysaccharides, organic acids and fatty acids, which contribute to the therapeutic effects (e.g., immunomodulatory, antioxidant), and for reducing blood lipids and sugar, facilitating defaecation, and decreasing blood pressure.[58,59]

Anti-inflammatory Actions

The *in vitro* and/or *in vivo* anti-inflammatory activities of *che qian zi* have been well described. The *in vitro* anti-inflammatory activity of the methanol, ethanol and aqueous extracts of the leaves of *Plantago major* has been proven by the lipoxygenase assay, which is usually used to examine the anti-inflammatory activity. This potential to attenuate the inflammatory response was further confirmed on acetaminophen-induced liver injury in rats showing an inhibitory effect on leukotrienes, which play a key role in inflammatory diseases through reducing the levels of pro-inflammatory cytokines of IL-1, IL-6 and TNF-α.[60] Moreover, the anti-inflammatory activity on carrageenan-induced paw oedema in rats was also reported with methanol extract from seeds of *Plantago major,* although the effect was less than the reference drug of indomethacin, a commercially available non-steroidal anti-inflammatory drug.[61] It has been stated that the anti-inflammatory activity of *Plantago major* was contributed to by flavonoids (such as baicalein and hispidulin) and iridoid glycosides (such as aucubin).[58,62–64] Other studies pointed out that hispidulin was effective as a 5-lipoxygenase inhibitor and inhibition of COX-2-catalysed prostaglandin biosynthesis might also be responsible for the anti-inflammatory action.[65]

Antimicrobial Actions

Pre-challenge administration of the soluble pectin polysaccharide (PMII) isolated from *Plantago major* leaves demonstrated defensive effects against systemic *S. pneumoniae* serotype 6B infection in inbred NIH/OlaHsd and Fox Chase SCID mice. This protective effect was attributed to its possible immuno-stimulatory activity.[66] Moreover, the antibacterial activities of *Plantago major* have been proven with leaves and seeds in different extracts (including aqueous, methanol, chloroform and hexane) to be positive against *E. coli, B. subtilis* and *Candida albicans* (*C. albicans*) cultures;[67] with leaves extracted in acetone to be effective on all nine species of bacteria: *E. coli, B. cereus, B. subtilis, Staphylococcus epidermidis* (*S. epidermidis*), *S. aureus, P. aeruginosa, K. pneumonia, Salmonella enteritidis* and

P. mirabilis.[68] Furthermore, the whole-plant aqueous, methanol and ethanol extracts of *Plantago major* demonstrated the ability to supress the bacterial growth of *B. subtilis, S. aureus, C. albicans, Candida tropicalis* and *E. coli.* In particular, methanol and ethanol extracts could inhibit both Gram-positive and Gram-negative bacteria by damaging Gram-positive bacteria cell walls and forming blebs on Gram-negative bacteria.[69]

Antiadhesive Actions

In addition to the most common causes of UTI, such as UPEC, *K. pneumonia, P. mirabilis, P. aeruginosa, E. faecalis, Enterobacter cloacae* and *Streptococcus bovis,* the fungus *Candida albicans* can also cause UTI. On the other hand, biofilm formation is a key factor in the colonisation by UPEC that enhances bacteria/fungus adherence to epithelium. By attaching to mucous surfaces, bacteria can resist the cleansing action of fluids such as urine.[44]

It was recently reported that the extract of *Plantago major* and its two active components, aucubin and baicalein, demonstrated inhibitory effects *in vitro* on growth, biofilm formation, metabolic activity and cell surface hydrophobicity of *C. albicans* in a dose-dependent manner. All three reagents demonstrated the inhibition of the total growth of *C. albicans* determined by MIC. Aucubin showed a strong fungicidal activity against *C. albicans* growth examined by the minimum fungicidal concentration (MFC), whereas aucubin and baicalein inhibited growth of *C. albicans* biofilm as assessed by the minimum biofilm inhibitory concentration (MBIC). This suggests that the extracts of *Plantago major,* aucubin and baicalein could effectively inhibit fungus growth and biofilm-related infections.[70]

Immunomodulatory Actions

Based on the traditional claims of *Plantago*-based natural products used in treating inflammation, cancers and infectious diseases, the immunomodulatory activity of the *Plantago* genus have been investigated. Its five chemical classes (flavonoids, monoterpenoids, triterpenoids, iridoid glycosides and phenolic compounds) of pure compounds were tested on human peripheral blood mononuclear cells (PBMC) with lymphocyte transformation by BrdU immunoassay and secretion of IFN-γ by enzyme-linked immunosorbent assay (ELISA). The aqueous aucubin, chlorogenic acid, ferulic acid, p-coumaric acid and vanillic acid were found to increase the activity of human lymphocyte proliferation and secretion of IFN-γ; both baicalein and baicalin demonstrated an enhancement of human PBMCs. Similar to oleanolic acid and ursolic acid of the triterpenoids, linalool of the monoterpenoids displayed strong stimulation of IFN-γ secretion. The data suggested that these active compounds were attributed to *Plantago* genus' possible immuno-stimulatory activity.[71]

Experimental Studies on *Hua Shi* 滑石

Hua shi 滑石 (hydrated magnesium silicate, commonly known as talc) is a white to greyish-white, very fine crystalline powder. Pure talc has the formula $Mg_3Si_4O_{10}(OH)_2$. Talc contains variable amounts of associated minerals, among which chlorites (hydrated aluminium and magnesium silicate), magnesite (magnesium carbonate), calcite (calcium carbonate) and dolomite (calcium and magnesium carbonate) are predominant. In CM, *hua shi* is thought to target the Bladder and the Stomach. *Hua shi* belongs to the category of herbs that drain dampness; these are typically diuretics to promote the increased production of urine in order to remove excessive damp from the body.[72]

Antimicrobial Actions

As talc contains a large amount of minerals, one study found that a mix of minerals consisting mainly of talc, sericite and halloysite had antibacterial effects. The mix of minerals could inhibit total bacterial growth, including the Gram-negative bacteria *E. coli* and *P. aeruginosa*, and the Gram-positive bacteria *S. aureus subsp.*

aureus, S. epidermidis and *B. cereus*, as well as the anaerobic bacterium *Propionibacterium acnes* (*P. acnes*).[72]

Antiadhesive Actions

It has been extensively proven that a herbal formula which consists of talc (*hua shi*), *Tetrapanax papyrifer* (Hook.) K. Koch (*tong cao* 通草), *Paeoniae* species (*chi shao* 赤芍), *Foeniculum vulgare* Mill (*xiao hui xiang* 小茴香), *Cinnamomum cassia* Presl (*gui zhi* 桂枝), *Litchi chinensis* Sonn. (*li zhi he* 荔枝核), *Semiaquilegia adoxoides* (DC.) Makino (*tian kui zi* 天葵子), *Viola yedoensis* Makino (*zi hua di ding* 紫花地丁), *Dianthus* species (*qu mai* 瞿麦), *Portulaca oleracea* L. (*ma chi xian* 马齿苋) and *Taraxacum* species (*pu gong ying* 蒲公英) possessed antimicrobial and antiadherent effects *in vitro* and *in vivo*.[73–76]

In patients with UTI caused by fluoroquinolone-resistant strains, clean-voided midstream urine samples during, and after, administration of the herbal formula were cultured and plated on blood agar plates followed by quantitation with pour plates or calibrated wire loops.[73] Its mode of action, particularly with respect to the adhesive activity of a uropathogenic strain of *E. coli* C16 to uroepithelial cells in the presence of the herbal formula, was further examined. The herbal formula showed significant effect on the rate of bacterial growth and markedly decreased the adherence of strain C16 in a dose-dependent way, demonstrated by the loss of half of hemagglutination abilities of the strain C16 at herb MIC (0.05g/ml). This indicates anti-adhesion may be one mode of action for the herbal formula used against pathogens.[74] Moreover, the preventive effect of the herbal formula on the clinical *E. coli* 11128 strain carrying Dr fimbriae was tested in experimental C3H/HeJ mice with ascending UTI. The herbal formula significantly reduced bacterial counts in urine, colonisation densities in the kidneys, neutrophilic infiltrates and renal lesions.[76] In addition to *in vivo* studies, the same research group defined Chinese herb-resistant UPEC and susceptible strains in isolated human urothelial cells, and adhesion of *E. coli* to urothelial cells *in vitro*. They found isolates of Chinese herb-resistant UPEC with haemolytic activity and virulence-related genes encoding PapC,

Hly and Cnf1 to have stronger uropathogenic activity and to be more adherent to urothelial cells.[75]

Experimental Studies on *Huang Bai* 黄柏

Huang bai 黄柏 is derived from two main species: *Phellodendron amurense Rupr* (PAR) and *Phellodendron chinense Schneid* (PCS). Its dried trunk bark has been traditionally used to treat various diseases, such as meningitis, cirrhosis, dysentery, pneumonia and tuberculosis.[77] So far, 140 compounds have been identified from *huang bai*, including alkaloids, isoquinoline alkaloid, limonoids, phenolic acid, quinic acid, lignans and flavonoids. Among them, alkaloids such as berberine, palmatine and jatrorrhizine are the major constituents of *huang bai*. It has been reported that the content of berberine, the major active ingredient of *huang bai*, is much higher in PCS than in PAR.[78,79] The crude bark of *huang bai* and/or its compounds exerts a wide range of pharmacological effects on inflammation, microbial (and bacterial) activity, cancer, hypotension, arrhythmia and gastric ulcers, as well as having antioxidant, antipyretic and immunomodulatory actions.[77,80]

Anti-inflammatory Actions

Huang bai has been widely used as an anti-inflammatory drug in CM. *In vitro* anti-inflammation effect of the methanol extract of *huang bai* has been shown to significantly decrease the release of TNF-α, IL-1β and NO from LPS-stimulated BV2 cells, a mouse microglia cell line and from LPS-stimulated primary mouse microglia. This occurred in a dose-dependent manner through suppression of LPS-stimulated phosphorylation of extracellular regulated protein kinases (ERK) and activation of NF-κB.[81] The *in vivo* anti-inflammation effect was further examined in LPS-induced acute airway inflammation in BALB/c mice. The methanol extract of *huang bai* attenuates LPS-induced infiltration of inflammatory cells (macrophages and neutrophils) and reduces the release of inflammatory mediators (TNF-α, macrophage inflammatory protein [MIP-2], IL-10, and

NO).[82] Besides the crude extracts of *huang bai*, the mixed ethanol extract of PCS and PAR at 2:1, named RAH13, demonstrated a stronger anti-inflammatory potency, as potent as the effects of celecoxib or dexamethasone in both acute and chronic animal inflammation models, when compared with the size of oedema in TPA-treated mice.[83] In addition, comparison of the anti-inflammatory effect of PAR and PCS has revealed that ethanol extracts of PCS were more effective than PAR on TPA-induced inflammation in mouse ears.[84] The active compounds responsible for the anti-inflammatory actions have been further identified from the alkaloid constituents,[85] such as berberine and coptisine, and from the non-alkaloid constituents,[86] such as limonoids including limonin and obakunone, through suppression of the activity of NF-κB, which is a key transcription factor involved in the inflammation process.

Antimicrobial Actions

Numerous studies have indicated that both the aqueous and ethanol extracts of *huang bai* possess an antimicrobial effect. *In vitro* studies using antimicrobial susceptibility tests showed 93% of 30 clinical isolates of *Mycoplasma hominis,* which causes infections in the genital tracts of humans adults, could be inhibited by *huang bai*.[87] It has also been reported that the extract of *huang bai* exerted a strong antibacterial effect on *Porphyromonas gingivalis,* a moderate effect on *Streptococcus mutans* and a partial effect on *Streptococcus sanguis in vitro.*[88]

Phellodendron amurense Rupr extracts have been shown to inhibit Gram-positive bacteria more effectively than Gram-negative bacteria with the most sensitive bacteria being *S. pyogenes*. Meanwhile, ethanol extracts of PAR demonstrated higher antimicrobial activity than aqueous extracts which might relate to the higher content of both total phenolic and flavonoid in ethanol extracts than in aqueous extracts.[89] As *P. aeruginosa* is one of the most common causative agents for both uncomplicated and complicated UTIs, it has been reported that berberine could inhibit aminoglycoside resistance in

P. aeruginosa in a MexXY-dependent manner as the resistance to aminoglycosides in *P. aeruginosa* is determined by the MexXY multidrug efflux system. Berberine was also observed to sufficiently reduce aminoglycoside MICs in *Achromobacter xylosoxidans* and *Burkholderia cepacia*, suppress MexXY/MexVW-mediated resistance of *P. aeruginosa* mutants, regulate MexXY-mediated gentamicin resistance in *P. aeruginosa* mutants and promote the synergistic effect of piperacillin and amikacin in multidrug-resistant *P. aeruginosa* strains. This indicates that the extract of *huang bai* and berberine have an ability to restore aminoglycoside activity in multi-medication resistant *P. aeruginosa*.[90]

In addition to antimicrobial activity, the monomers of *huang bai*, particularly berberine and palmatine, also showed antifungal activity *in vitro* and *in vivo*. *In vitro*, the ability of berberine hydrochloride and palmatine hydrochloride to inhibit the growth of *Microsporum canis*, known to cause UTI, has been assessed with MICs and growth curves. *In vivo*, berberine and palmatine have been tested in cyclophosphamide-induced dermatophytosis in the middle of the back of rabbits. This antifungal activity was suggested to occur through destruction of the fungal cell wall and cell membrane integrity, and through increasing expression of energy metabolic genes.[91]

Antiadhesive Actions

The main antibacterial substance of *huang bai*, berberine, has been found to have an effect on the adhesion to MRSA and intracellular invasion into HGFs. The lower concentration of berberine was sufficient to provide greater suppression of MRSA than ampicillin and oxacillin, but with a synergistic effect between berberine and ampicillin, and berberine and oxacillin against MRSA.[92]

Experimental Studies on *Huang Qi* 黄芪

The root of *Astragalus membranaceus* (Fisch.) and variants, known as *huang qi* 黄芪, is a traditional CM herb that has been widely used to treat conditions associated with tissue ischaemia, including cardiovascular and cerebrovascular diseases. More than 200 compounds have been isolated and identified from *huang qi*. Saponins, polysaccharides, flavonoids and amino acids are regarded as the significant bioactive constituents. Among them, the saponin astragaloside IV (AS-IV) is a principal active component of the herb known to be the qualitative control biomarker.[93,94] In pharmacological studies, crude extracts of *huang qi* and its isolated constituents have multiple pharmacologic effects including anti-inflammatory, antioxidant, antiasthma, anticancer, antidiabetic, antihyperglycemic, antiaging, antitumour and antiviral activities, and immunoregulatory, cardioprotective and hepatoprotective effects via numerous signalling pathways in vital organs and systems.[93,95]

Anti-inflammatory Actions

The anti-inflammatory activities of *huang qi* and its main bioactive compounds have been comprehensively studied *in vitro* and *in vivo*. It has been reported that *huang qi* could reduce the expression of iNOS, COX-2, IL-6, IL-1β and TNF-α in LPS-treated RAW 264.7 cells through mitogen-activated protein kinase phosphatase-1 (MKP-1)-dependent inactivation of p38 and the suppression of NF-κB-mediated transcription.[96,97] In addition, astragaloside IV (AS-IV) has demonstrated a powerful anti-inflammatory effect through modulating the NO, NF-κB and c-Jun N-terminal kinases (JNK) signalling pathway and suppression of the expression of inflammatory cytokines (such as ILs, chemokines, TNF-α and intracellular cell adhesion molecule-1 [ICAM-1) and inhibition of neutrophils' adhesion-related molecules (such as CD11b/CD18).[95,98] Furthermore, it has been shown that *Astragalus* polysaccharides (APS) possessed strong inhibitory effects on LPS- and palmitate-induced inflammation by inhibiting the production of TNF-α, IL-1, IL-8, p65 and ICAM via suppression of NF-κB and antimicrobial peptide (AMP)-activated protein kinase (AMPK) activity, the phosphorylation of ERK and JNK, and Rho/Rho-associated protein kinase (ROCK) signal pathways.[99,100]

Antimicrobial Actions

Astragalus polysaccharides have been shown to possess *in vitro* antibacterial activity. Synthesised silver nanoparticles (AgNPs) with a water-soluble fraction of polysaccharides extracted from the roots of *Astragalus membranaceus* (AMWP) (AMWP-AgNPs) could inhibit four reference bacterial strains (*S. aureus, S. epidermidis, E. coli* and *P. aeruginosa*) at comparatively low concentration. Furthermore, four clinical isolated drug-resistant strains (MRSA, MRSE, *E. coli* and *P. aeruginosa*) which are resistant to ampicillin, levofloxacin and cefoxitin were also inhibited by AMWP-AgNPs. Inhibition was assessed using the inhibition zone diameters and MICs using modified agar disk diffusion and tetrazolium methods.[101]

Furthermore, the human cathelicidin AMP LL-37 together with epithelial cells have been well known to be the first line of the host defence against pathogens, capable of protecting the mucosa against bacterial infection.[102,103] *Astragalus* polysaccharides could induce the production of the peptide LL-37 in airway epithelial HBE16 and A549 cells and resist bacterial infection through p38 MAPK/JNK and NF-κB signalling pathways.[104]

Immunomodulatory Actions

The immune system plays a fundamental role in the host defence against pathogens. As an immune-enhancing agent, an increasing number of *in vivo* and *in vitro* studies have demonstrated that *huang qi* and its compounds could enhance the immune system by both humoral and cellular immune responses.

It has been reported that *huang bai* could potentiate immunity through increasing thymus weight and proliferation of splenocytes, enhancing phagocytic function, stimulating natural killer (NK)-cell activity of peripheral blood lymphocytes, restoring steroid-inhibited NK-cell activity and increasing superoxide anion production by peritoneal macrophages via activation of the TLR4 signalling pathway.[96,97] In addition, AS-IV could dramatically enhance the proliferation and response of T and B lymphocytes, increase the level of IFN-r and the production of antibodies, and suppress the expression of IL-1, TNF-α, transforming growth factor (TGF)-β and thymic stromal lymphopoietin.[95,98] Furthermore, APS exhibited significant immunomodulating effects on both the specific immunity and the non-specific immunity to activate a series of immune cells (such as lymphocytes, macrophages and dendritic cells) but also potentiate the proliferation and differentiation of T and B lymphocytes, and the production of cytokines and immunoglobulins. *Astragalus* polysaccharides also exhibited immunorestorative effects both *in vitro* and *in vivo,* restoring the lymphocyte blastogenic response to normal levels in older mice and in tumour-bearing and cyclophosphamide-treated mice.[99,100]

Experimental Studies on *Qu Mai* 瞿麦

Qu mai 瞿麦 (*Dianthus superbus* L. or *Dianthus chinensis* L.), the biggest genus of family *Caryophyllaceae* consisting of over 600 species native from Asia and Europe, is popularly known as Chinese pink. It has been used in traditional CM as a diuretic, a contraceptive and an anti-inflammatory agent in the treatment of urinary infection. The bioactive compounds have been identified from *Dianthus* species including triterpenoid saponins, flavones, phenols, diantho-saponins, dianthramide, fatty acid derivatives and cyclic peptides. Among them, triterpenoid saponins such as dianosides A-I are considered as the major bioactive compounds of *Dianthus* species with a variety of bioactivities, as well as antioxidative, cytotoxic and neuroprotective properties.[105,106]

Anti-inflammatory Actions

The ethanolic extract of *Dianthus superbus* has demonstrated anti-inflammatory effects in an ovalbumin (OVA)-induced murine asthma model. It could significantly supress the levels of Th2-type cytokines including IL-4, IL-13, eotaxin and immunoglobulin (Ig) E in bronchoalveolar lavage fluid (BALF), reduce inflammatory cell infiltration and mucus production, and attenuate the overproduction of iNOS induced by OVA challenge.[107] More recently, *Dianthus superbus*-EtOAc soluble fraction (DS-EA) has been reported to have protective effects against renal inflammation and fibrosis in db/db mice through suppression of ICAM-1 and monocyte chemoattractant protein-1, reducing the translocation of NF-κB in angiotensin II (Ang II)-stimulated mesangial cells, and downregulating TGF-β/Smad signalling.[108]

Antimicrobial and Antiadherent Actions

A herbal formula comprising *hua shi* 滑石, *tong cao* 通草, *chi shao* 赤芍, *xiao hui xiang* 小茴香, *gui zhi* 桂枝, *li zhi he* 荔枝核, *tian kui zi* 天葵子, *zi hua di ding* 紫花地丁, *qu mai* 瞿麦, *ma chi xian* 马齿苋 and *pu gong ying* 蒲公英 has been extensively studied to have antimicrobial and antiadherent effects *in vitro* and *in vivo* (see section on *hua shi* 滑石).[73–76]

Summary of Pharmacological Actions of the Common Herbs

Each of these ten herbs has attracted research attention in experimental models of relevance to UTI. Anti-inflammatory and immunomodulatory actions were observed in most of the herbs including *di huang* 地黄, *fu ling* 茯苓, *gan cao* 甘草, *shan yao* 山药, *bian xu* 萹蓄, *che qian zi* 车前子, *huang bai* 黄柏, *huang qi* 黄芪 and *qu mai* 瞿麦 via the suppression of the production of pro-inflammatory cytokines and inflammatory mediators for anti-inflammation, enhancing the production of immune stimulators (IL-1β, IL-6, and TNF-α), and inhibiting the production of an immune suppressor (TGF-β) for immunomodulation. These overall anti-inflammatory and immunomodulatory effects have been well known to enhance the innate immune system against bacterial infection and invasions, although there are few studies focusing on bladder inflammation and immune responses resulting from bacterial infections of the urinary tract and bladder epithelium.

Antimicrobial actions were observed in all herbs except *fu ling* 茯苓. The herbs *gan cao* 甘草, *bian xu* 萹蓄, *che qian zi* 车前子, *huang bai* 黄柏 and *huang qi* 黄芪 showed strong antibacterial effect against uropathogenic bacteria such as Gram-negative *E. coli*, *K. pneumonia*, *E. aerogenes*, *P. vulgaris* and *P. aeruginosa*, and the Gram-positive *S. aureus subsp. aureus, S. epidermidis* and *B. cereus*, as well as the anaerobic bacterium *P. acnes*.

The antimicrobial actions of the abovementioned herbs were largely attributed to their secondary metabolites and their derivatives, including phenolics and polyphenols (such as flavones, flavonoids, flavonols, tannins, quinones and coumarins), terpenoids, essential oils and alkaloids. Among them, phenolics, polyphenols and alkaloids have demonstrated strong antimicrobial activity. As polyphenols and alkaloids contain numerous groups of secondary metabolites, it is not surprising that herbs with these metabolites are found to have effective antimicrobial activity *in vitro* against a wide array of microorganisms. However, *in vitro* findings have not been confirmed in animal and human studies of whole organism systems.[44,109,110] The mode of antimicrobial action is through different mechanisms, such as flavonoids through binding to adhesions and the multilayered cell wall complex; polyphenols and tannins through inhibiting bacterial enzymes, depriving substrate, disrupting bacterial membrane, and metal ion complexation; and terpenoids and essential oils through disrupting bacterial membrane and alkaloids through intercalating into the cell wall, respectively.[111,112]

One of the main strategies for protection against UPEC infection is to prevent adherence of the bacteria/fungus to the uroepithelium.[44,113] Such actions were observed in *gan cao* 甘草, *che qian zi* 车前子 and *huang bai* 黄柏 through inhibition of adhesin FimH, Dr fimbriae and biofilm formation by their bioactive compounds carbenoxolone, quercetin-3-glucoside and ethyl caffeate, aucubin, baicalein and berberine.

However, the number of available *in vitro* and *in vivo* studies relevant to UTI is limited and there is a lack of direct evidence for the ten selected herbs in UTI. One exception is a series of studies from one research group using a herbal formula which included *hua shi* 滑石 and *qu mai* 瞿麦. These studies demonstrated antimicrobial and antiadherent effects *in vitro* on UPEC from patients with UTI, and *in vivo* in experimental ascending UTI in mice. However, this effective treatment for UTI might not be due solely to herbs *hua shi* 滑石 and *qu mai* 瞿麦. The formula tested was a multi-herb formula, and it is possible that actions may be due to synergy of herbs and/or their constituent compounds.

Animal models of human UTI are vital experimental tools to investigate and assess the therapeutic effects of the herbs and/or compounds on UTI and underlying mechanisms.[114,115] Various animal models of UTI have been well established, such as chemicals or bacterial (particularly LPS)-induced cystitis by intravesical instillation, and prostatic inflammation initiated by transurethral instillation of bacteria. Further investigation to determine the effect of these, and other herbs and/or main compound alone, or in combination, in UTI animal models is highly recommended. Such studies could provide more effective guidance for the use of CHM in clinical practice.

These *in vitro* and *in vivo* studies that examined herb actions generally, as well as actions specific to UTI, provide potential explanations of the clinical benefits of some of the common herbs. The findings highlight that CHM have multiple components which can act on multiple pathways relevant to UTI. This fully reflects the multiple-targets synergy characteristics of CM generally.

References

1. Sihra N, Goodman A, Zakri R, *et al.* (2018) Nonantibiotic prevention and management of recurrent urinary tract infection. *Nat Rev Urol* **15**(12): 750–776.

2. Flower A, Wang LQ, Lewith G, *et al.* (2015) Chinese herbal medicine for treating recurrent urinary tract infections in women. *Cochrane Database Syst Rev* **(6)**: Cd010446.

3. Liu C, Ma R, Wang L, *et al.* (2017) *Rehmanniae radix* in osteoporosis: A review of traditional Chinese medicinal uses, phytochemistry, pharmacokinetics and pharmacology. *J Ethnopharmacol* **198**: 351–362.

4. Zhang RX, Li MX, Jia ZP. (2008) *Rehmannia glutinosa*: Review of botany, chemistry and pharmacology. *J Ethnopharmacol* **117**(2): 199–214.

5. Kim SH, Yook TH, Kim JU. (2017) *Rehmanniae radix*, an effective treatment for patients with various inflammatory and metabolic diseases: Results from a review of Korean publications. *J Pharmacopuncture* **20**(2): 81–88.

6. Viljoen A, Mncwangi N, Vermaak I. (2012) Anti-inflammatory iridoids of botanical origin. *Curr Med Chem* **19**(14): 2104–2127.

7. Choi YH. (2019) Catalpol attenuates lipopolysaccharide-induced inflammatory responses in BV2 microglia through inhibiting the TLR4-mediated NF-kappaB pathway. *Gen Physiol Biophys* **38**(2): 111–122.

8. Park KS. (2016) Catalpol reduces the production of inflammatory mediators via PPAR-gamma activation in human intestinal Caco-2 cells. *J Nat Med* **70**(3): 620–626.

9. Modaressi M, Delazar A, Nazemiyeh H, *et al.* (2009) Antibacterial iridoid glucosides from Eremostachys laciniata. *Phytother Res* **23**(1): 99–103.

10. Kim HM, An CS, Jung KY, *et al.* (1999) *Rehmannia glutinosa* inhibits tumour necrosis factor-alpha and interleukin-1 secretion from mouse astrocytes. *Pharmacol Res* **40**(2): 171–176.

11. Huang Y, Jiang C, Hu Y, *et al.* (2013) Immunoenhancement effect of *Rehmannia glutinosa* polysaccharide on lymphocyte proliferation and dendritic cell. *Carbohydr Polym* **96**(2): 516–521.

12. Huang Y, Qin T, Huang Y, *et al.* (2016) *Rehmannia glutinosa* polysaccharide liposome as a novel strategy for stimulating an efficient immune response and their effects on dendritic cells. *Int J Nanomedicine* **11:** 6795–6808.

13. Wang Y, Kwak M, Lee PC, *et al.* (2018) *Rehmannia glutinosa* polysaccharide promoted activation of human dendritic cells. *Int J Biol Macromol* **116:** 232–238.

14. Rios JL. (2011) Chemical constituents and pharmacological properties of *Poria cocos. Planta Med* **77**(7): 681–691.

15. Sun Y. (2014) Biological activities and potential health benefits of polysaccharides from *Poria cocos* and their derivatives. *Int J Biol Macromol* **68:** 131–134.

16. Lee KY, Jeon YJ. (2003) Polysaccharide isolated from *Poria cocos* sclerotium induces NF-kappaB/Rel activation and iNOS expression in murine macrophages. *Int Immunopharmacol* **3**(10–11): 1353–1362.

17. Fuchs SM, Heinemann C, Schliemann-Willers S, *et al.* (2006) Assessment of anti-inflammatory activity of *Poria cocos* in sodium lauryl sulphate-induced irritant contact dermatitis. *Skin Res Technol* **12**(4): 223–227.

18. Cuella MJ, Giner RM, Recio MC, *et al.* (1996) Two fungal lanostane derivatives as phospholipase A2 inhibitors. *J Nat Prod* **59**(10): 977–979.

19. Cuellar MJ, Giner RM, Recio MC, *et al.* (1997) Effect of the basidiomycete *Poria cocos* on experimental dermatitis and other inflammatory conditions. *Chem Pharm Bull (Tokyo)* **45**(3): 492–494.

20. Jain MK, Yu BZ, Rogers JM, *et al.* (1995) Specific competitive inhibitor of secreted phospholipase A2 from berries of *Schinus terebinthifolius. Phytochemistry* **39**(3): 537–547.

21. Kaminaga T, Yasukawa K, Kanno H, *et al.* (1996) Inhibitory effects of lanostane-type triterpene acids, the components of *Poria cocos*, on tumor promotion by 12-O-tetradecanoylphorbol-13-acetate in two-stage carcinogenesis in mouse skin. *Oncology* **53**(5): 382–585.

22. Lu MK, Chen JJ, Lin CY, Chang CC. (2010) Purification, structural elucidation, and anti-inflammatory effect of a water-soluble 1,6-branched 1,3-a-D-galactan from cultured mycelia of *Poria cocos. Food Chem* **118**(2): 349–356.

23. Spelman K, Burns J, Nichols D, *et al.* (2006) Modulation of cytokine expression by traditional medicines: A review of herbal immunomodulators. *Altern Med Rev* **11**(2): 128–150.

24. Yu SJ, Tseng J. (1996) Fu-Ling, a Chinese herbal drug, modulates cytokine secretion by human peripheral blood monocytes. *Int J Immunopharmacol* **18**(1): 37–44.

25. Chang HH, Yeh CH, Sheu F. (2009) A novel immunomodulatory protein from *Poria cocos* induces Toll-like receptor 4-dependent activation within mouse peritoneal macrophages. *J Agric Food Chem* **57**(14): 6129–6139.

26. Chen X, Zhang L, Cheung PC. (2010) Immunopotentiation and anti-tumor activity of carboxymethylated-sulfated beta-(1→3)-d-glucan from *Poria cocos. Int Immunopharmacol* **10**(4): 398–405.

27. Kaper JB, Nataro JP, Mobley HL. (2004) Pathogenic *Escherichia coli. Nat Rev Microbiol* **2**(2): 123–140.

28. Lee SM, Lee YJ, Yoon JJ, *et al.* (2012) Effect of *Poria cocos* on hypertonic stress-induced water channel expression and apoptosis in renal collecting duct cells. *J Ethnopharmacol* **141**(1): 368–376.

29. Zhao YY, Feng YL, Du X, *et al.* (2012) Diuretic activity of the ethanol and aqueous extracts of the surface layer of *Poria cocos* in rat. *J Ethnopharmacol* **144**(3): 775–778.

30. Feng YL, Lei P, Tian T, *et al.* (2013) Diuretic activity of some fractions of the epidermis of *Poria cocos. J Ethnopharmacol* **150**(3): 1114–1118.

31. Asl MN, Hosseinzadeh H. (2008) Review of pharmacological effects of *Glycyrrhiza* sp. and its bioactive compounds. *Phytother Res* **22**(6): 709–724.

32. Ji S, Li Z, Song W, *et al.* (2016) Bioactive constituents of *Glycyrrhiza uralensis* (Licorice): Discovery of the effective components of a traditional herbal medicine. *J Nat Prod* **79**(2): 281–292.

33. Zhang Q, Ye M. (2009) Chemical analysis of the Chinese herbal medicine Gan-Cao (licorice). *J Chromatogr A* **1216**(11): 1954–1969.

34. Peng F, Du Q, Peng C, *et al.* (2015) A review: The pharmacology of isoliquiritigenin. *Phytother Res* **29**(7): 969–977.

35. Yang R, Yuan BC, Ma YS, *et al.* (2017) The anti-inflammatory activity of licorice, a widely used Chinese herb. *Pharm Biol* **55**(1): 5–18.

36. Onkarappa R SK, Chaya K. (2005) Efficacy of four medicinally important plant extracts (crude) against pathogenic bacteria. *Asian J Microbiol Biotech Env Sci* **7**: 281–284.

37. Hatano T, Shintani Y, Aga Y, *et al.* (2000) Phenolic constituents of licorice. VIII. Structures of glicophenone and glicoisoflavanone, and effects of licorice phenolics on methicillin-resistant *Staphylococcus aureus. Chem Pharm Bull (Tokyo)* **48**(9): 1286–1292.

38. Hatano T, Kusuda M, Inada K, *et al.* (2005) Effects of tannins and related polyphenols on methicillin-resistant *Staphylococcus aureus. Phytochemistry* **66**(17): 2047–2055.

39. Fukai T, Marumo A, Kaitou K, *et al.* (2002) Antimicrobial activity of licorice flavonoids against methicillin-resistant *Staphylococcus aureus. Fitoterapia* **73**(6): 536–539.

40. Fukai T, Oku Y, Hano Y, *et al.* (2004) Antimicrobial activities of hydrophobic 2-arylbenzofurans and an isoflavone against vancomycin-resistant enterococci and methicillin-resistant *Staphylococcus aureus. Planta Med* **70**(7): 685–687.

41. Gaur R, Gupta VK, Singh P, *et al.* (2016) Drug resistance reversal potential of isoliquiritigenin and liquiritigenin isolated from *Glycyrrhiza glabra* against methicillin-resistant *Staphylococcus aureus* (MRSA). *Phytother Res* **30**(10): 1708–1715.

42. He J, Chen L, Heber D, *et al.* (2006) Antibacterial compounds from Glycyrrhiza uralensis. *J Nat Prod* **69**(1): 121–124.

43. Singh V, Pal A, Darokar MP. (2015) A polyphenolic flavonoid glabridin: Oxidative stress response in multidrug-resistant *Staphylococcus aureus. Free Radic Biol Med* **87**: 48–57.

44. Terlizzi ME, Gribaudo G, Maffei ME. (2017) UroPathogenic Escherichia coli (UPEC) infections: Virulence factors, bladder responses, antibiotic, and non-antibiotic antimicrobial strategies. *Front Microbiol* **8:** 1566.

45. Mooreville M, Fritz RW, Mulholland SG. (1983) Enhancement of the bladder defense mechanism by an exogenous agent. *J Urol* **130**(3): 607–609.

46. Jaiswal SK, Sharma NK, Bharti SK, *et al.* (2018) Phytochemicals as uropathognic *Escherichia coli* fimH antagonist: *In vitro* and *in silico* approach. *Curr Mol Med* **18**(9): 640–653.

47. Ma F, Wang D, Zhang Y, *et al.* (2018) Characterisation of the mucilage polysaccharides from *Dioscorea opposita* Thunb. with enzymatic hydrolysis. *Food Chem* **245:** 13–21.

48. Zhang Y, Chao L, Ruan J, *et al.* (2016) Bioactive constituents from the rhizomes of *Dioscorea septemloba* Thunb. *Fitoterapia* **115:** 165–172.

49. Zhang Y, Yu HY, Chao LP, *et al.* (2016) Anti-inflammatory steroids from the rhizomes of *Dioscorea septemloba* Thunb. *Steroids* **112:** 95–102.

50. Yang W, Wang Y, Li X, *et al.* (2015) Purification and structural characterization of Chinese yam polysaccharide and its activities. *Carbohydr Polym* **117:** 1021–1027.

51. Zhao GH, Kan JQ, Li ZX, *et al.* (2005) Structural features and immunological activity of a polysaccharide from *Dioscorea opposita* Thunb roots. *Carbohydr Polym* **61:** 125–131.

52. Gonzalez Begne M, Yslas N, Reyes E, *et al.* (2001) Clinical effect of a Mexican sanguinaria extract (*Polygonum aviculare* L.) on gingivitis. *J Ethnopharmacol* **74**(1): 45–51.

53. Granica S. (2015) Quantitative and qualitative investigations of pharmacopoeial plant material polygoni avicularis herba by UHPLC-CAD and UHPLC-ESI-MS methods. *Phytochem Anal* **26**(5): 374–382.

54. Walker JM, Maitra A, Walker J, *et al.* (2013) Identification of *Magnolia officinalis* L. bark extract as the most potent anti-inflammatory of four plant extracts. *Am J Chin Med* **41**(3): 531–544.

55. Granica S, Czerwinska ME, Zyzynska-Granica B, *et al.* (2013) Antioxidant and anti-inflammatory flavonol glucuronides from *Polygonum aviculare* L. *Fitoterapia* **91:** 180–188.

56. Seo SH, Lee SH, Cha PH, *et al.* (2016) *Polygonum aviculare* L. and its active compounds, quercitrin hydrate, caffeic acid, and rutin, activate the Wnt/beta-catenin pathway and induce cutaneous wound healing. *Phytother Res* **30**(5): 848–854.

57. Salama HM, Marraiki N. (2010) Antimicrobial activity and phytochemical analyses of *Polygonum aviculare* L. (Polygonaceae), naturally growing in Egypt. *Saudi J Biol Sci* **17**(1): 57–63.

58. Samuelsen AB. (2000) The traditional uses, chemical constituents and biological activities of *Plantago major* L: A review. *J Ethnopharmacol* **71**(1–2): 1–21.

59. Wang D, Qi M, Yang Q, *et al.* (2016) Comprehensive metabolite profiling of *Plantaginis Semen* using ultra high performance liquid chromatography with electrospray ionization quadrupole time-of-flight tandem mass spectrometry coupled with elevated energy technique. *J Sep Sci* **39**(10): 1842–1852.

60. Hussan F, Mansor AS, Hassan SN, *et al.* (2015) Anti-inflammatory property of *Plantago major* leaf extract reduces the inflammatory reaction in experimental acetaminophen-induced liver injury. *Evid Based Complement Alternat Med* **2015:** 347861.

61. Turel I, Ozbek H, Erten R, *et al.* (2009) Hepatoprotective and anti-inflammatory activities of *Plantago major* L. *Indian J Pharmacol* **41**(3): 120–124.

62. Beara IN, Lesjak MM, Jovin ED, *et al.* (2009) Plantain (*Plantago* L.) species as novel sources of flavonoid antioxidants. *J Agric Food Chem* **57**(19): 9268–9273.

63. Havsteen BH. (2002) The biochemistry and medical significance of the flavonoids. *Pharmacol Ther* **96**(2–3): 67–202.

64. Middleton E, Jr., Kandaswami C, Theoharides TC. (2000) The effects of plant flavonoids on mammalian cells: Implications for inflammation, heart disease and cancer. *Pharmacol Rev* **52**(4): 673–751.

65. Ringbom T, Segura L, Noreen Y, *et al.* (1998) Ursolic acid from *Plantago major*, a selective inhibitor of cyclooxygenase-2 catalyzed prostaglandin biosynthesis. *J Nat Prod* **61**(10): 1212–1215.

66. Hetland G, Samuelsen AB, Lovik M, *et al.* (2000) Protective effect of *Plantago major* L. Pectin polysaccharide against systemic Streptococcus pneumoniae infection in mice. *Scand J Immunol* **52**(4): 348–355.

67. Velasco-Lezama R, Tapia-Aguilar R, Roman-Ramos R, *et al.* (2006) Effect of *Plantago major* on cell proliferation *in vitro*. *J Ethnopharmacol* **103**(1): 36–42.

68. Metiner K, Ozkan O, Ak S. (2012) Antibacterial effects of ethanol and acetone extract of *Plantago major* L. on gram positive and gram negative bacteria. *Kafkas Univ Vet Fak Derg* **18**(3): 503–505.

69. Sharifa AA, Amaludin JJ, Kiong LS, *et al.* (2012) Anti-urolithiatic terpenoid compound from *Plantago major* Linn. *Sains Malaysiana* **41**(1): 33–39.

70. Shirley KP, Windsor LJ, Eckert GJ, *et al.* (2017) *In vitro* effects of *Plantago major* extract, aucubin, and baicalein on *Candida albicans* biofilm formation, metabolic activity, and cell surface hydrophobicity. *J Prosthodont* **26**(6): 508–515.

71. Chiang LC, Ng LT, Chiang W, *et al.* (2003) Immunomodulatory activities of flavonoids, monoterpenoids, triterpenoids, iridoid glycosides and phenolic compounds of *Plantago* species. *Planta Med* **69**(7): 600–604.

72. Park SK, Lee CW, Lee MY. (2009) Antibacterial effects of minerals from ores indigenous to Korea. *J Environ Biol* **30**(1): 151–4.

73. Tong Y, Jing Y, Zhao D, *et al.* (2011) Fluoroquinolone-resistant uncomplicated urinary tract infections, Chinese herbal medicine may provide help. *Afr J Tradit Complement Altern Med* **8**(5 Suppl): 108–114.

74. Tong Y, Wu Q, Zhao D, *et al.* (2011) Effects of Chinese herbs on the hemagglutination and adhesion of *Escherichia coli* strain *in vitro*. *Afr J Tradit Complement Altern Med* **8**(1): 82–87.

75. Tong Y, Xin B, Chi Y. (2014) Chinese herb-resistance and adherence to human uroepithelial cells of uropathogenic *Escherichia coli*. *Afr J Tradit Complement Altern Med* **11**(1): 109–115.

76. Tong YQ, Sun M, Chi Y. (2016) Prophylactic herbal therapy prevents experimental ascending urinary tract infection in mice. *Chin J Integr Med* **22**(10): 774–777.

77. Ryuk JA, Zheng MS, Lee MY, *et al.* (2012) Discrimination of *Phellodendron amurense* and *P. chinense* based on DNA analysis and the simultaneous analysis of alkaloids. *Arch Pharm Res* **35**(6): 1045–1054.

78. Chan CO, Chu CC, Mok DK, *et al.* (2007) Analysis of berberine and total alkaloid content in cortex phellodendri by near infrared spectroscopy (NIRS) compared with high-performance liquid chromatography coupled with ultra-visible spectrometric detection. *Anal Chim Acta* **592**(2): 121–131.

79. Chen ML, Xian YF, Ip SP, *et al.* (2010) Chemical and biological differentiation of *Cortex Phellodendri Chinensis* and *Cortex Phellodendri Amurensis*. *Planta Med* **76**(14): 1530–1535.

80. Sun Y, Lenon GB, Yang AWH. (2019) *Phellodendri cortex*: A phytochemical, pharmacological, and pharmacokinetic review. *Evid Based Complement Alternat Med* **2019:** 7621929.

81. Park YK, Chung YS, Kim YS, *et al.* (2007) Inhibition of gene expression and production of iNOS and TNF-alpha in LPS-stimulated microglia by methanol extract of *Phellodendri cortex*. *Int Immunopharmacol* **7**(7): 955–962.

82. Mao YF, Li YQ, Zong L, *et al.* (2010) Methanol extract of *Phellodendri cortex* alleviates lipopolysaccharide-induced acute airway inflammation in mice. *Immunopharmacol Immunotoxicol* **32**(1): 110–115.

83. Park EK, Rhee HI, Jung HS, *et al.* (2007) Antiinflammatory effects of a combined herbal preparation (RAH13) of *Phellodendron amurense* and *Coptis chinensis* in animal models of inflammation. *Phytother Res* **21**(8): 746–750.

84. Xian YF, Mao QQ, Ip SP, *et al.* (2011) Comparison on the anti-inflammatory effect of *Cortex Phellodendri Chinensis* and *Cortex Phellodendri Amurensis* in 12-O-tetradecanoyl-phorbol-13-acetate-induced ear edema in mice. *J Ethnopharmacol* **137**(3): 1425–1430.

85. Wu J, Zhang H, Hu B, *et al.* (2016) Coptisine from *Coptis chinensis* inhibits production of inflammatory mediators in lipopolysaccharide-stimulated RAW 264.7 murine macrophage cells. *Eur J Pharmacol* **780**: 106–114.

86. Fujii A, Okuyama T, Wakame K, *et al.* (2017) Identification of anti-inflammatory constituents in *Phellodendri Cortex* and *Coptidis Rhizoma* by monitoring the suppression of nitric oxide production. *J Nat Med* **71**(4): 745–756.

87. Che YM, Mao SH, Jiao WL, *et al.* (2005) Susceptibilities of *Mycoplasma hominis* to herbs. *Am J Chin Med* **33**(2): 191–196.

88. Wong RW, Hagg U, Samaranayake L, *et al.* (2010) Antimicrobial activity of Chinese medicine herbs against common bacteria in oral biofilm: A pilot study. *Int J Oral Maxillofac Surg* **39**(6): 599–605.

89. Wang W, Zu Y, Fu Y, *et al.* (2009) In vitro antioxidant, antimicrobial and anti-herpes simplex virus type 1 activity of *Phellodendron amurense* Rupr. from China. *Am J Chin Med* **37**(1): 195–203.

90. Morita Y, Nakashima K, Nishino K, *et al.* (2016) Berberine is a novel type efflux inhibitor which attenuates the MexXY-mediated aminoglycoside resistance in *Pseudomonas aeruginosa*. *Front Microbiol* **7**: 1223.

91. Xiao CW, Ji QA, Wei Q, *et al.* (2015) Antifungal activity of berberine hydrochloride and palmatine hydrochloride against *Microsporum canis*-induced dermatitis in rabbits and underlying mechanism. *BMC Complement Altern Med* **15**: 177.

92. Yu HH, Kim KJ, Cha JD, *et al.* (2005) Antimicrobial activity of berberine alone and in combination with ampicillin or oxacillin against methicillin-resistant *Staphylococcus aureus*. *J Med Food* **8**(4): 454–461.

93. Fu J, Wang Z, Huang L, *et al.* (2014) Review of the botanical characteristics, phytochemistry, and pharmacology of *Astragalus membranaceus* (Huangqi). *Phytother Res* **28**(9): 1275–1283.

94. Li X, Qu L, Dong Y, *et al.* (2014) A review of recent research progress on the *Astragalus* genus. *Molecules* **19**(11): 18850–18880.

95. Li L, Hou X, Xu R, *et al.* (2017) Research review on the pharmacological effects of astragaloside IV. *Fundam Clin Pharmacol* **31**(1): 17–36.

96. Auyeung KK, Han QB, Ko JK. (2016) *Astragalus membranaceus*: A review of its protection against inflammation and gastrointestinal cancers. *Am J Chin Med* **44**(1): 1–22.

97. Qi Y, Gao F, Hou L, *et al.* (2017) Anti-inflammatory and immunostimulatory activities of astragalosides. *Am J Chin Med* **45**(6): 1157–1167.

98. Ren S, Zhang H, Mu Y, *et al.* (2013) Pharmacological effects of astragaloside IV: A literature review. *J Tradit Chin Med* **33**(3): 413–416.

99. Jin M, Zhao K, Huang Q, *et al.* (2014) Structural features and biological activities of the polysaccharides from *Astragalus membranaceus*. *Int J Biol Macromol* **64**: 257–266.

100. Xie JH, Jin ML, Morris GA, *et al.* (2016) Advances on bioactive polysaccharides from medicinal plants. *Crit Rev Food Sci Nutr* **56**(Suppl 1): S60–S84.

101. Ma Y, Liu C, Qu D, *et al.* (2017) Antibacterial evaluation of silver nanoparticles synthesized by polysaccharides from *Astragalus membranaceus* roots. *Biomed Pharmacother* **89**: 351–357.

102. Lai Y, Gallo RL. (2009) AMPed up immunity: How antimicrobial peptides have multiple roles in immune defense. *Trends Immunol* **30**(3): 131–141.

103. Xhindoli D, Pacor S, Benincasa M, *et al.* (2016) The human cathelicidin LL-37: A pore-forming antibacterial peptide and host-cell modulator. *Biochim Biophys Acta* **1858**(3): 546–566.

104. Zhao L, Tan S, Zhang H, *et al.* (2018) *Astragalus* polysaccharides exerts anti-infective activity by inducing human cathelicidin antimicrobial peptide LL-37 in respiratory epithelial cells. *Phytother Res* **32**(8): 1521–1529.

105. The Pharmacopoeia Commission of PRC China. (1992) *Pharmcopoeia of the People's Republic of China (English edition)*. Guandong Science and Technology Press, Guangzhou.

106. Kim DH, Park GS, Nile AS, *et al.* (2019) Utilization of *Dianthus superbus* L and its bioactive compounds for antioxidant, anti-influenza and toxicological effects. *Food Chem Toxicol* **125:** 313–321.

107. Shin IS, Lee MY, Ha H, *et al.* (2012) *Dianthus superbus fructus* suppresses airway inflammation by downregulating of inducible nitric oxide synthase in an ovalbumin-induced murine model of asthma. *J Inflamm (Lond)* **9**(1): 41.

108. Yoon JJ, Park JH, Kim HJ, *et al.* (2019) *Dianthus superbus* improves glomerular fibrosis and renal dysfunction in diabetic nephropathy model. *Nutrients* **11**(3): 553.

109. Othman L, Sleiman A, Abdel-Massih RM. (2019) Antimicrobial activity of polyphenols and alkaloids in Middle Eastern plants. *Front Microbiol* **10:** 911.

110. Cowan MM. (1999) Plant products as antimicrobial agents. *Clin Microbiol Rev* **12**(4): 564–582.

111. Pandey AK, Kumar, S. (2013) Perspective on plant products as antimicrobial agents: A review. *Pharmacologia* **4**(7): 469–480.

112. Subramani R, Narayanasamy M, Feussner KD. (2017) Plant-derived antimicrobials to fight against multi-drug-resistant human pathogens. *3 Biotech* **7**(3): 172.

113. Rafsanjany N, Lechtenberg M, Petereit F, *et al.* (2013) Antiadhesion as a functional concept for protection against uropathogenic *Escherichia coli*: *In vitro* studies with traditionally used plants with antiadhesive activity against uropathognic *Escherichia coli*. *J Ethnopharmacol* **145**(2): 591–597.

114. Bjorling DE, Wang ZY, Bushman W. (2011) Models of inflammation of the lower urinary tract. *Neurourol Urodyn* **30**(5): 673–682.

115. Carey AJ, Tan CK, Ipe DS, *et al.* (2016) Urinary tract infection of mice to model human disease: Practicalities, implications and limitations. *Crit Rev Microbiol* **42**(5): 780–799.

7

Clinical Evidence for Acupuncture and Related Therapies

OVERVIEW

Acupuncture and related therapies are a non-pharmacological treatment option for urinary tract infection. This chapter describes the evidence of acupuncture and related therapies used in six randomised controlled trials, one controlled clinical trial, and one non-controlled study. Overall, the evidence is limited, and clinicians should use their clinical judgment regarding the use of these therapies.

Introduction

Acupuncture is part of a family of techniques which stimulate acupuncture points to correct imbalances of energy and restore health to the body. Methods of stimulating acupuncture points include the following:

- Acupuncture: Insertion of an acupuncture needle into acupuncture points;
- Acupressure: Application of pressure to acupuncture points;
- Moxibustion: Burning of a herb (usually *ai ye* 艾叶, *Artemesia vulgaris* L.) close to, or on, the skin to induce a warming sensation.

While many of these therapies have ancient roots, several have emerged as new techniques in the last century. Ear acupuncture/ acupressure has increased in popularity in recent years and is a cost-effective treatment option. With ear acupuncture/acupressure, patients are able to stimulate the ear acupuncture points themselves outside of the clinical encounter, giving them greater flexibility to manage their own health care.

Identification of Clinical Studies

A comprehensive search of English and Chinese language databases identified 22,053 citations (Fig. 7.1). Many of these were duplicates, which were excluded. A further 9,218 citations were excluded after reading the title and abstracts. Full text was retrieved for 1,954 articles, most of which were excluded for not meeting the inclusion criteria. Two studies were identified as interventions not commonly practised outside of China, but they will not be presented here. Eight clinical studies met the inclusion criteria for this review. Six randomised controlled trials (RCTs; one of which reported results in two papers), one controlled clinical trial (CCT) and one non-controlled study were included.

Acupuncture

Five studies meeting the inclusion criteria evaluated acupuncture alone or as integrative medicine (IM). Three studies were RCTs (A1–A3), one was a non-randomised CCT (A4) and one was a non-controlled study (A5).

Randomised Controlled Trials of Acupuncture

Three RCTs (A1–A3), involving 241 participants, evaluated acupuncture for adults with recurrent urinary tract infection (UTI). One study (A3) focused on postmenopausal women, one study (A1) included adult women of any age and the remaining study included adult participants aged 18 to 60 years.

Two studies (A1, A2) were conducted in Norway and the third study (A3) was conducted in China. Participants had a history of UTI between 1.5 and 13 years in one study (A3), had their first UTI at the

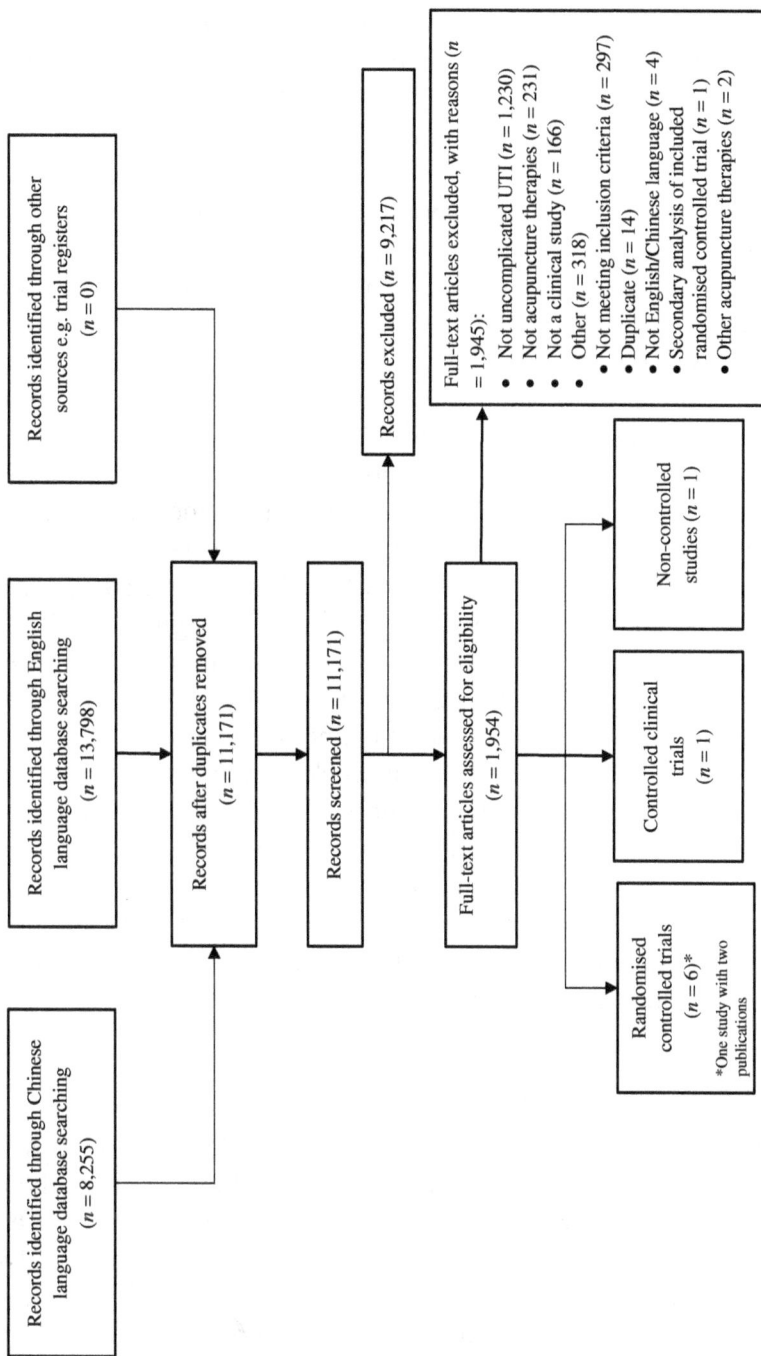

Fig. 7.1. Flowchart of study selection process: Acupuncture and related therapies.

Records identified through Chinese language database searching
(*n* = 8,255)

Records identified through English language database searching
(*n* = 13,798)

Records identified through other sources e.g. trial registers
(*n* = 0)

Records after duplicates removed
(*n* = 11,171)

Records screened (*n* = 11,171)

Records excluded (*n* = 9,217)

Full-text articles assessed for eligibility
(*n* = 1,954)

Full-text articles excluded, with reasons (*n* = 1,945):

- Not uncomplicated UTI (*n* = 1,230)
- Not acupuncture therapies (*n* = 231)
- Not a clinical study (*n* = 166)
- Other (*n* = 318)
- Not meeting inclusion criteria (*n* = 297)
  - Duplicate (*n* = 14)
  - Not English/Chinese language (*n* = 4)
  - Secondary analysis of included randomised controlled trial (*n* = 1)
  - Other acupuncture therapies (*n* = 2)

Non-controlled studies (*n* = 1)

Controlled clinical trials
(*n* = 1)

Randomised controlled trials
(*n* = 6)*

*One study with two publications

mean age of 14 years (A1) or reported more than 14 UTIs in the previous five years (A2). Pathogens identified from urine culture included 19 cases of *Escherichia coli* (*E. coli*), five cases of *Staphylococcus saprophyticus*, five cases of *Enterococci* and one case of *Klebsiella* (A2).

Chinese medicine (CM) syndrome differentiation was used to guide treatment in one study (A1). Syndromes were reported in a secondary paper, and included Spleen *qi/yang* deficiency, Kidney *qi/yang* deficiency, Liver *qi* stagnation, Kidney *yin* deficiency, Blood deficiency and damp-heat in the Lower Energiser. One study compared acupuncture with no treatment and with a second control arm that received sham acupuncture (A2). The other studies were two arm trials comparing acupuncture to no treatment (A1), and the combination of acupuncture plus infrared radiation of the abdomen to levofloxacin capsules (A3). Two acupuncture points were common to all three studies: KI3 *Taixi* 太溪 and SP6 *Sanyinjiao* 三阴交. Five points were common to two studies: CV3 *Zhongji* 中极, BL23 *Shenshu* 肾俞, BL28 *Pangguangshu* 膀胱俞, SP9 *Yinlingquan* 阴陵泉 and LR3 *Taichong* 太冲. The study by Hong *et al.* (2013; A3) used abdominal acupuncture theory in selecting points.

Treatment was provided for four weeks in the two studies from Norway, and for three months in the study from China. Follow-up assessment six months after the end of treatment was conducted in two studies (A1, A2), with both studies reporting losing four and six participants to follow-up, respectively. Follow-up data were reported in a second publication for the RCT by Alraek *et al.* (2003; A1), and this was considered a secondary paper for the main study.

Risk of Bias

All three RCTs were described as randomised. One study (A2) posed 'low' risk of bias as randomisation was made in blocks of five. There was insufficient information about the methods for generating the randomisation sequence in the other RCTs, which were judged to be of 'unclear' risk. One study used closed envelopes to conceal allocation ('low' risk). Insufficient information was reported for allocation concealment in the other studies.

The three-arm trial by Aune *et al.* (1998; A2) that compared acupuncture with sham acupuncture, was considered to be 'low' risk for blinding of participants, but 'high' risk for this domain when acupuncture was compared with no treatment. Two RCTs (A1, A3) were judged 'high' risk for participant blinding as it was likely the blinding would have been broken due to the nature of interventions and comparators. All studies were judged 'high' risk for blinding of personnel. Outcome assessors were unaware of group allocation in two RCTs ('low' risk; A1, A2), and there was insufficient information in the third RCT ('unclear' risk; A3).

One RCT (A3) was judged 'low' risk for the domain incomplete outcome data as no data were missing. In the remaining two studies, the number of participant withdrawals was low and balanced across groups, but it was unclear whether missing data would have influenced the results. All trials were judged as 'unclear' risk for selective outcome reporting as no trial protocols or trial registrations were reported or identified.

Outcomes

All three RCTs involved participants with recurrent UTI. Recurrence was the outcome in two studies (A1, A2). The third RCT (A3) provided treatment during the acute infection stage of participants with recurrent UTI and reported short-term composite cure (assessed six weeks or less after the end of treatment).

Acupuncture versus No Treatment

Meta-analysis of two studies found acupuncture was more effective than no treatment in reducing UTI recurrence (135 participants, risk ratio [RR] 0.39 [0.26, 0.58], $I^2 = 0\%$; A1, A2).

Acupuncture versus Sham Acupuncture

Results from one study found the chance of recurrence at six months was lower with acupuncture than sham acupuncture (53 participants, RR 0.45 [0.22, 0.92]; A2).

Acupuncture plus Infrared Radiation versus Antibiotics

The chance of achieving a short-term composite cure based on symptoms and urine tests with acupuncture plus infrared radiation was greater than that with antibiotics in one study (70 participants, RR 2.88 [1.49, 5.53]; A3).

Frequently Reported Acupuncture Points in Meta-analyses Showing Favourable Effect: Acupuncture

One meta-analysis was conducted for the comparison of acupuncture versus no treatment. Seven acupuncture points were common to both studies, which was not surprising as both RCTs were conducted by the same research group. Acupuncture points CV3 *Zhongji* 中极, BL23 *Shenshu* 肾俞, BL28 *Pangguangshu* 膀胱俞, KI3 *Taixi* 太溪, SP6 *Sanyinjiao* 三阴交, SP9 *Yinlingquan* 阴陵泉 and LR3 *Taichong* 太冲 were used in both studies. These acupuncture points may contribute to the reduction of UTI recurrence, although few studies were included in the meta-analysis.

Assessment using Grading of Recommendations Assessment, Development and Evaluation

The strength and quality ('certainty') of evidence was assessed using the Grading of Recommendations Assessment, Development and Evaluation (GRADE) approach. As described in Chapter 4, a consensus on important interventions, comparators and outcomes was reached through consultation with content experts and clinical advisers. Acupuncture was considered to be an important intervention. As such, GRADE assessments were planned for three comparisons:

- Acupuncture versus sham acupuncture;
- Acupuncture versus antibiotics;
- Acupuncture plus antibiotics versus antibiotics alone.

As none of the included studies tested the second and third comparisons, GRADE assessments were unable to be made. The certainty of evidence for these two comparisons is unknown.

Table 7.1. GRADE: Acupuncture versus Sham Acupuncture

Outcome	Absolute Effect		Relative Effect (95% CI) No. of Participants (Studies)	Certainty of the Evidence (GRADE)
	With Acupuncture	With Sham Acupuncture		
Recurrence, treatment duration: 4 w	58 per 100	26 per 100	RR 0.45* (0.22 to 0.92) 53 (1 RCT)	⊕⊕⊕○ MODERATEᵃ
	Difference: 32 fewer per 100 patients (95% CI: 5 to 45 fewer per 100 patients)			

*Statistically significant result.
ᵃSmall sample size.
Abbreviations: CI, confidence interval; GRADE, Grading of Recommendations Assessment, Development and Evaluation; RCT, randomised controlled trial; RR, risk ratio.

Acupuncture versus Sham Acupuncture

One study (A2) tested the comparison of acupuncture versus sham acupuncture in 53 people with recurrent UTI. Acupuncture may have been superior to sham acupuncture in reducing the chance of recurrence (Table 7.1). The study also reported on safety, with similar numbers of adverse events reported in both groups. Adverse events in the acupuncture group were three cases of warm sensation in the legs, two cases of gastrointestinal discomfort, two cases of more frequent menstruation and one case of dizziness. Adverse events in the sham acupuncture group were two cases of warm sensation in the legs, two cases of gastrointestinal discomfort, and one case each of pain, less frequent menstruation and less climacteric discomfort.

Controlled Clinical Trials of Acupuncture

One controlled clinical trial was included that evaluated electroacupuncture as IM (A4). Eighty postmenopausal women (at least one year since the final menstrual period) with persistent UTI were recruited from a community clinic in China. The mean duration of symptoms was 6.5 months, and the mean age of women was 68.9 years. The study did not report CM syndrome differentiation. Women were allocated to 14 days of treatment with acupuncture plus levofloxacin, or with levofloxacin alone. Electroacupuncture was administered to BL28 *Pangguangshu* 膀胱俞, three times per week, and levofloxacin tablets were taken daily.

The study reported composite cure, which was defined as all symptoms disappearing and two normal urine tests. Data were available for 71 participants. The chance of achieving a short-term composite cure with electroacupuncture as IM was 1.84 that of levofloxacin alone (RR 1.84 [1.01, 3.35]). The study did not report on adverse events.

Non-controlled Studies of Acupuncture

One non-controlled study combined acupuncture with moxibustion, using the warm needle technique (A5). The case series included 32 adult participants from China. The study did not report whether participants had an acute, recurrent or persistent UTI. However, as the duration was a mean of 1.5 years, it was considered unlikely to be an acute UTI.

Participants received a standardised treatment, and no CM syndrome differentiation was described. Acupuncture points included CV3 *Zhongji* 中极, CV4 *Guanyuan* 关元, SP9 *Yinlingquan* 阴陵泉, SP6 *Sanyinjiao* 三阴交, KI3 *Taixi* 太溪, BL20 *Pishu* 脾俞 and BL23 *Shenshu* 肾俞. Treatment was administered daily for 20 days and participants were followed up for six months. There was no mention of adverse events in the study report.

Safety of Acupuncture

Adverse events were reported in one RCT (A2). In the acupuncture group, three cases of feeling warm in the legs were reported, as well as two cases each of gastrointestinal discomfort and more frequent menstruation, and one case of dizziness. Among participants who received sham acupuncture, adverse events included two cases of feeling warm in the legs, two cases of gastrointestinal discomfort and one case each of pain, less frequent menstruation and less climacteric discomfort.

Ear Acupressure

One RCT (A6) evaluated ear acupressure as IM. Sixty adult participants with pyelonephritis and cystitis participated in the study. The infection stage was not reported but was likely to be in the acute stage as patients were recruited from inpatient hospital departments in China. The mean age of participants was 43.4 years in the treatment group, and 42.9 years in the control group. More females were included than males (55 females compared to five males). Signs and symptoms ranged from one to 26 days duration and all patients completed the study.

Standardised ear acupressure was used and CM syndrome differentiation was not described. People in the intervention group received ear acupressure to points: CO10 Kidney 肾, CO9 Bladder 膀胱, CO13 Spleen 脾, CO9,10i Ureter 输尿管, HX3 Urethra 尿道, AH6a Sympathetic 交感 and CO18 Endocrine 内分泌. Participants with cystitis received daily ear acupressure plus intravenous administration of levofloxacin and/or amoxicillin for seven days, and people with pyelonephritis received ear acupressure with intravenous administration of cefoperazone-sulbactam for 14 days. Patients in the control group received the same antibiotic treatment as the intervention group.

Risk of bias assessment found several potential sources of bias. The study was described as randomised but the method was not described. No information was reported for how allocation was concealed and both sequence generation and allocation concealment were judged to be of 'unclear' risk. The participants and personnel were unlikely to be blind to group allocation due to the nature of the intervention and comparator. Both were judged as 'high' risk. There was insufficient information as to whether outcome assessors were blind. Data were available for all participants, posing 'low' risk of bias for the domain incomplete outcome data. No trial registration or protocol was identified and the study was assessed as 'unclear' risk for selective outcome reporting.

Outcomes included short-term composite cure and UTI signs and symptoms. Criteria for composite cure were (1) no symptoms of UTI one month after the end of treatment; and (2) negative urine culture. Participants who received ear acupressure as IM were as likely to achieve a short-term composite cure as participants who received antibiotics alone (RR 1.08 [0.59, 1.97]).

Ear acupressure as IM did result in faster resolution of symptoms from the time of randomisation. This was seen for the duration of urinary frequency (mean difference [MD] –3.20 days [–3.88, –2.52]), increased urinary urgency (MD –3.80 days [–4.74, –2.86]), dysuria (MD –4.60 days [–5.40, –3.80]) and flank pain (MD –3.20 days [–4.14, –2.26]). The number of patients with urine tests positive for microorganisms at end of treatment was not different between the two groups (RR 0.40 [0.08, 1.90]). The study did not report on adverse events.

Moxibustion

Moxibustion was combined with antibiotic therapy in one RCT (A7). Sixty adult participants were recruited from both inpatient and outpatient hospital departments in China. Participants were those who reported recurrent infections of the urinary tract, and the location of infection was not reported. The mean age of study participants was 45.3 years.

Treatment was provided for three months during, and after, acute UTI and participants were followed up for a further six weeks. No CM syndromes were reported. Moxibustion treatment was standardised for all participants, who received moxibustion to BL23 *Shenshu* 肾俞, CV4 *Guanyuan* 关元, CV6 *Qihai* 气海, ST36 *Zusanli* 足三里 and BL22 *Sanjiaoshu* 三焦俞. Treatment was provided daily for ten days, which constituted one course of treatment. Three treatment courses were provided, totalling 30 moxibustion sessions.

Participants in both groups also received treatment with antibiotics. Antibiotic selection was made based on drug sensitivity tests. Antibiotics were provided for two weeks initially. On return of a negative urine culture, a further two to four antibiotics were selected. Each antibiotic was used for one week before changing to the next antibiotic. After two to four weeks of alternating antibiotic use, low-dose antibiotics were used nightly for three months.

Methodological quality of the study was 'low'. The study was described as using random group allocation, yet the details were not described. Furthermore, no information was found on how group allocation was concealed. A judgment of 'unclear' risk of bias was made for the domains sequence generation and allocation concealment. Participants were unlikely to be blind to the use of moxibustion or antibiotics alone, and personnel were not blind to group allocation. Both domains were considered 'high' risk of bias. Insufficient information was available for whether outcome assessors were blind to group allocation ('unclear' risk). All participants completed the study and outcome data were available for all, posing 'low' risk of bias. No trial registration or trial protocol was identified for the RCT, which was judged as 'unclear' risk for selective outcome reporting.

The study reported on medium-term composite cure (assessed between six weeks and six months after the end of treatment). Criteria for cure were (1) symptoms disappeared; (2) urine white cell count less than five units/high power field (HPF); and (3) negative urine culture. The chance of achieving a composite cure with moxibustion plus antibiotics was not statistically different to that of antibiotics alone (RR 2.33 [0.67, 8.18]). The RCT did not report on adverse events.

Ultrashort Wave Therapy

One study (A8) evaluated ultrashort wave therapy as IM. Ultrashort wave therapy using a specialised machine is a technique to treat inflammation and is frequently used for pelvic inflammation. Purported benefits of this technique include regulation of the nervous, cardiovascular, endocrine and immune systems, and improved kidney function. The ultrashort wave therapy machine uses two pads (a positive and a negative) to deliver Chinese herbal medicine (CHM) to acupuncture points. The RCT did not describe the CHM used.

Participants with acute UTI were recruited from the inpatient department of a hospital in China. Sixty participants were enrolled, all of whom completed the study. The participants' ages ranged from 31 to 72 years; the mean age of participants was 45.6 years in the intervention group and 50.3 years in the control group. More females than males were included (53 females compared to seven males).

Chinese medicine syndromes were not described. Treatment was provided daily for 14 days to treat the acute infection, using a standardised treatment. Acupuncture points were CV4 *Guanyuan* 关元, ST28 *Shuidao* 水道, BL23 *Shenshu* 肾俞 (used on the left side only), BL28 *Pangguangshu* 膀胱俞 (right side), SP9 *Yinlingquan* 阴陵泉 (right side), SP6 *Sanyinjiao* 三阴交 (left side), ST36 *Zusanli* 足三里 (right side) and KI1 *Yongquan* 涌泉 (left side). Both groups received conventional antibiotics. The study did not report whether follow-up assessment was made after the end of treatment.

The RCT had similar methodological shortcomings to those found in other RCTs included in this chapter. A lack of detail about sequence generation and allocation concealment led to a judgment of 'unclear' risk of bias. Participants were unlikely to be blind to their group allocation, and personnel were not blind, posing 'high' risk of bias. There was insufficient information reported as to whether outcome assessors were blind to group allocation. No data were missing, posing 'low' risk of bias for incomplete outcome data. The paper did not report trial registration and no protocol was identified, resulting in a judgment of 'unclear' risk for selective outcome reporting.

Composite cure was assessed at the end of treatment. Cure was defined as (1) resolution of symptoms; (2) three separate negative urine cultures; and (3) negative urine indices. At the end of treatment, the chance of achieving a composite cure with ultrashort wave therapy as IM was not statistically different to conventional antibiotics (RR 1.21 [1.00, 1.46], $p = 0.05$). A second outcome related to length of hospital stay. The mean length of hospital stay was reported for both groups, and the length of stay was 3.3 days less with ultrashort wave therapy as IM (10.6 days versus 13.3

days). Data were not able to be analysed to determine statistical significance as the standard deviation was not reported. The study did not report adverse events.

Clinical Evidence for Commonly Used Acupuncture and Related Therapies

Three acupuncture therapies are recommended in clinical guidelines and textbooks that have been included in Chapter 2: acupuncture,[1,2] ear acupuncture[1,2] and ultrashort wave therapy.[2] No studies meeting the inclusion criteria evaluated ear acupuncture. One RCT (A3) combined acupuncture with infrared radiation of the abdomen, one CCT (A4) used electrical stimulation of acupuncture points (electroacupuncture), and one non-controlled study (A5) combined acupuncture with moxibustion. As these acupuncture treatment techniques and combinations were not described in Chapter 2, they will not be discussed further in this section.

The evidence for acupuncture when used alone comes from two RCTs (A1, A2). Acupuncture points used in these studies were CV3 *Zhongji* 中极, CV4 *Guanyuan* 关元, BL23 *Shenshu* 肾俞, BL28 *Pangguangshu* 膀胱俞, KI3 *Taixi* 太溪, SP6 *Sanyinjiao* 三阴交, SP9 *Yinlingquan* 阴陵泉, ST36 *Zusanli* 足三里, LR3 *Taichong* 太冲 and LR2 *Xingjian* 行间. With the exception of KI3 *Taixi* 太溪 and LR2 *Xingjian* 行间, these points are recommended in clinical textbooks and guidelines. Practitioners may consider selecting from these points to address an individual patient's syndrome differentiation.

Both studies evaluated the effect of acupuncture on recurrence, with meta-analysis showing acupuncture to be more effective than no treatment in reducing the chance of recurrence. Furthermore, acupuncture was superior to sham acupuncture in reducing recurrence. The number and type of adverse events were similar between those who received acupuncture and those who received sham acupuncture (see the section 'Safety of Acupuncture').

Ultrashort wave therapy is recommended in one guideline.[2] Ultrashort wave therapy was tested as IM to antibiotics in one RCT (A8). The technique was applied to the points CV4 *Guanyuan* 关元,

ST28 *Shuidao* 水道, BL23 *Shenshu* 肾俞, BL28 *Pangguangshu* 膀胱俞, SP9 *Yinlingquan* 阴陵泉, SP6 *Sanyinjiao* 三阴交, ST36 *Zusanli* 足三里 and KI1 *Yongquan* 涌泉. Ultrashort wave therapy as IM was not statistically different to antibiotics alone in increasing the changes of a composite cure. The authors reported that the duration of hospital stay was less in participants who received ultrashort wave therapy.

Summary of Acupuncture and Related Therapies Clinical Evidence

The use of acupuncture therapies for acute, persistent or recurrent UTI was less frequently tested than CHM. Eight clinical studies met the inclusion criteria for this review and evaluated acupuncture (including electroacupuncture), ear acupressure, moxibustion and a more modern technique, ultrashort wave therapy. Treatment duration was two weeks to 20 days in three studies of acute UTI, which reflects the short duration of acute infection. Treatment duration in studies of people with recurrent infection ranged from four weeks to three months. One CCT provided treatment to people with recurrent UTI for two weeks, which may not be reflective of clinical practice.

Syndrome differentiation was reported in only one study (A1). Syndromes had a greater emphasis on organ dysfunction, for example Spleen *qi/yang* deficiency, Kidney *qi/yang* deficiency, Liver *qi* stagnation and Kidney *yin* deficiency. These syndromes are more commonly seen in cases of persistent and recurrent UTI, and this study included women with recurrent UTI.

The most frequently used acupuncture point was BL23 *Shenshu* 肾俞 (used in five studies), followed by BL28 *Pangguangshu* 膀胱俞, CV4 *Guanyuan* 关元, SP6 *Sanyinjiao* 三阴交 and SP9 *Yinlingquan* 阴陵泉 (four studies each). The acupuncture points BL28 *Pangguangshu* 膀胱俞, SP6 *Sanyinjiao* 三阴交 and SP9 *Yinlingquan* 阴陵泉 are recommended as the main points to be used for UTI and are used for the syndrome dampness-heat in the Bladder. Both BL23 *Shenshu*

肾俞 and CV4 *Guanyuan* 关元 are recommended for the syndrome of dual deficiency of Spleen and Kidney and retention of dampness-heat. In this way, the acupuncture points frequently used in clinical studies appear to be aligned with the syndromes described in guidelines and textbooks.

Due to the small number of included studies, only one meta-analysis was able to be conducted. Meta-analysis of two studies showed acupuncture may be superior to no treatment in reducing the chance of recurrence in people with recurrent UTI. Results from individual studies showed the following:

- Acupuncture was superior to sham acupuncture in reducing recurrence;
- Acupuncture plus infrared radiation produced a greater chance of composite cure than antibiotics;
- Electroacupuncture plus antibiotics increased the chance of a short-term cure, compared to antibiotics alone;
- Ear acupressure plus antibiotics hastened resolution of urinary frequency, urgency, dysuria and flank pain.

Risk of bias assessment revealed that none of the studies were free from bias, which may lower confidence in the results. Few studies evaluated safety, and the adverse events that were reported in one RCT were mild in nature. Overall, there is insufficient evidence for acupuncture therapies in people with acute, persistent or recurrent UTI; clinicians should use their clinical experience to determine the suitability of acupuncture therapies for UTI.

References

1. 中华中医药学会. (2008) 中医内科常见诊疗指南—中医病证部分. 北京: 中国中医药出版社, pp. 111–113.
2. 杨霓芝, 刘旭生. (2013) 中医临床诊治泌尿科专病 (第 3 版). 北京: 人民卫生出版社.

References for Included Acupuncture Therapies Clinical Studies

Study No.	Reference
A1	Alraek T, Soedal LI, Fagerheim SU, *et al.* (2002) Acupuncture treatment in the prevention of uncomplicated recurrent lower urinary tract infections in adult women. *Am J Public Health* **92**(10): 1609–1611.
	Alraek T, Baerheim A. (2003) The effect of prophylactic acupuncture treatment in women with recurrent cystitis: Kidney patients fare better. *J Altern Complement Med* **9**(5): 651–658.
A2	Aune A, Alraek T, LiHua H, *et al.* (1998) Acupuncture in the prophylaxis of recurrent lower urinary tract infection in adult women. *Scand J Prim Health Care* **16**(1): 37–9.
A3	洪建云, 李福, 梁肖清, *et al.* (2013) 腹丛刺为主治疗女性慢性肾盂肾炎疗效观察. 中国针灸 **33**(4): 303–305.
A4	许文漪, 金晓晓, 邝海东, *et al.* (2015) 电针膀胱俞联合抗生素治疗绝经后妇女慢性尿路感染疗效观察. 上海医药 **36**(22): 30–31, 34.
A5	姜曼, 刘颖, 谭奇纹. (2014) 温针灸治疗尿路感染临床疗效观察. 山东中医杂志 **33**(4): 287–288.
A6	朱文胜, 刘孝琼. (2015) 耳穴贴压联合西药治疗非复杂性尿路感染 30 例临床观察. 河北中医 **37**(2): 224–225.
A7	于思明, 郭丹丹. (2010) 灸法联合抗生素治疗成年女性慢性尿路感染 30 例. 山东中医杂志 **29**(9): 621–622.
A8	周桂芬, 刘红玲, 张彤霞, *et al.* (2007) 超短波中药穴位导入治疗尿路感染的临床观察与护理. 护理研究 **(30):** 2751–2752.

8

Clinical Evidence for Combination Therapies

OVERVIEW

Chinese medicine interventions are frequently used in combination in clinical practice. This chapter reviews the evidence of studies that tested combinations of Chinese medicine therapies. All three included studies combined Chinese herbal medicine with an acupuncture therapy. Some promising benefits were seen in achieving cure and reducing duration of urinary symptoms, but more research is needed to confirm these findings.

Introduction

Combination Chinese medicine (CM) therapies are defined as two or more CM interventions from different categories administered together, for example, Chinese herbal medicine (CHM) plus acupuncture. This approach is common in clinical practice. This chapter reviews the evidence from eligible clinical studies. Previous systematic reviews of combination therapies were not identified in the database searches.

Identification of Clinical Studies

Search of electronic databases identified more than 22,000 results (Fig. 8.1). After removal of duplicates, the title and abstracts of citations were read and more than 10,000 irrelevant citations were excluded. The full texts of the remaining articles were retrieved and

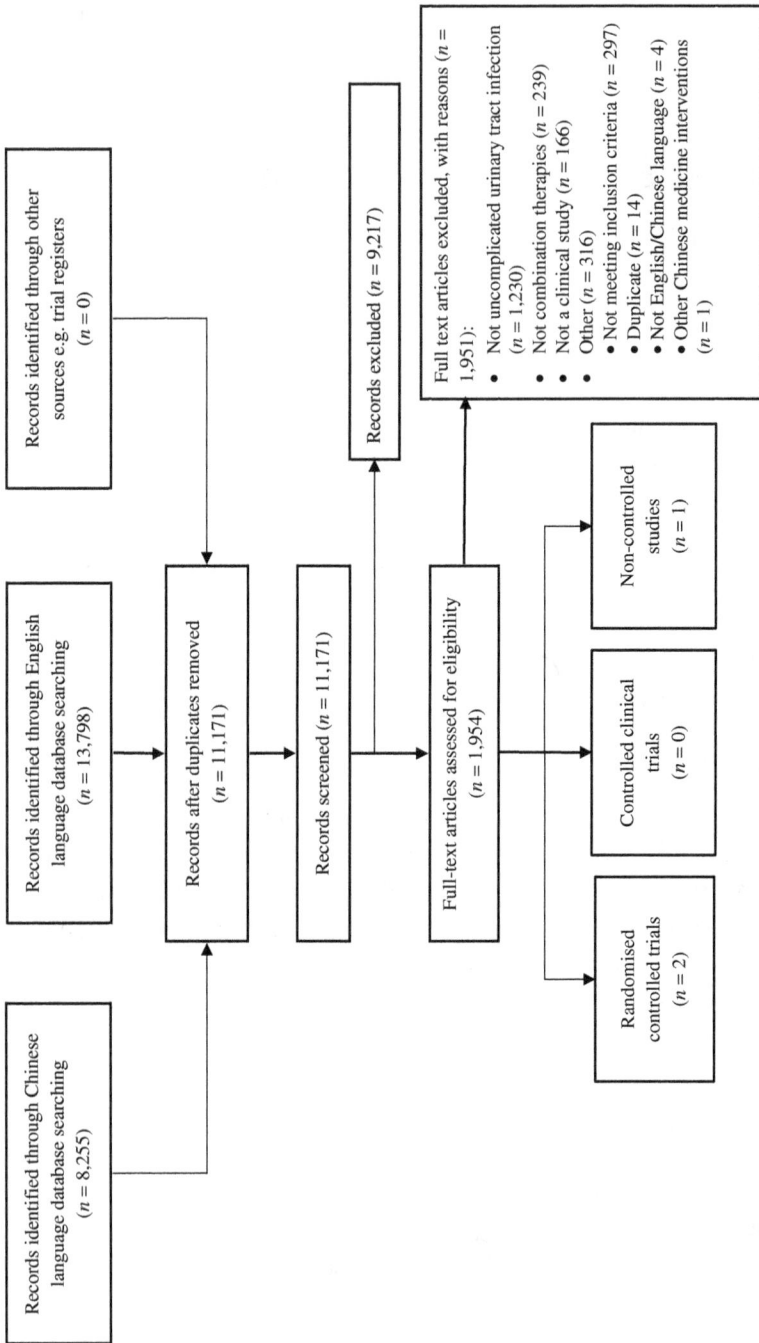

Fig. 8.1. Flowchart of study selection process: Combination therapies.

Records identified through Chinese language database searching (*n* = 8,255)

Records identified through English language database searching (*n* = 13,798)

Records identified through other sources e.g. trial registers (*n* = 0)

Records after duplicates removed (*n* = 11,171)

Records screened (*n* = 11,171)

Records excluded (*n* = 9,217)

Full-text articles assessed for eligibility (*n* = 1,954)

Full text articles excluded, with reasons (*n* = 1,951):
- Not uncomplicated urinary tract infection (*n* = 1,230)
- Not combination therapies (*n* = 239)
- Not a clinical study (*n* = 166)
- Other (*n* = 316)
  - Not meeting inclusion criteria (*n* = 297)
  - Duplicate (*n* = 14)
  - Not English/Chinese language (*n* = 4)
  - Other Chinese medicine interventions (*n* = 1)

Randomised controlled trials (*n* = 2)

Controlled clinical trials (*n* = 0)

Non-controlled studies (*n* = 1)

four clinical studies that evaluated combinations of CM therapy met the eligibility criteria. One study tested an intervention not commonly used outside of China and will not be presented here. Two studies were randomised controlled trials (RCTs) (C1, C2) and one was a non-controlled case series (C3).

Randomised Controlled Trials of Combination Therapies

Two RCTs (C1, C2) evaluated combinations of CM therapies in people with uncomplicated urinary tract infections (UTIs). Both studies were conducted in China, recruiting 192 adult participants with recurrent UTI from hospital inpatient and outpatient departments. Participants had an active infection at the time of study enrolment. One study (C2) included women with both upper and lower UTI and the site of infection was not reported in the other study. One RCT (C2) provided treatment during acute infection which continued after infection resolved and the other (C1) provided treatment during acute infection only. Age ranged from 20 to 75 years in the study by Gao *et al.* (2013; C1), and the mean age of postmenopausal women was 62.7 years (C2).

Chinese medicine syndrome differentiation was used as an inclusion criterion in one study. The RCT by Gao *et al.* (C1) included people with Spleen and Kidney *yang* deficiency. Treatment was tailored towards additional CM diagnoses, which included damp-heat, Blood stasis and *yang* deficiency. The second study stated that CM syndrome differentiation was used to guide treatment, but the details of syndromes were not reported.

Treatment was provided for four weeks in one study (C1) and for up to ten weeks in the other (C2). Follow-up assessment was conducted at one year (C2). All participants completed the studies. Both studies combined CHM with an acupuncture therapy. Gao *et al.* (C1) evaluated the combination of CHM and indirect moxibustion with ginger. This technique involves placing slices of ginger (approximately 0.5 cm thick) on acupuncture points, and small cones of moxibustion are burned on top.[1] This technique is often used for *yang* deficiency.[1] This RCT applied ginger moxibustion to CV12 *Zhongwan* 中脘, CV4 *Guanyuan* 关元, CV6 *Qihai* 气海, BL23 *Shenshu* 肾俞 and BL20 *Pishu* 脾俞 daily for five days, followed by two days' break. This was repeated for four weeks, with 20 treatments administered. Participants in the comparator arm received nitrofurantoin.

The second study (C2) used a more complex treatment regimen. In the acute phase, women allocated to the treatment group received oral *Yin qiao ba zheng san* 银翘八正散 and topical wash *Ku shen tang* 苦参汤 plus antibiotics, followed by oral *Zhi bai di huang tang* 知柏地黄汤 plus moxibustion for an additional one to two months. Ginger moxibustion was applied to points CV4 *Guanyuan* 关元, CV6 *Qihai* 气海, BL23 *Shenshu* 肾俞, BL20 *Pishu* 脾俞, SP6 *Sanyinjiao* 三阴交 and ST36 *Zusanli* 足三里 three times weekly for four weeks.

One herb was used in three CHM formulas in the two studies: *huang qi* 黄芪. Herbs used in two CHM formulas were *bai hua she she cao* 白花蛇舌草, *bai jiang cao* 败酱草, *che qian cao* 车前草, *fu ling* 茯苓, *huang bai* 黄柏, *qu mai* 瞿麦, *tai zi shen* 太子参 and *tu si zi* 菟丝子. Acupuncture points that were common to multiple studies were BL20 *Pishu* 脾俞, BL23 *Shenshu* 肾俞, CV4 *Guanyuan* 关元 and CV6 *Qihai* 气海 (two studies each).

Risk of Bias

Both RCTs were reviewed to determine potential sources of bias. Neither study reported details of how the randomisation sequence was generated or how group allocation was concealed. Both were assessed as 'unclear' risk of bias for sequence generation and allocation concealment. Participants in the studies were unlikely to be blind due to the nature of the interventions and comparators and personnel were not blind to group allocation. The studies were judged to pose 'high' risk for blinding of participants and personnel. As neither described whether outcome assessors were blind to group allocation, both studies were judged as 'unclear' risk. All participants completed the trials and data were available for measured outcomes, posing 'low' risk of bias. No trial registrations or published protocols were identified. Both studies were assessed as 'unclear' risk for selective outcome reporting.

Clinical Evidence for Combination Therapies

Both RCTs reported on composite cure. One RCT (C2) reported the number of episodes of recurrence in one year and one RCT (C2) reported the duration of all urinary symptoms.

Chinese Herbal Medicine plus Moxibustion versus Antibiotics

Short-term cure was evaluated in one study of CHM plus moxibustion (C1). Treatment during acute infection did not result in a greater chance of cure than antibiotics (72 participants, risk ratio [RR] 1.21 [0.71, 2.07]).

Chinese Herbal Medicine plus Moxibustion and Antibiotics versus Antibiotics Alone

In women with recurrent UTI, the combination of CHM, moxibustion and antibiotics increased the chance of achieving a long-term cure (six or more months after the end of treatment) more than antibiotics alone (74 participants, RR 3.53 [2.04, 6.12]; C2). The mean number of recurrent episodes was 1.1 episodes lower in people who received CHM plus moxibustion and antibiotics (74 participants, [−1.32, −0.88]). The combination also reduced the duration of all urinary symptoms (1.8 days) more than antibiotics (74 participants, [−2.37, −1.23]).

Non-Controlled Studies of Combination Therapies

One non-controlled study (C3) met the inclusion criteria described in Chapter 4. The case series was conducted in China, with participants recruited from hospital inpatient and outpatient departments. Sixty adult participants with persistent UTI were included and the mean duration of symptoms was 4.62 years.

The case series included participants with Spleen and Kidney *yang* deficiency. In the intervention group, participants received *Yi qi qing lin hua yu san* 益气清淋化瘀汤 for oral use and applied as a CHM fomentation to acupuncture points. In addition, a cloth was soaked in the *Yi qi qing lin hua yu san* 益气清淋化瘀汤 decoction while still warm, and the warm cloth was applied to the acupuncture point CV8 *Shenque* 神阙. This technique was applied twice daily for two weeks during the active infection stage (one course of treatment). Participants received two courses, totalling 56 treatments. The study reported on adverse events, with none occurring during the course of the study.

Safety of Combination Therapies

Two of the three included clinical studies reported on adverse events, with none occurring during one case series (C3) and the details not being adequately reported in one RCT (C2). There is insufficient evidence to describe the safety of combinations of CM therapies in people with uncomplicated UTI.

Summary of Combination Therapies Evidence

Few studies have evaluated the combination of different CM interventions for people with acute, persistent or recurrent UTI, despite this being a common strategy in clinical practice. Evaluating combinations of interventions in clinical studies can be more challenging, particularly when the evidence for separate interventions is not clear. Both RCTs tested combinations of therapies for people with recurrent UTI, while the case series tested combinations of therapies for people with persistent UTI. There is no evidence from studies included in this chapter for the role of combination therapies for the treatment of acute UTI and insufficient evidence for persistent and recurrent UTI.

All studies described CM syndromes. One RCT (C1) and the case series (C3) selected participants with Spleen and Kidney *yang* deficiency. Both RCTs described using syndrome differentiation to guide treatment, which included Spleen and Kidney *yang* deficiency, combined with damp-heat, Blood stasis or *yang* deficiency in one study (C1) and was not specified in the other. Syndromes were consistent with those described for persistent and recurrent UTI in Chapter 2, including *yang* deficiency generally, and damp-heat.

All studies combined CHM with an acupuncture therapy. Herbs common to both RCTs included *huang qi* 黄芪, *bai hua she she cao* 白花蛇舌草, *bai jiang cao* 败酱草, *che qian cao* 车前草, *fu ling* 茯苓, *huang bai* 黄柏, *qu mai* 瞿麦, *tai zi shen* 太子参 and *tu si zi* 菟丝子. *Huang qi* 黄芪, *fu ling* 茯苓, *huang bai* 黄柏 and *qu mai* 瞿麦 were among the most frequently used oral herbs for recurrent UTI in Chapter 5 (see Chapter 5, Table 5.36). Common acupuncture points in studies testing combination therapies included BL20 *Pishu* 脾俞, BL23 *Shenshu* 肾俞, CV4 *Guanyuan* 关元 and CV6 *Qihai* 气海. Both BL23 *Shenshu* 肾俞 and CV4 *Guanyuan* 关元 were frequently used in acupuncture therapy studies described in Chapter 7. Practitioners may consider these when formulating a treatment plan according to syndrome differentiation.

As no combination of interventions was tested in multiple studies, meta-analyses were unable to be conducted. Benefits from individual RCTs suggest that oral and topical CHM plus moxibustion and antibiotics may:

- Increase the chance of a long-term cure;
- Reduce recurrence;
- Reduce the duration of all urinary symptoms.

While evidence from individual studies may appear promising, there is insufficient evidence to be able to make any suggestions for approaches that could be adopted in clinical practice. Future research will shed more light on the potential benefits of different combinations of CM interventions.

Reference

1. Wang Y. (2009) Micro-system techniques. In: Wang Y (ed), *Micro-Acupuncture in Practice*. Churchill Livingstone, Saint Louis, pp. 7–22.

References for Included Combination Therapies Clinical Studies

Study No.	Reference
C1	高碧峰, 雷根平, 李小会, *et al.* (2013) 温肾健脾方配合隔姜灸治疗复发性尿路感染疗效观察. 陕西中医 **34**(8): 956–957.
C2	刘麒, 全宇, 文光, *et al.* (2015) 中西医结合联合外治对中老年女性复发性尿路感染的疗效影响研究. 辽宁中医杂志 **42**(2): 358–361.
C3	曲健. (2012) 益气清淋化瘀汤加神阙穴药熨治疗慢性尿路感染脾肾两虚型临床观察. 学位论文.

9

Summary and Conclusions

OVERVIEW

Urinary tract infections cause considerable discomfort. Antibiotic treatments are effective, but antibiotic resistance poses a challenge for effective long-term management. Interest in complementary and alternative treatments, including Chinese medicine, is increasing and many studies have examined the efficacy and safety of Chinese herbal medicine, acupuncture and related therapies for acute, persistent and recurrent urinary tract infections. This chapter provides a 'whole-evidence' analysis of Chinese medicine treatments for urinary tract infections. Evidence from classical and contemporary literature and clinical research are compared. The implications for clinical practice and future research are described.

Introduction

Uncomplicated urinary tract infections (UTIs) are common in community and healthcare settings.[1] Antibiotics are an effective and affordable treatment for bacterial UTIs but resistance to uropathogens is increasing.[2] Non-pharmacological treatments may offer benefit. Acupuncture has been suggested as a treatment option in the clinical practice guideline of the Society of Obstetricians and Gynaecologists of Canada for women with recurrent infections who are not responsive to, or are intolerant of, antibiotic prophylaxis.[3] A Cochrane systematic review found that Chinese herbal medicine (CHM) may be beneficial for women with recurrent UTI.[4] The published evidence for key Chinese medicine (CM) treatments is promising.

This book provides a 'whole-evidence' analysis of the potential role of CM treatments for uncomplicated UTI. Clinical practice guidelines and textbooks have recommended traditional CHM formulas and manufactured products, acupuncture, ear acupuncture, ultrashort wave therapy, and diet and lifestyle recommendations (Chapter 2). The analysis of the classical literature identified that CHM, acupuncture therapies and dietary therapy have been used in past eras to treat symptoms of UTI (Chapter 3). Methods used to evaluate evidence from clinical studies are described in Chapter 4. Findings from clinical studies have revealed promising benefits of oral CHM and acupuncture in improving clinical outcomes (Chapter 5, Chapter 7 and Chapter 8).

Chinese Medicine Syndrome Differentiation

Syndrome differentiation is a key feature of CM. Chinese medicine clinical practice guidelines and textbooks described in Chapter 2 suggest four key syndromes relating to UTI: dampness-heat in the Bladder, *yin* deficiency and dampness-heat, dual deficiency of Spleen and Kidney with retention of dampness-heat, and Liver depression and *qi* stagnation. The acute infection stage is considered an excess pattern, with dampness-heat in the Bladder as the key syndrome. In patients who develop persistent or recurrent infections, both excess and deficiency patterns exist. The chronic nature of these infections can be seen in depletion of Spleen and Kidney, and stagnation of Liver *qi*.

Search of the classical literature (Chapter 3) was conducted based on symptoms experienced during the acute infection stage. Accordingly, the syndrome described in many citations was (damp) heat in the Bladder. While it was possible that some citations may have described UTI in people who experienced recurrent infections, it was difficult to determine this due to limited descriptions in the included citations and complexity of the language used in classical texts. Some of the citations that appear most typical of UTI also described Kidney deficiency, which may suggest recurrent UTI.

However, it is difficult to be certain about whether citations described acute, recurrent or persistent infections.

Many clinical studies described CM syndromes. Among the 188 CHM clinical studies reviewed in Chapter 5, 114 studies (60.6%) described using CM syndrome differentiation as an inclusion criterion or for guiding treatment (Chapter 5). The most common syndromes/diagnoses described in studies of acute UTI included Lower Energiser dampness-heat/heat strangury *re lin* 热淋/Bladder dampness-heat/dampness-heat syndrome (20 studies), *yin* deficiency and dampness-heat (three studies), and fatigue strangury (*lao lin* 劳淋, two studies).

Syndromes reported in studies of people with persistent UTI more frequently involved organ dysfunction. Syndromes reported in multiple studies included Spleen and Kidney (*yang*) deficiency syndrome alone (seven studies) or combined with retained pathogen (two studies) and Blood stasis (one study), Kidney deficiency and damp-heat (four studies), Liver and Kidney *yin* deficiency (two studies), damp-heat in the Lower Energiser (two studies), Spleen and Kidney dual deficiency of *qi* and Blood (two studies), *yin* deficiency and damp-heat (two studies), and retention of damp-heat (two studies).

Syndromes seen in CHM studies of people with recurrent UTI were similar to those seen for persistent UTI. Syndromes described in multiple studies included retained dampness-heat/ Bladder dampness-heat/dampness-heat syndrome (13 studies), *yin* deficiency and dampness-heat (four studies), Spleen and Kidney deficiency syndrome (four studies), Kidney *yin* deficiency (three studies), Kidney deficiency and dampness-heat (three studies), dual deficiency of *qi* and *yin* (three studies), cold-heat complex syndrome (two studies) and Kidney *yang* deficiency (two studies).

While variance was seen in the syndrome names, the key concepts for syndromes in clinical studies were consistent with those seen in Chapter 2. These included damp-heat, impaired functioning of the Spleen and Kidney, and *yin* deficiency. One syndrome, Liver depression and *qi* stagnation, was found in only one included CHM study, although three studies did describe *qi* stagnation combined with Blood stasis. Liver depression and *qi* stagnation are caused by emotions such as anger. This impairs the Liver's function of regulating *qi*, Blood and emotions, and often presents with Bladder dampness-heat in the acute infection stage. This syndrome is less common in clinical practice.

Few studies of acupuncture and related therapies described CM syndromes (one of the eight included studies; Chapter 7). Syndromes in people with recurrent UTI included Spleen *qi/yang* deficiency, Kidney *qi/yang* deficiency, Liver *qi* stagnation, Kidney *yin* deficiency, Blood deficiency and damp-heat in the Lower Energiser. Chinese medicine syndromes were reported in all three studies that tested combinations of CM therapies, and included Spleen and Kidney *yang* deficiency, damp-heat, *yang* deficiency and Blood heat. Syndromes in studies of acupuncture therapies and combination therapies were consistent with those described in Chapter 2 for persistent and recurrent UTI.

While many of the studies reported using CM syndromes to guide treatment, results for clinical outcomes were typically reported in aggregate for all participants, regardless of syndrome. This poses a challenge in translating evidence into clinical practice. While combining results of all studies can provide a clear picture about the effectiveness of CM treatments generally, reporting of additional analyses according to syndrome differentiation will improve potential for translation of evidence into clinical practice.

Chinese Herbal Medicine

This section summarises the evidence from Chapter 2, Chapter 3, Chapter 5 and Chapter 8. Chinese herbal medicine is an important CM treatment option for acute, persistent and recurrent UTI. Clinical practice guidelines and textbooks included in Chapter 2 describe oral use of traditional CHM formulas and manufactured products. These treatments are prescribed according to syndrome differentiation and may be used to provide symptomatic relief. Chinese herbal medicine may also be used as a steam wash applied to the genital area.

Chinese herbal medicine was the mainstay of treatment in classical literature citations (Chapter 3). In total, 488 citations described treatment with CHM. The vast majority of treatments prescribed CHM for oral use (480 citations; 98.4%). Diversity was seen in oral CHM formulas. One hundred and twenty-three different formulas were described in the 488 citations, with 51 formulas found in two or more citations. Topical CHM was used in eight citations that described topical application of herbs to the lower abdomen or genital area.

The focus on oral CHM treatments seen in classical literature continued in clinical studies. Oral CHM was used in 185 of the 188 clinical studies, and four studies tested the combination of oral and topical CHM (one study tested both oral CHM alone and oral plus topical CHM). The preference to test oral CHM was irrespective of the UTI type (acute, persistent or recurrent). There appeared to be a preference to test oral CHM as integrative medicine to antibiotic treatment in clinical studies: 82 studies tested oral CHM and 111 studies tested the combination of oral CHM with antibiotics. Several three-arm studies tested oral CHM alone and as an integrative medicine.

Some formulas tested in multiple studies were common to all three categories of UTI. *Ba zheng san* 八正散 was the most frequently tested oral CHM formula in acute UTI randomised controlled trials (RCTs; eight studies) and persistent UTI RCTs (three studies). The manufactured product, *San jin pian* 三金片, was the second most frequently evaluated oral CHM in acute UTI RCTs (used in six RCTs) and was used in two RCTs for recurrent UTI. *Zhi bai di huang tang* 知柏地黄汤 was tested in two persistent UTI RCTs and *Zhi bai di huang tang* (decoction)/*wan* (pill) 知柏地黄汤/丸 was tested in two recurrent UTI RCTs. The overlap for *Ba zheng san* 八正散 and *San jin pian* 三金片 is likely to be due to persistent UTI studies enrolling participants during the acute infection stage. Both *Ba zheng san* 八正散 and *San jin pian* 三金片 are recommended for acute infection where the main syndrome is dampness-heat in the Bladder (see Chapter 2).

The finding that *Zhi bai di huang tang/wan* 知柏地黄汤/丸 was used in both persistent and recurrent UTI is likely due to the long-term duration of these UTI types. In CM, long-term conditions can deplete *yin*, and *Zhi bai di huang tang/wan* 知柏地黄汤/丸 is recommended in clinical guidelines and textbooks in Chapter 2 for the syndrome *yin* deficiency and dampness-heat.

Studies were analysed according to the population under investigation: acute UTI, persistent UTI or recurrent UTI. Meta-analyses were possible for outcomes relating to cure, recurrence and duration of symptoms. Results from meta-analyses of acute UTI studies showed benefits of oral CHM, compared to antibiotic-based treatment, in improving the chance of short-term (six weeks or less) and long-term (six months or more) composite cure. Benefits appeared to be greater when oral CHM was combined with antibiotic-based therapy, with improvements in the chance of short-term, medium-term (between six weeks and six months) and long-term cure. The combination also reduced the overall duration of urinary frequency, urinary urgency, dysuria, fever, suprapubic pain and haematuria, and fewer people had pyuria at the end of treatment.

Fewer studies tested oral CHM for persistent UTI compared to acute and recurrent UTI (52 studies versus 67 and 66, respectively). Similar findings were seen in terms of achieving a cure: oral CHM provided greater chance of short-term and long-term cure than antibiotics, and oral CHM combined with antibiotic-based treatment increased the chance of short-term, medium-term and long-term cure. In addition, the chance of recurrence was reduced when oral CHM was compared to antibiotics. Oral CHM used alone, or with antibiotics, produced greater reduction in the biological outcome measure beta-2 microglobulin (β2-MG), while oral CHM alone resulted in a greater reduction in serum creatinine than antibiotics.

In people with recurrent UTI, results for composite cure followed the same trend as for acute UTI: benefits with oral CHM in achieving a cure in the short-term and long-term, and benefits when oral CHM was combined with antibiotic-based therapy in achieving a short-term, medium-term and long-term cure. In addition, oral CHM alone reduced the duration of urinary symptoms, and when combined with antibiotics, reduced the chance of recurrence between six and 12 months and the number of UTI episodes within one year.

Clinical experts in nephrology and CM were consulted to identify important clinical questions relating to the evidence for CHM. Two comparisons were considered the most important: (1) oral CHM versus antibiotics; and (2) oral CHM plus antibiotics versus antibiotics alone. Important outcomes were cure, recurrence, duration of symptoms, health-related quality of life and adverse events. The strength and quality of evidence ('certainty') was assessed using the Grading of Recommendations Assessment, Development and Evaluation (GRADE) and is summarised in Table 9.1. Many results came from 'low' certainty evidence, which limits confidence in the results.

Chinese herbal medicine is often viewed as a natural treatment and therefore considered safer to use than conventional medicine.[5] However, Chinese herbal medicine is not free of side effects. Approximately one-third of all clinical studies reported on safety, and no serious adverse events were reported. Adverse events were frequently gastrointestinal events, were mild, and resolved with treatment. Research from longitudinal studies designed to assess safety will provide valuable information about the safety of CHM for people with acute, persistent and recurrent UTI.

Table 9.1. Summary of Certainty of Evidence for Oral Chinese Herbal Medicine Randomised Controlled Trials

	Acute UTI		Persistent UTI		Recurrent UTI	
Outcomes	CHM Alone	CHM IM	CHM Alone	CHM IM	CHM Alone	CHM IM
Short-term cure	Very low	Moderate	Moderate	Low	Low	Moderate
Medium-term cure	Low	Low	NA	Low	Low	Low
Long-term cure	Low	Moderate	Low	Low	Moderate	Moderate
Recurrence	Low	Low	Low	Low	Low	Low
Duration of symptoms	Low	Low	Low	Low	Low	Low

Abbreviations: CHM, Chinese herbal medicine; IM, integrative medicine; NA, not applicable; UTI, urinary tract infection.
For further details of the magnitude of the effect, see Chapter 5, Tables 5.16, 5.17, 5.30, 5.31, 5.44 and 5.45.

Chinese Herbal Medicine Formulas in Key Clinical Guidelines and Textbooks, Classical Literature and Clinical Studies

The CHM treatments used for UTI in clinical practice and research, and those cited in classical literature, are diverse. An analysis was undertaken of the CHM treatments mentioned in each of these sources of evidence. Chinese herbal medicine treatments described in Chapter 2 were prescribed according to syndrome differentiation. While one syndrome, dampness-heat in the Bladder, is considered the key syndrome for acute infection, there is no direct correlation between CM deficiency syndromes and conventional medicine categories of persistent or recurrent UTI. Analysis of formulas used in clinical studies in Chapter 5 is based on all formulas reported in all included studies (regardless of UTI category).

Assessment was based on the formula name rather than formula ingredients. It is likely that formulas with the same, or similar, herb ingredients but with different formula names were included. Assessing similarity of formulas is challenging and was not undertaken. Thus, it is likely that the actual number for each formula is higher than those listed in Tables 9.2 and 9.3. Traditional formulas recommended in

Table 9.2. Summary of Chinese Herbal Medicine Traditional Formulas

Formula Name	Clinical Guidelines and Textbooks	No. of Classical Literature Citations	CHM Clinical Studies (Chapter 5)*			Combination Therapies (Chapter 8)
			No. of RCTs	No. of CCTs	No. of Non-controlled Studies	
Ba zheng san 八正散	Yes	16	14	1	1	0
Chen xiang san 沉香散	Yes	12	1	0	0	0
Wu bi shan yao wan 无比山药丸	Yes	0	1	0	0	0
Zhi bai di huang tang 知柏地黄汤	Yes	0	6	1	0	1

Table 9.2. (*Continued*)

Formula Name	Clinical Guidelines and Textbooks	No. of Classical Literature Citations	CHM Clinical Studies (Chapter 5)*			Combination Therapies (Chapter 8)
			No. of RCTs	No. of CCTs	No. of Non-controlled Studies	
Bu shen jian pi qing ling tang 补肾健脾清淋汤	No	0	2	1	0	0
Bu zhong yi qi tang 补中益气汤	No	2	2	0	1	0
Er ding er xian tang 二丁二仙方	No	0	3	0	0	0
Er xian tang 二仙汤	No	0	4	0	0	0
He fa tong lin tang 和法通淋汤	No	0	2	0	0	0
Qing xin lian zi yin 清心莲子饮	No	0	6	0	1	0
Shen qi di huang tang 参芪地黄汤	No	0	3	0	0	0
Si miao san 四妙散	No	0	2	1	0	0
Xie re san yu tong ling tang 泻热散瘀通淋汤	No	0	2	0	0	0
Yi qi zi shen qing li fang 益气滋肾清利方	No	0	2	0	0	0
Yi shen xie zhuo hua yu tang 益肾泄浊化瘀汤	No	0	3	0	0	0
Zi shen qing gan tong lin tang 滋肾清肝通淋汤	No	0	2	0	0	0
Zi shen tong lin fang 滋肾通淋方	No	0	2	0	0	0
Zhu ling tang 猪苓汤	No	1	2	0	0	0

*Some studies used more than one CHM formula or selected formulas according to syndrome differentiation. Abbreviations: CCTs, controlled clinical trials; CHM, Chinese herbal medicine; RCTs, randomised controlled trials.

clinical guidelines and textbooks (Chapter 2) are summarised in Table 9.2 and commercially available manufactured products are summarised in Table 9.3. The CHM treatments that have been tested in multiple RCTs have also been included in these tables.

Two of the four traditional formulas described in Chapter 2 were found in classical literature citations and were tested in at least one clinical study: *Ba zheng san* 八正散 and *Chen xiang san* 沉香散.

Table 9.3.   Summary of Chinese Herbal Medicine Manufactured Products

| Formula Name | Clinical Guidelines and Textbooks | No. of Classical Literature Citations | CHM Clinical Studies (Chapter 5)* | | | |
			No. of RCTs	No. of CCTs	No. of Non-controlled Studies	Combination Therapies (Chapter 8)
Ba zheng he ji 八正合剂	Yes	0	1	0	0	0
Jin gui shen qi wan 金匮肾气丸	Yes	0	0	0	0	0
Niao gan ning ke li 尿感宁颗粒	Yes	0	1	0	0	0
Re lin qing ke li 热淋清颗粒	Yes	0	3	0	0	0
San jin pian 三金片	Yes	0	8	3	2	0
Shen shu ke li 肾舒颗粒	Yes	0	2	0	1	0
Zhi bai di huang wan 知柏地黄丸	Yes	0	2	1	0	0
Jin qian cao ke li 金钱草颗粒	No	0	3	0	0	0
Long qing pian 癃清片	No	0	2	0	0	0
Ning mi tai jiao nang 宁泌泰胶囊	No	0	5	1	0	0
Yin hua mi yan ling pian 银花泌炎灵片	No	0	2	0	0	0

*Some studies used more than one CHM formula or selected formulas according to syndrome differentiation. Abbreviations: CHM, Chinese herbal medicine; RCTs, randomised controlled trials; CCTs, controlled clinical trials.

Ba zheng san 八正散 is recommended in contemporary literature for the syndrome dampness-heat in the Bladder. *Ba zheng san* 八正散 was used in 16 clinical studies (nine acute UTI, three persistent UTI and four recurrent UTI). The use of this formula in persistent and recurrent UTI is likely to relate to the inclusion of participants during the acute infection stage. The evidence for *Ba zheng san* 八正散 suggests benefit in improving short-term cure when used alone and when combined with antibiotics for people with acute UTI. This formula was not different to antibiotics in preventing recurrence in people with acute UTI. Findings from one RCT showed a greater chance of cure and lower risk of recurrence when *Ba zheng san* 八正散 was used with antibiotics.

Chen xiang san 沉香散 can be used for the syndrome Liver depression and *qi* stagnation. Analysis of classical literature showed the earliest citation of the use of *Ba zheng san* 八正散 was in *Yu Ji Wei Yi* 玉机微义 (c. 1396), while the earliest citation of *Chen xiang san* 沉香散 was in *Tai Ping Sheng Hui Fang* 太平圣惠方 (c. 992). These formulas have a consistent history of use for UTI. The RCT that tested *Chen xiang san* 沉香散 also tested other formulas according to syndrome differentiation. Results were reported in aggregate, preventing analysis of the effectiveness of this formula alone. The lack of evidence suggests that further research on the effectiveness of this formula is warranted.

Two other formulas that have been tested in multiple RCTs also have a long history of use. *Bu zhong yi qi tang* 补中益气汤 was used for UTI symptoms in *Zhang Shi Yi Tong* 张氏医通 (c. 1695) and is used in clinical practice to tonify the Stomach and Spleen and benefit *qi*. Although not directly acting to resolve dampness and clear heat in the Bladder, this formula may assist in improving digestive function to prevent formation of damp. The second formula, *Zhu ling tang* 猪苓汤, was found in one citation from *Shen Ju Ren Yi An* 沈菊人医案 (c. 1875), a more recent book. *Zhu ling tang* 猪苓汤 has actions that clear heat, nourish *yin* and promote urination. This formula appears to be more targeted towards UTI, and actions of nourishing *yin* suggest it may be more suitable for persistent or recurrent UTI.

Of the four guideline-recommended formulas, two appear to be frequently tested in clinical studies: *Ba zheng san* 八正散 and *Zhi bai di huang tang* 知柏地黄汤. Several studies evaluated the combination of these two formulas. Only one of the four formulas recommended in textbooks/guidelines has been tested when combined with other CM therapies. This occurred in one study that used *Zhi bai di huang tang* 知柏地黄汤 and moxibustion after the initial infection had been treated with oral *Yin qiao ba zheng san* 银翘八正散, topical *Ku shen tang* 苦参汤 and antibiotics.

Fourteen different formulas have been tested in multiple RCTs that have not been recommended in clinical textbooks and guidelines included in Chapter 2. As highlighted above, two of these have been used for UTI symptoms in past eras. The majority of these formulas were tested in RCTs.

Analysis of the use of manufactured products was also undertaken (Table 9.3). Commercially available manufactured products have also been recommended in clinical textbooks and guidelines. Advances in manufacturing processes have allowed for production of CHM products on a large scale. Thus, it was not surprising that none of the formulas included in Chapter 2, or tested in multiple RCTs, were found in the classical literature.

Six of the seven manufactured products that were included in Chapter 2 have been tested in clinical studies. *Jin gui shen qi wan* 金匮肾气丸 is recommended in the *National Standard for Manufactured Products of Chinese Herbal Medicine* 中药成方制剂国家标准,[6] but was not evaluated in the clinical studies included in Chapter 5. Its absence in the included clinical studies may be due to the traditional indication for *Jin gui shen qi wan* 金匮肾气丸. This formula is recommended for the CM syndrome dual deficiency of Spleen and Kidney with retention of dampness-heat, which is more commonly related to persistent and recurrent UTI. As many of the studies of persistent and recurrent UTI recruited participants during the acute infection stage, treatments tested may have been more targeted to the acute CM syndrome e.g. *San jin pian* 三金片 and *Re lin qing ke li* 热淋清颗粒 (see Chapter 2 for full list of manufactured products for dampness-heat in the Bladder).

The most frequently tested of the seven products was *San jin pian* 三金片, evaluated in 14 studies (eight acute UTI, two persistent UTI and four recurrent UTI). *San jin pian* 三金片 is prescribed for the CM syndrome dampness-heat in the Bladder, usually in the acute infection stage. Few benefits over antibiotics were seen when *San jin pian* 三金片 was used alone in people with acute UTI. In RCTs for acute UTI, *San jin pian* 三金片 plus antibiotics increased the chance of short-term cure and reduced the chance of recurrence, compared to antibiotics alone. No such difference in short-term cure was seen in CCTs. More people with persistent UTI who received *San jin pian* 三金片 and antibiotics achieved a short-term cure than those who received antibiotics alone. In people with recurrent UTI, *San jin pian* 三金片 alone was not statistically different to antibiotics in preventing recurrence but was superior to antibiotics alone when used as integrative medicine. The evidence for *San jin pian* 三金片 appears to be conflicting, and clinicians should use their clinical judgment about the suitability of this product for acute or recurrent UTI.

In addition to oral and topical use, CHM can also be applied as a steam wash. This treatment has been recommended in two clinical guidelines.[7,8] None of the included studies examined the effectiveness of this treatment alone. One CCT combined oral CHM and topical steam wash for people with persistent UTI,[9] which reduced the number of people with a microbiologically positive urine culture at the end of treatment. A second CCT combined oral CHM and topical steam wash for people with recurrent UTI.[10] This study showed a reduction in symptom duration, although it did not increase the chances of a short-term cure.

Acupuncture and Related Therapies

This section summarises the evidence from Chapter 2, Chapter 3, Chapter 7 and Chapter 8. Acupuncture and related therapies provide an alternative treatment option to CHM for people with acute, persistent or recurrent UTI. Three acupuncture therapies have been recommended in key clinical textbooks and guidelines: acupuncture, ear acupuncture and ultrashort wave therapy. Acupuncture was used for symptoms of UTI as early as the Song and Jin dynasties (961–1271; Chapter 3), showing a long history of use.

Compared to CHM, fewer clinical studies that evaluated acupuncture therapies met the criteria for inclusion in Chapter 7. Five studies tested acupuncture alone or as integrative medicine with antibiotics. Meta-analysis of two RCTs showed acupuncture could reduce the chance of recurrence in people with recurrent UTI, compared to no treatment. Grading of Recommendations Assessment, Development and Evaluation assessment was conducted for the comparison acupuncture versus sham acupuncture. Based on 'moderate' level evidence, findings from one study showed acupuncture was superior to sham acupuncture in reducing the chance of recurrence.

Evidence for other acupuncture therapies came from individual studies. One RCT evaluated ultrashort wave therapy as integrative medicine to antibiotics in people with acute UTI. A non-significant trend showed ultrashort wave therapy may improve composite cure, compared to antibiotics alone. Ear acupressure, used as integrative medicine, was not statistically different to antibiotics alone in improving the chance of a short-term cure, although symptoms such as dysuria, urinary frequency, urinary urgency and flank pain resolved faster in people who received ear acupressure plus antibiotics. Finally, moxibustion was also used as integrative medicine to antibiotics in one study of people with recurrent UTI. The combination did not increase the chance of a composite cure between six weeks and six months after the end of treatment. Few adverse events were reported in these studies, but further evidence on the safety of these interventions is required.

Acupuncture Therapies in Key Clinical Guidelines and Textbooks, Classical Literature and Clinical Studies

The intervention that was consistently used across all sources of evidence was acupuncture (Table 9.4). Acupuncture has been recommended in contemporary literature, was described in 24 classical literature citations and was tested in five clinical studies. The absence

Table 9.4. **Summary of Acupuncture and Related Therapies**

Intervention	Clinical Guidelines and Textbooks	No. of Classical Literature Citations	Clinical Studies (Chapter 7)				Combination Therapies (Chapter 8)
			RCTs (No. of Studies)	CCTs (No. of Studies)	Non-controlled Studies (No. of Studies)		
Acupuncture	Yes	24	3	1	1		0
Ear acupuncture	Yes	0	0	0	0		0
Ultrashort wave therapy	Yes	0	1	0	0		0

Abbreviations: CCTs, controlled clinical trials; RCTs, randomised controlled trials.

of acupuncture from studies testing combination CM therapies was interesting but is more likely to be related to the small number of studies included in this chapter than to any preferences for specific combinations of CM therapies.

The second intervention described in Chapter 2 that was tested in clinical studies included in Chapter 7 was ultrashort wave therapy. As this is a recently developed intervention, it was not surprising to find no mention of this treatment in classical literature citations. Similarly, ear acupuncture was a recent development in the 1950s[11] and was absent in the classical literature analysis. Despite being recommended in clinical guidelines and textbooks, none of the studies that were eligible for inclusion in Chapter 7 tested ear acupuncture. One RCT tested ear acupressure plus antibiotics and some benefit was seen in hastening symptom resolution. Whether the effects of ear acupressure and ear acupuncture are comparable is unclear. What is clear is that more evidence is needed for the interventions recommended for treatment of UTI.

Moxibustion was not recommended in clinical textbooks and guidelines used as references for Chapter 2. This may be due to concerns about introducing heat in the acute stage of UTI where the predominant CM syndrome is damp-heat. Moxibustion was tested in one RCT that included participants with recurrent UTI. The study did not report CM syndromes. Based on the acupuncture points used, it appears that the aim of treatment was to tonify the Spleen and

Kidney, a syndrome seen in people with persistent and recurrent UTI. However, it appeared that this study enrolled people during an acute infection. The rationale for testing moxibustion was unclear; clinicians should consider the suitability of moxibustion based on each individual's signs and symptoms. Due to the overall lack of evidence, CM clinicians should use their clinical judgment when selecting treatments for patients with acute, recurrent or persistent UTI.

A comparison of the acupuncture points used in each category of evidence was undertaken. Acupuncture points recommended in clinical guidelines and textbooks in Chapter 2 are described in Table 9.5. All of the main acupuncture points described in Chapter 2 were found in at least one other source of evidence, and two acupuncture points were found in contemporary literature, in classical literature and in clinical studies: SP6 *Sanyinjiao* 三阴交 and SP9 *Yinlingquan* 阴陵泉. Both of these acupuncture points have the functions of resolving damp and benefiting the Lower Energiser,[12] and their importance for acute, recurrent or persistent UTI is clear. Interestingly, the acupuncture point BL39 *Weiyang* 委阳, which regulates urination,[12] was not tested in any of the included acupuncture studies (Chapter 7), nor was it used in studies that tested combinations of CM therapies (Chapter 8). It appears that points on the Spleen

Table 9.5. Summary of Acupuncture Points

| Intervention | Clinical Guidelines and Textbooks | No. of Classical Literature Citations | Acupuncture Clinical Studies (Chapter 7) | | | Combination Therapies (Chapter 8) |
			No. of RCTs	No. of CCTs	No. of Non-controlled Studies	
BL28 *Pangguangshu* 膀胱俞	Yes	0	3	1	0	0
CV3 *Zhongji* 中级	Yes	0	3	0	1	0
SP9 *Yinlingquan* 阴陵泉	Yes	6	2	0	1	0
BL39 *Weiyang* 委阳	Yes	1	0	0	0	0
SP6 *Sanyinjiao* 三阴交	Yes	3	4	0	1	1

Abbreviations: CCTs, controlled clinical trials; RCTs, randomised controlled trials.

meridian and the back *shu* 俞 points on the Bladder meridian were tested in preference. Acupuncture points BL28 *Pangguangshu* 膀胱俞, CV3 *Zhongji* 中级, SP9 *Yinlingquan* 阴陵泉 and SP6 *Sanyinjiao* 三阴交 may be selected for patients with acute, persistent or recurrent UTI, in conjunction with other points to address individual syndrome differentiation.

Limitations of Evidence

Every effort has been made to ensure the accuracy of the contents included in this book. Highly authoritative CM textbooks and guidelines were sought and located to inform the content presented in Chapter 2. It is possible that other textbooks and guidelines not referred to for Chapter 2 describe different syndromes and treatments for UTI. The contents presented in Chapter 2 should not be considered as the only syndromes and treatments relevant to UTI. Chinese medicine clinicians should use their clinical knowledge and experience when making a CM diagnosis and prescribing treatments.

Classical Literature

The electronic database used for the classical literature analysis, the *Zhong Hua Yi Dian* (ZHYD) 中华医典, is a large and representative collection of classical CM texts.[13,14] Results identified in the ZHYD are dependent on the search terms selected. Search terms were identified after reviewing CM textbooks, guidelines and CM dictionaries, and through consulting with clinical experts. After testing terms and reviewing results for relevance, a group of 13 search terms was included in the final search. The Chinese term *lin* 淋 featured in all terms.

Work by Barrett *et al.* (2015)[15] has suggested that the term *long* 癃 was used for urinary disorders before the Han dynasty (202 BC–220 AD) and re-emerged in books published during the Song and Jin dynasties (961–1271). Pilot searches using this term identified that signs and symptoms in citations of *long* 癃 were not consistent with UTI, and this term was excluded from the final search. It is possible that other terms were used to describe UTI and related symptoms in the past that have not been included in this search. Furthermore, it is also possible that the meaning of some terms have changed over time. Thus, addition of other search terms may produce different results in analysis of the classical literature.

Selection criteria were developed to assist in identifying 'possible' and 'most likely' citations of UTI. Citations that described two or more of the four key symptoms of UTI (urinary frequency, urinary urgency, dysuria, and burning sensation or pain on urination) plus at least one secondary symptom were judged as most likely to relate to UTI. This criterion is based on the typical presentation of UTI. Some citations provided insufficient information to make a judgment about the likelihood of relating to UTI, although it is possible that these were in fact UTI cases. The application of different inclusion and classification criteria may alter the findings for classical literature presented in Chapter 3.

Clinical Studies

Clinical studies were identified through a comprehensive search of nine English- and Chinese-language biomedical databases. It is likely that research evaluating the role of CM treatments for UTI has been published in the Japanese and Korean literature; however, resource restraints prevented access to such information. More than 22,000 potentially relevant citations were located and reviewed. Due to the volume of records reviewed, it is possible that errors may have occurred during classification of studies that resulted in studies being excluded that may have been relevant for this review.

Inclusion criteria were developed in consultation with experts in nephrology. The decision was made to focus on uncomplicated UTIs in adults, and findings from analyses may not be applicable for patients with complicated UTI. Eligibility criterion for controlled trials was the use of a clinical practice guideline-recommended treatment, sham/placebo, or no treatment as the comparator. Clinical practice guidelines of the European Association of Urology,[16] Canadian Urological Association (CUA),[17] Society of Obstetricians and Gynaecologists of Canada,[3,18] American College of Obstetricians and Gynaecologists,[19] Infectious Diseases Society of America and the European Society for Microbiology and Infectious Diseases,[20] German Urological Society,[21] National Institute for Health and Care Excellence (NICE),[22,23] Scottish Intercollegiate Guidelines Network (SIGN),[24] the Korean guideline for UTI,[25] the joint guideline of the American Urological Association (AUA), CUA and Society of Urodynamics, Female Pelvic Medicine & Urogenital Reconstruction (SUFU),[26] and the Japanese Society of Chemotherapy and Japanese Association for Infectious Diseases guideline for clinical research of antimicrobial agents on urogenital infections[27] were reviewed in considering selection of comparators. However, we may not have identified all relevant clinical guidelines that describe conventional medical management of uncomplicated UTI. Minor differences in clinical guidelines were noted, and the comparators used in clinical studies may not reflect practice in any given geographical location.

Analysis of results hinged on data presented in included studies. We attempted to obtain information about location of infection, but this was not always specified. Subgroup analysis of studies was undertaken for studies which reported the location of infection, which was grouped broadly as lower UTI, upper UTI, both upper and lower UTI, and not specified. This may allow for greater translation of the findings into clinical practice. However, this information was not always reported and results for overall meta-analyses may not be applicable for every clinical scenario.

Studies testing CM interventions in adults with uncomplicated UTI were evaluated. Additional information about population subgroups was extracted from the included studies. Several studies focused on postmenopausal women and UTI in the elderly. While subgroup analyses were conducted for these factors, it was not possible to present all analyses undertaken. Again, results of meta-analyses may not be applicable for different clinical populations.

Studies were grouped according to the characteristics of UTI (acute, persistent or recurrent) for analysis. In studies of persistent and recurrent UTI, participants were frequently enrolled during an acute infection, although this was not always clear. Some of these studies provided treatment only during the acute infection while others continued treatment after the infection had resolved. This is reflected in the outcomes reported by these studies. Among RCTs, all studies of acute UTI reported cure; 34 of 39 persistent UTI RCTs reported cure; and 38 of 47 recurrent UTI RCTs reported cure. As most studies reported composite cure (based on resolution of signs/symptoms and biological tests), as opposed to clinical cure (resolution of signs/symptoms only), it appears that most studies were targeting the acute infection stage in people with persistent and recurrent infection.

Recurrence is an important outcome in UTI. Diversity in approaches for assessing recurrence was evident in included studies. We took the conservative view that recurrence was only certain in patients who achieved a cure at the end of treatment. We did not analyse results for studies that assessed recurrence in all participants, or in participants who achieved some improvement in symptoms. Thus, the findings from meta-analyses may underestimate or overestimate the true effect of CM treatments.

Recurrent UTIs have a significant personal impact.[28] Two CHM studies reported health-related quality of life (HRQoL) using the Medical Outcome Study 36-item Short Form Health Survey (SF-36),[29] which is a general wellbeing questionnaire. Results for these two studies were inconsistent with the scoring for the SF-36 and were excluded from analysis. There is insufficient evidence on the effect of CM treatments on disease-specific HRQoL. Similarly, there is insufficient evidence of the effect of CM treatment on health care costs for people with acute, persistent or recurrent UTI. Finally, none of the studies were free from bias, and the certainty of the evidence ranged from 'very low' to 'moderate'. Confidence in the results is lowered as a result of these assessments.

Implications for Practice

Chapter 2 describes the key CM syndromes and treatments recommended in clinical textbooks and CM guidelines. The key syndrome for acute UTI is dampness-heat in the Bladder, and syndromes more relevant for persistent and recurrent infections include *yin* deficiency and dampness-heat, dual deficiency of Spleen and Kidney with retention of dampness-heat, and Liver depression and *qi* stagnation. Dampness-heat was described in classical literature, as was deficiency of the Kidney. Two of the four traditional formulas described in contemporary literature have their origins in classical literature. Some of the treatments described in classical literature may no longer be in use and clinicians should adhere to local CM regulations and restrictions on use.

The syndromes described in contemporary and classical literature were also found in clinical studies, suggesting that treatments tested in clinical studies have relevance for clinical practice. Evidence for treatments that have been recommended in contemporary literature has been analysed as part of the overall pool of studies and separately to determine the effectiveness of individual treatment (see Chapter 5, Chapter 7 and Chapter 8). Many studies tested treatments that are not recommended in clinical practice guidelines. As results for studies were pooled for meta-analysis, it remains unclear whether treatments not yet included in clinical guidelines offer greater, or less, benefit than those recommended in clinical guidelines and textbooks.

In order to investigate which herbs may be contributing to the positive effects seen in meta-analyses, descriptive statistics were used to determine frequently used herbs. High-frequency herbs in positive meta-analyses for composite cure in acute UTI included *che qian zi* 车前子, *bian xu* 萹蓄 and *qu mai* 瞿麦. High-frequency herbs were similar in positive meta-analyses for composite cure in persistent and recurrent UTI. The herbs *gan cao* 甘草, *fu ling* 茯苓, *sheng di huang* 生地黄, *shan yao* 山药 and *qu mai* 瞿麦 were frequently used in studies included in these meta-analyses. Experimental studies have shown these herbs to have anti-inflammatory, antimicrobial, antiadhesive and immunomodulatory actions. Clinicians may consider prescribing formulas that include these herbs or may consider these herbs when modifying existing formulas according to each individual patient's syndrome.

Clinical guidelines and textbooks included in Chapter 2 recommend CHM steam wash applied to the genital area as a treatment for

UTI. This treatment was combined with oral CHM in two CCTs but was not evaluated alone. There appears to be insufficient evidence for this treatment based on the included studies. Given that it involves a topical application and is unlikely to have any systemic side effects, clinicians may consider this treatment based on clinical experience and in consultation with patient preferences.

There is limited evidence for acupuncture therapies and combinations of CM therapies. Acupuncture points BL28 *Pangguangshu* 膀胱俞, SP6 *Sanyinjiao* 三阴交 and SP9 *Yinlingquan* 阴陵泉 are recommended as main points for UTI in clinical guidelines and textbooks included in Chapter 2, and are among the most frequently used acupuncture points in clinical studies. The key actions of these points are to resolve dampness and heat, and to tonify the Spleen in order to regulate the water passages. Clinicians may consider using these in patients with the CM syndrome dampness-heat in the Bladder.

Patients who are unsatisfied with, or intolerant of, conventional pharmaceutical treatments often look to complementary and alternative medicine with the belief that these are safe to use.[5] Safety of CM treatments was assessed as part of this review of the evidence. No serious adverse events were reported in included studies. Adverse events were reported in approximately one-third of CHM studies. These were mild in nature and typically involved gastrointestinal events. Adverse events were reported in one acupuncture therapy clinical trial and included gastrointestinal events, dizziness, shortened menstrual cycle in women and warm sensations on the skin. Patients should be advised about the potential risks of CM treatment in order to make an informed choice about their care.

Implications for Research

The emphasis on evidence-based medicine continues to grow in both conventional and complementary medicines. Many clinical studies have evaluated CM interventions for UTI, but more work is needed. Rigorous high-quality studies are needed that use patient-centred validated outcomes. Chinese medicine syndromes incorporated into the trial design will facilitate translation of findings into clinical practice. Trial registration in clinical trial registries is critical to improve transparency in trial reporting. Study reports should provide details required by the Consolidated Standards of Reporting Trials (CONSORT)[30] and extensions for herbal medicine,[31] acupuncture[32] and moxibustion.[33] Adequate reporting of trial design increases the possibility for study replication.

Blinding participants to group allocation is considered important to reduce performance bias. A small number of included studies compared CM interventions with a placebo or sham intervention, and an even smaller number used a 'double dummy' design to ensure both participants and personnel were blinded to group allocation. As most studies compared a CM intervention with antibiotic therapy, blinding was considered unlikely to have occurred. In any case, it has been argued that the 'gold standard' of double-blinded RCT is becoming impractical and irrelevant, and does not meet the needs of clinicians and policy makers.[34] Designing clinical trials that cater for the nuances of CM while enabling real-world decision making is a challenge that needs consideration in future research.

Most studies reported cure based on clinical signs/symptoms alone, or in conjunction with biological tests, and many assessed UTI recurrence. The issues relating to assessment of recurrence in included studies have been highlighted above. Diversity was seen in other outcomes relevant to this review, which included both objective and subjective outcomes. Work is underway to determine a core outcome set for uncomplicated acute UTI in adults.[35] Once established, the core outcome set will reduce variability in outcome measures and increase the ability to synthesise results of studies to estimate the effect of interventions.

Safety of CM therapies was reported in many studies included in this review. Reports were typically limited to descriptions of the nature and number of adverse events, with few studies assessing severity or likelihood of relating to the intervention or control. Study designs other than RCTs are better suited for collection of safety data. Nevertheless, improved reporting of adverse events in clinical studies may help to identify any potential safety concerns.

All of the included studies of CHM tested oral administration of CHM, with none testing topical application of CHM alone. As topical CHM steam wash is recommended in clinical guidelines and textbooks included in Chapter 2, it is important that this practice is tested in clinical studies. Few studies evaluated the effects of acupuncture and related therapies on UTI. Given the promising results seen, these interventions are worthy of further exploration. One interesting result of study selection was that no studies of other CM interventions, such as cupping or dietary therapy, met the inclusion criteria for this review. As diet and lifestyle advice are discussed in Chapter 2, research would provide evidence for the role of these interventions.

Clinical studies are important to test efficacy and effectiveness of interventions. Equally important is understanding the mechanism of action relevant to the disease. The herbs used in studies that contributed to meta-analysis favouring CHM may provide promising avenues for drug discovery. Experimental studies of some of the key herbs were reviewed and several herbs have anti-inflammatory, antimicrobial, antiadhesive and immunomodulatory actions that are relevant for UTI. Authentication of CHM formulas and herb ingredients should be undertaken as part of the quality assurance process in clinical trials and the process used should be clearly reported. Efforts should be made to quantify the amounts of active constituents in herbal preparations. Study reports that include such information will contribute to improved reporting of CHM studies as outlined in the CONSORT extension for herbal medicines.[31]

References

1. Tandogdu Z, Wagenlehner FM. (2016) Global epidemiology of urinary tract infections. *Curr Opin Infect Dis* **29**(1): 73–79.
2. Foxman B. (2010) The epidemiology of urinary tract infection. *Nat Rev Urol* **7**(12): 653–660.
3. Epp A, Larochelle A, SOGC Urogynaecology Committee, *et al.* (2010) Recurrent urinary tract infection. SOGC Clinical Practice Guideline No. 250. *J Obstet Gynaecol Can* **32**(11): 1082–1090.

4. Flower A, Wang LQ, Lewith G, *et al.* (2015) Chinese herbal medicine for treating recurrent urinary tract infections in women. *Cochrane Database Syst Rev* **(6):** Cd010446.

5. Chung VC, Ma PH, Lau CH, *et al.* (2014) Views on traditional Chinese medicine amongst Chinese population: A systematic review of qualitative and quantitative studies. *Health Expect* **17**(5): 622–636.

6. 国家药典委员会. (2008) 中华人民共和国卫生部药品标准—中药成方制剂. 中华人民共和国卫生部药典委员会.

7. 中华中医药学会. (2017) 中医药单用/联合抗生素治疗常见感染性疾病临床实践指南-单纯性下尿路感染(中华中医药学会团体标准). 中国中医药出版社; 北京.

8. 杨霓芝, 刘旭生. (2013) 中医临床诊治泌尿科专病 (第3版). 人民卫生出版社; 北京.

9. 卢巧珍. (2004) 健脾利水通淋方治疗慢性尿路感染疗效观察. 辽宁中医杂志 **31**(6): 493–494.

10. 禹宏. (2009) 清热补肾汤内服外洗治疗绝经后妇女复发性尿路感染临床观察. 中医药临床杂志 **21**(4): 306–308.

11. Gori L, Firenzuoli F. (2007) Ear acupuncture in European traditional medicine. *Evid Based Complement Alternat Med* **4**(Suppl 1): 13–16.

12. Deadman P, Al-Khafaji M, Baker K. (2000) *A Manual Of Acupuncture.* Journal of Chinese Medicine Publications, East Sussex, England.

13. May B, Lu C, Xue C. (2012) Collections of traditional Chinese medical literature as resources for systematic searches. *J Altern Complement Med* **18**(12): 1101–1107.

14. May B, Lu Y, Lu C, *et al.* (2013) Systematic assessment of the representativeness of published collections of the traditional literature on Chinese Medicine. *J Altern Complement Med* **19**: 403–409.

15. Barrett P, Flower A, Lo V. (2015) What's past is prologue: Chinese medicine and the treatment of recurrent urinary tract infections. *J Ethnopharmacol* **167**: 86–96.

16. Bonkat G, Bartoletti R, Bruyere F, *et al.* (2018) Urological infections guidelines: European Association of Urology. Available from: https://uroweb.org/guideline/urological-infections/.

17. Dason S, Dason JT, Kapoor A. (2011) Guidelines for the diagnosis and management of recurrent urinary tract infection in women. *Can Urol Assoc J* **5**(5): 316–322.

18. Epp A, Larochelle A. (2017) No. 250: Recurrent urinary tract infection. *J Obstet Gynaecol Can* **39**(10): e422–e431.

19. American College of Obstetricians and Gynecologists. (2008) ACOG Practice Bulletin No. 91: Treatment of urinary tract infections in non-pregnant women. *Obstet Gynecol* **111**(3): 785–794.

20. Gupta K, Hooton TM, Naber KG, *et al.* (2011) International clinical practice guidelines for the treatment of acute uncomplicated cystitis and pyelonephritis in women: A 2010 update by the Infectious Diseases Society of America and the European Society for Microbiology and Infectious Diseases. *Clin Infect Dis* **52**(5): e103–e120.

21. Kranz J, Schmidt S, Lebert C, *et al.* (2017) Uncomplicated bacterial community-acquired urinary tract infection in adults. *Dtsch Arztebl Int* **114**(50): 866–873.

22. National Institute for Health and Care Excellence. (2018) Pyelonephritis (acute): Antimicrobial prescribing: NICE. Available from: https://www.nice.org.uk/guidance/ng111.

23. National Institute for Health and Care Excellence. (2018) Urinary tract infection (lower): Antimicrobial prescribing: NICE. Available from: https://www.nice.org.uk/guidance/ng109.

24. Scottish Intercollegiate Guidelines Network. (2012) SIGN 88: Management of suspected bacterial urinary tract infection in adults: Scottish Intercollegiate Guidelines Network. Available from: https://www.sign.ac.uk/assets/sign88.pdf.

25. Kang CI, Kim J, Park DW, *et al.* (2018) Clinical practice guidelines for the antibiotic treatment of community-acquired urinary tract infections. *Infect Chemother* **50**(1): 67–100.

26. Anger J, Lee U, Ackerman AL, *et al.* (2019) Recurrent uncomplicated urinary tract infections in women: AUA/CUA/SUFU guideline. *J Urol* **202**(2): 282–289.

27. Yasuda M, Muratani T, Ishikawa K, *et al.* (2016) Japanese guideline for clinical research of antimicrobial agents on urogenital infections: Second edition. *J Infect Chemother* **22**(10): 651–661.

28. Medina M, Castillo-Pino E. (2019) An introduction to the epidemiology and burden of urinary tract infections. *Ther Adv Urol* **11**: 1756287219832172.

29. Ware JJ, Sherbourne C. (1992) The MOS 36-item short-form health survey (SF-36). I. Conceptual framework and item selection. *Med Care* **30**: 473–483.

30. Schulz KF, Altman DG, Moher D. (2010) CONSORT 2010 statement: Updated guidelines for reporting parallel group randomised trials. *PLoS Med* **7**(3): e1000251.

31. Gagnier JJ, Boon H, Rochon P, *et al.* (2006) Reporting randomized, controlled trials of herbal interventions: An elaborated CONSORT statement. *Ann Intern Med* **144**(5): 364–367.
32. MacPherson H, Altman DG, Hammerschlag R, *et al.* (2010) Revised STandards for Reporting Interventions in Clinical Trials of Acupuncture (STRICTA): Extending the CONSORT statement. *J Evid Based Med* **3**(3): 140–155.
33. Cheng CW, Fu SF, Zhou QH, *et al.* (2013) Extending the CONSORT Statement to moxibustion. *J Integr Med* **11**(1): 54–63.
34. Armstrong K. (2012) Methods in comparative effectiveness research. *J Clin Oncol* **30**(34): 4208–4214.
35. Duane S, Vellinga A, Murphy AW, *et al.* (2019) COSUTI: A protocol for the development of a core outcome set (COS) for interventions for the treatment of uncomplicated urinary tract infection (UTI) in adults. *Trials* **20**(1): 106.

Glossary

Terms	Acronym	Definition	Reference
95% confidence interval	95% CI	A measure of the uncertainty around the main finding of a statistical analysis. Estimates of unknown quantities, such as the odds ratio comparing an experimental intervention with a control, are usually presented as a point estimate and a 95% confidence interval. This means that if someone were to keep repeating a study in other samples from the same population, 95% of the confidence intervals from those studies would contain the true value of the unknown quantity. Alternatives to 95%, such as 90% and 99% confidence intervals, are sometimes used. Wider intervals indicate lower precision; narrow intervals, greater precision.	https://training.cochrane.org/handbook
Acupressure	—	Application of pressure on acupuncture points.	—
Acupuncture	—	The insertion of needles into humans or animals for remedial purposes.	World Health Organization (2007) WHO International Standard Terminologies of Traditional Medicine in the Western Pacific Region.

(Continued)

(Continued)

Terms	Acronym	Definition	Reference
Allied and Complementary Medicine Database	AMED	Alternative medicine bibliographic database.	https://www.ebsco.com/products/research-databases/allied-and-complementary-medicine-database-amed
Australian New Zealand Clinical Trial Registry	ANZCTR	Clinical trial registry based in Australia.	www.anzctr.org.au/
China National Knowledge Infrastructure	CNKI	Chinese language bibliographic database.	www.cnki.net
Chinese Biomedical Literature Database	CBM	Chinese language bibliographic database.	www.imicams.ac.cn
Chinese Clinical Trial Registry	ChiCTR	Chinese clinical trial registry.	http://www.chictr.org.cn/
Chinese herbal medicine	CHM	—	—
Chinese medicine	CM	—	—
Chongqing VIP Information Company	CQVIP	Chinese language bibliographic database.	www.cqvip.com
ClinicalTrials.gov	—	Clinical trial registry based in the United States.	https://clinicaltrials.gov/
Cochrane Central Register of Controlled Trials	CENTRAL	Bibliographic database that provides a highly concentrated source of reports of controlled trials.	https://community.cochrane.org/editorial-and-publishing-policy-resource/overview-cochrane-library-and-related-content/databases-included-cochrane-library/cochrane-central-register-controlled-trials-central

(Continued)

Terms	Acronym	Definition	Reference
Combination therapies	—	Two or more Chinese medicines from different therapy groups (e.g., Chinese herbal medicine, acupuncture therapies or other Chinese medicine therapies) administered together.	—
Controlled clinical trials	CCT	A study in which people are allocated to different interventions using methods that are not random.	https://training.cochrane.org/handbook
Convention on International Trade in Endangered Species of Wild Fauna and Flora	CITES	International convention aimed at preventing or regulating trade in threatened and endangered species of plants and animals.	https://www.cites.org/eng/disc/text.php
Cumulative Index of Nursing and Allied Health Literature	CINAHL	Bibliographic database.	https://www.ebscohost.com/nursing/products/cinahl-databases
Effect size	—	A generic term for the estimate of the effect of a treatment in a study.	http://handbook.cochrane.org/
Effective rate	—	A measure of the proportion of participants who achieved an improvement, as outlined in Chapter 4.	—
Electroacupuncture	—	Electric stimulation of the acupuncture needle following insertion.	World Health Organization (2007) WHO International Standard Terminologies of Traditional Medicine in the Western Pacific Region.
European Union Clinical Trials Register	EU-CTR	European clinical trial registry.	https://www.clinicaltrialsregister.eu
Excerpta Medica database	Embase	Bibliographic database.	http://www.elsevier.com/solutions/embase

(Continued)

(Continued)

Terms	Acronym	Definition	Reference
Grading of Recommendations Assessment, Development and Evaluation	GRADE	Approach used to grade quality of evidence and strength of recommendations.	http://www.gradeworkinggroup.org/
Health-related quality of life	HR-QoL	A conceptual or operational measurement that is commonly used in a health care setting as a means to assess the impact of disease on the person.	—
Heterogeneity	—	Used in a general sense to describe the variation in, or diversity of, participants, interventions and measurement of outcomes across a set of studies, or the variation in internal validity of those studies. Used specifically, as statistical heterogeneity, to describe the degree of variation in the effect estimates from a set of studies. Also used to indicate the presence of variability among studies beyond the amount expected due solely to the play of chance.	https://training.cochrane.org/handbook
Homogeneity	—	Used in a general sense to mean that the participants, interventions and measurement of outcomes are similar across a set of studies. Used specifically to describe the effect estimates from a set of studies where they do not vary more than would be expected by chance.	https://training.cochrane.org/handbook

(*Continued*)

Terms	Acronym	Definition	Reference
I^2	—	A measure of study heterogeneity; indicates the percentage of variance in a meta-analysis.	https://training.cochrane.org/handbook
Integrative medicine	—	Chinese herbal medicine combined with pharmacotherapy or other conventional therapy.	—
Mean difference	MD	In meta-analysis, a method used to combine measures on continuous scales, where the mean, standard deviation and sample size in each group are known. The weight given to the difference in means from each study (e.g. how much influence each study has on the overall results of the meta-analysis) is determined by the precision of its estimate of effect; mathematically this is equal to the inverse of the variance. This method assumes that all of the trials have measured the outcome on the same scale.	https://training.cochrane.org/handbook
Meta-analysis	—	The use of statistical techniques in a systematic review to integrate the results of included studies. Sometimes misused as a synonym for systematic reviews, where the review includes a meta-analysis.	—
Moxibustion	—	A therapeutic procedure involving ignited material (usually moxa) to apply heat to certain points or areas of the body surface for managing disease.	World Health Organization (2007) WHO International Standard Terminologies of Traditional Medicine in the Western Pacific Region.

(*Continued*)

(Continued)

Terms	Acronym	Definition	Reference
Non-controlled studies	—	Observations made on individuals, usually receiving the same intervention, before and after the intervention but with no control group.	https://training.cochrane.org/handbook
PubMed	PubMed	Bibliographic database.	http://www.ncbi.nlm.nih.gov/pubmed
Randomised controlled trial	RCT	Clinical trial that uses a random method to allocate participants to treatment and control groups.	—
Risk of bias	—	Assessment of clinical trials to indicate if the results may overestimate or underestimate the true effect because of bias in study design or reporting.	https://training.cochrane.org/handbook
Risk ratio (relative risk)	RR	The ratio of risks in two groups. In intervention studies, it is the ratio of the risk in the intervention group to the risk in the control group. A risk ratio of 1 indicates no difference between comparison groups. For undesirable outcomes, a risk ratio that is less than 1 indicates that the intervention was effective in reducing the risk of that outcome.	https://training.cochrane.org/handbook
Standardised mean difference	SMD	In meta-analysis, a method used to combine results for continuous scales which measure the same outcome, but measure it in different ways (e.g. with different scales). The results of studies are standardised to a uniform scale to allow data to be combined.	https://training.cochrane.org/handbook

(*Continued*)

Terms	Acronym	Definition	Reference
Summary of findings	SoF	Presentation of results and rating the quality of evidence based on the GRADE approach.	http://www.gradeworkinggroup.org/
Transcutaneous electrical nerve stimulation	TENS	Application of transdermal electrical current to acupuncture points via conducting pads.	—
Urinary tract infection	UTI	Infection of the upper or lower urinary tract.	—
Wanfang database	Wanfang	Chinese language bibliographic database.	www.wanfangdata.com
World Health Organization	WHO	World Health Organization is the directing and coordinating authority for health within the United Nations system. It is responsible for providing leadership on global health matters, shaping the health research agenda, setting norms and standards, articulating evidence-based policy options, providing technical support to countries and monitoring and assessing health trends.	http://www.who.int/about/en/
Zhong Hua Yi Dian 中华医典	ZHYD	The *Zhong Hua Yi Dian* [*Encyclopaedia of Traditional Chinese Medicine*] is a comprehensive series of electronic books on compact disc. The collection was put together by the Hunan Electronic and Audio-visual Publishing House. It is the largest collection of Chinese electronic books and includes the major Chinese ancient works, many of which are from rare manuscripts and are the only	Hu R, ed. (2014) *Zhong Hua Yi Dian* [*Encyclopaedia of Traditional Chinese Medicine*], 5th ed. Hunan Electronic and Audio-Visual Publishing House, Chengsha.

(*Continued*)

(*Continued*)

Terms	Acronym	Definition	Reference
		existing copies. These books cover the period from ancient times up to the period of the Republic of China (1911—1948).	
Zhong Yi Fang Ji Da Ci Dian 中医方剂大辞典	ZYFJDCD	Compendium of Chinese herbal formulas with over 96,592 entries derived from classical Chinese books. The Nanjing Chinese Medicine Institute compiled the *Zhong Yi Fang Ji Da Ci Dian* and first published it in 1993.	Peng HR, ed. (1994) *Zhong Yi Fang Ji Da Ci Dian* [*Great Compendium of Chinese Medical Formulae*]. People's Medical Publishing House, Beijing.

Index

www.ingramcontent.com/pod-product-compliance
Lightning Source LLC
Chambersburg PA
CBHW050537190326
41458CB00007B/1822